Radiation Therapy for Benign Disorders

Kanika Sood Sharma
Editor

Radiation Therapy for Benign Disorders

Applications and Emerging Trends

Springer

Editor
Kanika Sood Sharma
Department of Radiation Oncology
Dharamshila Narayana Superspeciality Hospital
New Delhi, Delhi, India

ISBN 978-981-95-6634-1 ISBN 978-981-95-6635-8 (eBook)
https://doi.org/10.1007/978-981-95-6635-8

This Springer imprint is published by the registered company Springer Nature Singapore Pte Ltd.
The registered company address is: 152 Beach Road, #21-01/04 Gateway East, Singapore 189721, Singapore

This work is respectfully dedicated to the patients who have entrusted us with their care, inspiring advances in the therapeutic application of radiation beyond oncologic indications. Their enduring strength and cooperation have been central to expanding the scope of radiation therapy.

It is further dedicated to the distinguished pioneers of radiation medicine, whose visionary contributions identified and established the integral role of radiation in the management of benign diseases. With deep appreciation, this volume honours both the recipients of care and the trailblazers whose efforts have enriched the discipline.

Finally, this dedication is made with heartfelt gratitude to my father, the late Dr D R Sharma, whose lifelong teaching to never stop the journey of learning continues to inspire and motivate every step of this work.

Acknowledgements

I sincerely acknowledge the invaluable support and guidance from numerous individuals and institutions that have made this work possible. I remain profoundly indebted to the pioneers and mentors of radiation oncology, whose foundational research and clinical insights underpin this exploration. Their dedication and scholarship have been a constant source of motivation. I also extend my gratitude to my colleagues and collaborators for their critical insights and unwavering support throughout this endeavour.

I am deeply grateful to my spouse, Dr Gaurav Sood, and my children, Gaurika and Aayansh, for their steadfast patience and encouragement during the manuscript's preparation. My sincere appreciation also goes to my brother, Dr Vikas Sharma, for his invaluable assistance with citations, significantly enhancing the scholarly rigour of this work. Special thanks are due to my parents-in-law for their continuous encouragement and unwavering support. I acknowledge with appreciation Sanjeev Maggoo for his seamless coordination with the authors.

Finally, I gratefully acknowledge Narayana Health for fostering a fertile academic environment that has been instrumental in the successful completion of this book. I also take this opportunity to thank Springer and the production editor, Badrinath Parthasarathy, for their dedication in bringing this book to fruition.

Contents

Introduction of Radiation Therapy for Benign Diseases

1

Kanika Sood Sharma

1.1 Introduction

Radiotherapy (RT) is most widely recognized for its role in cancer treatment; however, its use in managing benign (non-malignant) conditions has a rich historical precedent. During the early to mid-twentieth century, RT was frequently applied to a variety of non-cancerous ailments, such as peptic ulcers, tinea capitis, and dysfunctional uterine bleeding [1]. With time, concerns about radiation-induced cancer (RIC)—particularly among pediatric and adolescent populations—led to a marked decline in its use for benign indications [2]. Whereas RT is utilized for cancer treatment, low-dose RT has been explored as a treatment for a variety of noncancerous inflammatory and degenerative musculoskeletal, orthopedic, and soft tissue diseases after conventional medical treatments are ineffective or feasible [3–9]. RT is commonly used for benign inflammatory and degenerative musculoskeletal diseases in Germany, where approximately 10–30% of RT is practiced in noncancer conditions [10]. Outside of Germany, RT is seldom used to treat benign conditions. In modern clinical practice, RT for benign diseases is confined to select hyperproliferative and inflammatory disorders, where high-quality evidence supports its effectiveness as a first- or second-line treatment [11]. The primary barrier to broader application remains the risk of RIC, highlighting the need for individualized, judicious risk-benefit assessments. This book offers a review of current literature, explores the ethical and clinical considerations surrounding RT for benign conditions, and reflects on the evolving role and future potential of radiotherapy in this domain.

RT for benign conditions utilizes two primary biological mechanisms [12, 13]:

K. Sood Sharma (✉)
Department of Radiation Oncology, Dharamshila Narayana Superspeciality Hospital, New Delhi, Delhi, India

K. Sood Sharma (ed.), *Radiation Therapy for Benign Disorders*,
https://doi.org/10.1007/978-981-95-6635-8_1

Antiproliferative effects target abnormal cell growth, making it effective for preventing pathological processes like heterotopic ossification after hip replacement surgery. In pigmented villonodular synovitis, this approach also shows utility in reducing recurrence rates following synovectomy procedures.

Anti-inflammatory effects form the second mechanism, particularly beneficial for managing inflammatory disorders. Graves' orbitopathy (GO) represents a key application where RT modulates immune-mediated tissue responses.

1.2 Historical Perspective

RT for benign conditions saw extensive use from the 1920s to the 1970s, driven by early successes in symptom management. Key applications included peptic ulcers, tinea capitis, excessive uterine bleeding, and musculoskeletal diseases like heterotopic calcification [3–9]. Early protocols, such as 14.8 Gy for gastric acid suppression in peptic ulcers, demonstrated efficacy with minimal acute toxicity. However, long-term follow-up revealed significant carcinogenic risks, particularly in pediatric populations. A cohort study of 10,834 individuals irradiated for tinea capitis (4.5–49.5 cGy) showed a 20.2 excess relative risk per Gray (ERR/Gy) for thyroid cancer, peaking 20–30 years post-exposure. Patients receiving gastric RT for peptic ulcers had a 2.77-fold increased risk of stomach cancer and a 1.87-fold risk of pancreatic cancer compared to non-irradiated counterparts. Meta-analyses indicated a 22% increased risk of non-breast cancers after breast irradiation, with lung and esophageal cancers showing dose-dependent latency [14–20]. These findings prompted a global decline in RT for benign conditions post-1970s, though Germany maintained its use, refining protocols for inflammatory/proliferative disorders. German studies contributed modern dose standards (e.g., 20–30 Gy in fractionated regimens) and demonstrated durable tumor control in unresectable soft-tissue lesions with 50–54 Gy.

In Central and Eastern Europe and Germany, the following indications are recognized [21]. However, a universally accepted definition of RT indication in benign diseases has not been mandated. General indications for RT identified by the German Working Group on Radiotherapy of Benign Diseases are listed in Table 1.1.

Application of RT for benign conditions shows regional variation. In the UK, North America and much of Europe; the utilization is minimal due to historical apprehensions, limited awareness among referring physicians, and policy-level obstacles. This disparity is largely driven by reimbursement structures, cultural attitudes toward radiation, and the organization of specialist referral pathways. Contemporary practice now reserves RT for select cases where benefits outweigh carcinogenic risks, particularly in older patients or refractory conditions.

Table 1.1 Indications for RT in benign diseases (German Working Group on Radiotherapy of Benign Diseases)

Category	Indications
Inflammatory disorders (acute/chronic)	Sweat gland abscess [in axilla] Furuncles and carbuncles Panaritium Infections unresponsive to antibiotics
Degenerative and painful musculoskeletal conditions	Acute or chronic insertion tendinitis Painful osteoarthritic changes in major joints (e.g., hip, knee)
Hyperproliferative soft tissue disorders	Early-stage prophylactic treatment for Morbus Dupuytren and Morbus Ledderhose Induratio penis plastica (Morbus Peyronie) Postoperative prevention of recurrence in keloids and pterygium
Functional disorders	Graves' orbitopathy Arteriovenous malformations Age-related macular degeneration Persistent lymphatic fistula
Other conditions	Prophylaxis of heterotopic ossification (e.g., at hip, elbow, shoulder) Post-angioplasty or stenting Prevention of neointimal hyperplasia Management of vascular anomalies such as hemangiomas
Dermatologic conditions	Chronic pruritus from refractory dermatoses or eczema Inaccessible psoriatic lesions (e.g., subungual sites) Basal cell carcinoma (superficial or inaccessible sites)

1.3 Current Clinical Indications

Contemporary treatment approaches prioritize the use of lower radiation doses and highly conformal techniques to enhance precision and minimize toxicity. Dose considerations differ significantly from oncological regimens. A common anti-inflammatory protocol delivers 20 Gray (Gy) in 10 fractions, with equivalent regimens achieving comparable biological effectiveness. These lower doses are generally well tolerated, with most patients experiencing minimal acute toxicity. Standard dose ranges span from 3 to 50 Gy, with an average total dose around 20 Gy, typically administered through hypofractionated regimens (fewer sessions with larger doses per fraction) [22–26]. These advancements aim to preserve therapeutic benefit while reducing the risk of long-term complications. Today, RT is considered a viable treatment option for several benign diseases, including:

- *Musculoskeletal disorders: heterotopic* ossification, plantar fasciitis, epicondylitis, arthritis, heel spurs, and Dupuytren's contracture [27–31]
- *Inflammatory conditions:* hidradenitis suppurativa, Graves' orbitopathy

- *Vascular malformations: arteriovenous* malformations, hemangiomas
- *Other indications: keloids,* Peyronie's disease, and certain neurodegenerative disorders

1.4 Efficacy and Safety

A substantial body of prospective studies and clinical reviews reflects the efficacy of radiotherapy (RT) in the management of select benign conditions. These include:

- *Heterotopic ossification:* RT is highly effective for both prevention and treatment, with response rates exceeding 85%.
- *Plantar fasciitis:* Clinically meaningful pain relief and functional improvement have been reported, with 92% of patients maintaining symptom stability compared to 62% in control groups.
- *Dupuytren's contracture:* RT can effectively halt disease progression in 70–87% of cases.
- *Graves' orbitopathy:* Approximately 60% of patients experience improved ocular motility and reduced orbital inflammation following RT.
- *Plantar fasciitis*—30 Gy/10 fractions achieving 92% stability vs. 62% controls.
- *Peyronie's disease*—12–18 Gy showing 65% curvature reduction.

Overall, the safety profile of RT in benign diseases is favorable. Acute side effects are generally mild, and late complications are infrequent when contemporary techniques and appropriate dose constraints are applied. Nevertheless, the primary concern remains the small, but measurable, risk of radiation-induced cancer (RIC), particularly in younger individuals and those with a longer anticipated lifespan. This risk underscores the importance of careful patient selection and individualized risk-benefit analysis. Collectively, data reinforce the need for individualized treatment decisions in benign disease, weighing the clinical benefits of RT against the long-term risk of RIC—especially in patients with longer life expectancy.

1.5 Modern Techniques and Risk Mitigation

Technological advancements in radiotherapy—particularly intensity-modulated radiotherapy (IMRT) and image-guided radiotherapy (IGRT)—have significantly enhanced treatment precision, enabling better tumor targeting while sparing surrounding healthy tissues. However, while IMRT reduces high-dose exposure to critical structures, it can inadvertently increase the volume of normal tissue exposed to low-dose radiation, potentially modifying the risk profile for radiation-induced cancers (RIC). Table 1.2 highlights the radiation therapy protocols and outcomes for benign conditions: dose, efficacy, and preferred techniques. To mitigate these risks, several strategies are employed:

Table 1.2 Radiation therapy protocols and outcomes for benign conditions: dose, efficacy, and preferred techniques

Condition	Typical dose	Efficacy (% response)	Preferred technique
Heterotopic ossification	7–10 Gy	85–92% prevention	IMRT/3D-CRT
Hidradenitis suppurativa	30–50 Gy	78% symptom control	Electron therapy
Dupuytren's contracture	15–21 Gy	70–87% disease arrest	Photon/electron therapy
Graves' orbitopathy	20 Gy/10 fractions	60% motility improvement	Photon therapy

- *Judicious patient selection,* prioritizing older individuals or those with limited therapeutic alternatives.
- *Dose minimization and hypofractionation* to reduce cumulative exposure while maintaining efficacy.
- *Effective shielding* of adjacent normal tissues during treatment.
- *Use of advanced planning systems and delivery techniques,* such as conformal RT and adaptive RT.
- *Follow-up and surveillance* to detect and manage late effects, including secondary malignancies.

1.6 Balancing Risks and Benefits

RT for benign diseases involves careful risk-benefit analysis. Although the risk of RIC is low, it is not negligible and must be considered alongside the potential for substantial symptomatic relief and improved quality of life—particularly when conventional therapies have failed or are unsuitable. In older patients, given their limited remaining life expectancy, the absolute risk of RIC is significantly reduced, making RT a more favorable option in this population. In younger patients, with a longer lifespan and increased susceptibility to late effects, the threshold for offering RT is higher. Non-radiation alternatives should be explored and exhausted before considering RT.

1.7 Conclusion

Radiotherapy for benign diseases represents a carefully considered therapeutic approach within a complex and evolving clinical landscape. Although the risk of radiation-induced cancer is low, it underscores the importance of judicious patient selection, thorough informed consent, and meticulous treatment planning. Advances in modern RT techniques have enhanced both safety and efficacy, supporting its use in well-defined indications—especially for older patients and those with limited treatment options. To broaden its acceptance, continued efforts in clinician education, evidence generation, and policy reform are essential. A balanced, patient-centered strategy—anchored in ethical practice and supported by high-quality data—will ensure that radiotherapy retains its value as a meaningful option in the management of select benign conditions.

References

1. Montero A, Alvarez B. The use of radiotherapy for non-malignant diseases: barriers and benefits. Clin Oncol. 2020;32(6):345–52.
2. Trott KR, Kamprad F. Estimation of cancer risks after radiotherapy of benign diseases. Strahlenthererapie und Onkologie. 2006;182(8):431–6.
3. Torres Royo L, Antelo Redondo G, Árquez Pianetta M, Arenas PM. Low-dose radiation therapy for benign pathologies. Rep Pract Oncol Radiother. 2020;25(2):250–4. https://doi.org/10.1016/j.rpor.2020.02.004.
4. Hu ZH, Chen W, Sun JN, et al. Radiotherapy for the prophylaxis of heterotopic ossification after total hip arthroplasty: a systematic review and meta-analysis of randomized controlled trials. Med Dosim Spring. 2021;46(1):65–73. https://doi.org/10.1016/j.meddos.2020.07.010.
5. Thompson AM, Seivright J, Atluri S, et al. Radiotherapy for Hidradenitis Suppurativa: a systematic review. Dermatology. 2021;237(3):357–64. https://doi.org/10.1159/000514027.
6. Shin JY, Lee JW, Roh SG, Lee NH, Yang KM. A comparison of the effectiveness of triamcinolone and radiation therapy for ear keloids after surgical excision: a systematic review and meta-analysis. Plast Reconstr Surg. 2016;137(6):1718–25.
7. Eng TY, Abugideiri M, Chen TW, et al. Radiation therapy for benign disease: keloids, macular degeneration, orbital Pseudotumor, Pterygium, Peyronie disease, trigeminal neuralgia. Hematol Oncol Clin North Am. 2020;34(1):229–51. https://doi.org/10.1016/j.hoc.2019.09.006.
8. Dove APH, Cmelak A, Darrow K, et al. The use of low-dose radiation therapy in osteoarthritis: a review. Int J Radiat Oncol Biol Phys. 2022;114(2):203–20. https://doi.org/10.1016/j.ijrobp.2022.04.029.
9. Canyilmaz E, Canyilmaz F, Aynaci O, et al. Prospective randomized comparison of the effectiveness of radiation therapy and local steroid injection for the treatment of plantar fasciitis. Int J Radiat Oncol Biol Phys. 2015;92(3):659–66. https://doi.org/10.1016/j.ijrobp.2015.02.009.
10. Seegenschmiedt M-H, Micke O, GCG-BD. Patterns-of-care study for non-malignant diseases in Germany; 2008. https://doi.org/10.1007/978-3-540-68943-0_7.
11. Nardone V, D'Ippolito E, Grassi R, et al. Non-oncological radiotherapy: a review of modern approaches. J Pers Med. 2022;12(10) https://doi.org/10.3390/jpm12101677.
12. Wang JS, Wang HJ, Qian HL. Biological effects of radiation on cancer cells. Mil Med Res. 2018;5(1):20. https://doi.org/10.1186/s40779-018-0167-4.
13. Hall EJ, Giaccia AJ. Radiobiology for the radiologist. 8th ed. Philadelphia: Lippincott Williams & Wilkins; 2018.
14. Travis LB, et al. Second malignant neoplasms and cardiovascular disease after radiotherapy. J Natl Cancer Inst. 2012;104(5):357–70.
15. Ron E, et al. Cancer incidence after radiotherapy for benign conditions. Radiat Res. 1995;142(1):1–11.
16. Shore RE. Radiation-induced non-cancer effects and risks: evidence and implications. Radiat Prot Dosim. 2011;143(2–4):365–9.
17. Ron E, Modan B, Boice JD Jr, et al. Tumors of the brain and nervous system after radiotherapy in childhood. N Engl J Med. 1988;319(16):1033–9.
18. Sadetzki S, Chetrit A, Freedman L, et al. Long-term follow-up for brain tumor development after childhood exposure to ionizing radiation for tinea capitis. Radiat Res. 2005;163(4):424–32.
19. Travis LB, Gospodarowicz M, Curtis RE, et al. Lung cancer following chemotherapy and radiotherapy for Hodgkin's disease. J Natl Cancer Inst. 2002;94(3):182–92.

20. Mazonakis M, Damilakis J. Cancer risk after radiotherapy for benign diseases. Phys Med. 2017;42:285–91. https://doi.org/10.1016/j.ejmp.2017.01.014. Epub 2017 Feb 8
21. Micke O, Seegenschmiedt MH, German Working Group on Radiotherapy of Benign Diseases. Consensus guidelines for radiation therapy of benign diseases: a multicenter approach in Germany. Int J Radiation Oncol Biol Phys. 2002;52(2):496–513.
22. Seegenschmiedt MH, Micke O, Muecke R. Radiotherapy for non-malignant disorders: state of the art and update of the evidence-based practice guidelines. Br J Radiol. 2015;88(1051):20150080. https://doi.org/10.1259/bjr.20150080.
23. Seegenschmiedt MH, Micke O, Niewald M, et al. DEGRO guidelines for the radiotherapy of non-malignant disorders: part III: hyperproliferative disorders. Strahlenther Onkol. 2015;191(7):541–8. https://doi.org/10.1007/s00066-015-0818-2.
24. Ott OJ, Niewald M, Weitmann HD, et al. DEGRO guidelines for the radiotherapy of non-malignant disorders. Part II: painful degenerative skeletal disorders. Strahlenther Onkol. 2015;191(1):1–6. https://doi.org/10.1007/s00066-014-0757-3.
25. Cuttino JT, Todor D, Rosenzweig J, et al. Radiotherapy for benign disease: current concepts and clinical practice. Radiographics. 2017;37(2):546–63.
26. Fornacon-Wood I, Hanna GG, Price GJ, et al. Radiotherapy for benign disease: a review of clinical practice and future directions. Clin Oncol. 2020;32(7):417–26.
27. Macaulay D, Ivanova J, Birnbaum H, Sorg R, Skodny P. Direct and indirect costs associated with Dupuytren's contracture. J Med Econ. 2012;15(4):664–71. https://doi.org/10.3111/13696998.2012.670678.
28. Hoyt BW, Pavey GJ, Potter BK, Forsberg JA. Heterotopic ossification and lessons learned from fifteen years at war: a review of therapy, novel research, and future directions for military and civilian orthopaedic trauma. Bone. 2018;109:3–11. https://doi.org/10.1016/j.bone.2018.02.009.
29. Porter KS, Harrington CJ, Babikian A, et al. Heterotopic ossification formation in military beneficiaries following hip- and pelvic-level amputations. Mil Med. 2023; https://doi.org/10.1093/milmed/usad129.
30. Potter BK, Burns TC, Lacap AP, Granville RR, Gajewski DA. Heterotopic ossification following traumatic and combat-related amputations. Prevalence, risk factors, and preliminary results of excision. J Bone Joint Surg Am. 2007;89(3):476–86. https://doi.org/10.2106/jbjs.F.00412.
31. Forsberg JA, Pepek JM, Wagner S, et al. Heterotopic ossification in high-energy wartime extremity injuries: prevalence and risk factors. J Bone Joint Surg Am. 2009;91(5):1084–91. https://doi.org/10.2106/jbjs.H.00792.

Principles of Radiation Therapy in Non-malignant Conditions

2

Poonam Goyal and Deepak Kumar Garg

2.1 Background

The role of radiation therapy in non-malignant conditions dates back to the early twentieth century [1]. With the expansion in the knowledge of radiobiology, its indications in benign conditions also increased. Empirical means with out biopsy or without any clear evidence radiation was used for benign conditions but now with studies we have definite role and mechanism of action.

The aim of radiation in non-malignant settings is modulation of inflammatory, proliferative, or aberrant vascular responses rather than cytotoxicity in malignant lesions.

Major indications include dermatological conditions (keloids), orthopedic conditions (heterotopic ossification), vascular malformations, and neurological disorders (trigeminal neuralgia). In recurrent, refractory cases or when surgery is contraindicated, its use is more relevant.

Key differences between malignant and non-malignant applications include the lower total dose, conservative fractionation, and greater emphasis on minimizing long-term toxicity in benign conditions. Importantly, patients' selection must be very strict, with consideration of life expectancy, age, and comorbidities, to ensure a favorable risk-benefit profile.

Modern techniques such as 3D conformal radiotherapy (3DCRT), intensity-modulated radiotherapy (IMRT), and stereotactic radiosurgery (SRS) allow for precise delivery, thus further reducing adverse effects. Due to crude methods of radiation treatment in past [lack of dose monitoring, poor shielding of radium sources] there were cases reported developing secondary malignancy like osteo sarcoma and leukemia after 10 to 15 years of radiation exposure.

P. Goyal (✉)
Narayana Hospital Jaipur, Jaipur, Rajasthan, India

D. K. Garg
Mahatma Gandhi Medical College, Jaipur, Rajasthan, India

K. Sood Sharma (ed.), *Radiation Therapy for Benign Disorders*,
https://doi.org/10.1007/978-981-95-6635-8_2

2.2 Pathogenesis

The pathogenesis of benign conditions treatable with radiation therapy varies depending on the disease type, but many involve aberrant cellular proliferation, chronic inflammation, or dysregulated vascular or connective tissue remodeling. In cases of keloids and hypertrophic scars, main causative mechanism is exaggerated fibroblast proliferation and excessive collagen deposition following dermal injury. Fibroblasts in these lesions exhibit prolonged survival and resistance to apoptosis, making them potential targets for radiotherapy [2]. Radiation suppresses fibroblast proliferation and disrupts the fibrotic cascade by modulating TGF-β and other cytokines.

Heterotopic ossification (HO), the formation of bone in non-skeletal tissues, often follows trauma or surgery. Mesenchymal progenitor cells in soft tissues undergo osteogenic differentiation under the influence of bone morphogenetic proteins (BMPs), leading to ectopic bone formation. Radiation interferes with this process by inhibiting mitosis in these precursor cells when administered within 72 h post-injury [3].

In arteriovenous malformations (AVMs), abnormal connections between arteries and veins lead to high-flow vascular shunts. RT induces endothelial damage and gradual vessel occlusion, thus reducing flow and minimizing hemorrhage risk [4].

Most common cause of secondary trigeminal neuralgia is compression of superior cerebellar artery [SCA]. Radiation through stereotactic radiosurgery (e.g., Gamma Knife) targets the trigeminal root entry zone, inducing focal necrosis and axonal degeneration to alleviate pain [5].

Inflammatory and autoimmune conditions such as Grave's ophthalmopathy or plantar fasciitis exhibit chronic immune activation and tissue remodeling. RT induces anti-inflammatory effects by modulating cytokine profiles (e.g., IL-1, TNF-α), suppressing macrophages and leukocyte infiltration, and promoting apoptosis of activated immune cells [6].

The common factor in these pathologies is dysregulated tissue response, via excessive cell proliferation, abnormal angiogenesis, or persistent inflammation—all of which are modifiable targets of radiation therapy at low doses. Requirement is to understand the specific pathogenesis causing that condition for designing an appropriate treatment protocol.

2.3 Role of Radiation Therapy

Radiation therapy (RT) in non-malignant diseases helps in multifactorial ways, offering therapeutic benefit across dermatologic, neurologic, vascular, musculoskeletal, and inflammatory conditions. Unlike its oncologic application, the aim here is modulation of aberrant cellular processes, not tumor eradication.

2.3.1 Inflammatory Conditions

Grave's orbitopathy, characterized by retro-orbital inflammation, responds to low-dose RT (20 Gy in 10 fractions) as it decreases edema and fibrosis. Similarly, plantar fasciitis and degenerative joint diseases have shown improvement with RT doses as low as 3–6 Gy in fractionated regimens [6].

2.3.2 Musculoskeletal Conditions

Heterotopic ossification (HO), especially following hip replacement or spinal trauma, is effectively prevented using a single RT fraction of 7–8 Gy delivered perioperatively. Randomized trials have demonstrated comparable efficacy to NSAIDs, with fewer gastrointestinal side effects [7].

2.3.3 Vascular Malformations

In cerebral arteriovenous malformations (AVMs), stereotactic radiosurgery (SRS) is employed when surgery poses high risk. Doses ranging from 16 to 25 Gy lead to gradual endothelial proliferation, thrombosis, and obliteration of the AVM nidus over months to years [4].

2.3.4 Neurologic Disorders

Trigeminal neuralgia unresponsive to medical therapy can be treated with SRS, typically using Gamma Knife. A dose of 80–90 Gy to the root entry zone yields pain relief in over 80% of patients [5]. Similarly, RT is used in acoustic neuromas and pituitary adenomas for tumor control and symptom relief.

2.3.5 Dermatological Applications

The most common benign conditions treated with RT are keloids. Post-excisional RT significantly reduces recurrence rates when administered within 24 h. Commonly used modalities since old age are electron beam therapy and superficial X-rays. The mechanism involves inhibition of fibroblast proliferation and suppression of collagen synthesis [2].

2.3.6 Rare Indications

Rare indications are Dupuytren's contracture, Peyronie's disease, and pigmented villonodular synovitis. Each indication involves tissue overgrowth or inflammation, with radiation offering a non-invasive alternative to surgery. It means radiation therapy can be applied in selected patients where conventional therapies have failed or are contraindicated.

2.4 Radiation Technique

Radiation techniques for non-malignant conditions must prioritize precision and tissue sparing, given the long-life expectancy of patients and the generally benign nature of the diseases being treated.

2.4.1 Selection of Modality

Choice of modality depends on target depth and anatomical location. Superficial lesions like keloids are effectively treated using electron beam therapy or superficial X-rays. Deeper targets such as AVMs or trigeminal nerve roots require high-precision techniques like stereotactic radiosurgery (SRS) using Gamma Knife, Cyber-Knife, or LINAC-based systems [4, 5].

2.4.2 Time, Dose, and Fractionation

Benign conditions need doses lower than those used in malignant ones. For example, keloids may be treated with 10–20 Gy in 2–3 fractions post-surgery [2]. HO prophylaxis involves a single fraction of 7–8 Gy. Chronic inflammatory conditions often respond to very low-dose RT (e.g., 3–6 Gy in 1–2 Gy/fraction) [6, 7].

2.4.3 Immobilization and Imaging

The use of immobilization devices and image guidance must be meticulous and repositionable with time. Accurate targeting in SRS procedures utilize stereotactic frames or frameless systems, CT/MRI fusion, and daily image guidance to ensure submillimeter accuracy.

2.4.4 Field Design and Planning

Fields selected are typically small, with tight margins to minimize exposure to adjacent healthy tissues. Treatment planning is individualized and can be done by 3D conformal RT or IMRT to conform to irregular shapes and spare critical structures.

2.4.5 Timing to Treatment

In certain conditions, timing is very critical. For example, in HO prevention, RT is most effective when given within 72 h post-operatively. In keloid treatment, initiation within 24 h of excision maximizes fibroblast suppression [3].

Advances in technology continue to improve the safety and efficacy of RT in benign conditions, allowing better conformity and fewer side effects.

2.5 Toxicity Profile and Strategies to Minimize Risk

A very cautious approach is required for radiation therapy in benign conditions as there are more chances for long-term toxicities in generally healthy individuals with long life expectancy.

2.5.1 Acute Toxicity

Acute side effects include mild erythema, edema, and local discomfort, which are typically self-limiting. In head and neck applications, mucositis and xerostomia may occur. Most of these resolve with supportive care.

2.5.2 Late Toxicity

Late effects include skin pigmentation, fibrosis, alopecia, and in rare cases, tissue necrosis. In CNS applications, neurological deficits or radio-necrosis can occur; use of SRS techniques minimizes such risks [5].

2.5.3 Carcinogenesis

The risk of radiation-induced secondary malignancies is a key concern. However, studies suggest that with low doses and limited fields, the risk remains very low (<0.1%) [8]. Proper patient selection and dose planning are the key factors to make benefit-risk ratio favorable.

2.6 Risk Reduction Strategies

Dose Reduction: Use of lowest effective dose with careful fractionation [principle of ALARA].

Precision Techniques: Online imaging [daily before treatment and correction done than and there] and offline imaging [weekly portal imaging].

Patient Selection: young individuals should be carefully selected for RT in benign conditions unless absolutely indicated.

Shielding and Margins: Narrow margin i.e. Gross Tumour Volume (GTV) to Clinical Target Volume (CTV) and CTV to Planning Target Volume (PTV) margins are minimum [3-5mm].

Close follow-up is essential for monitoring delayed toxicity and for promptly managing any arising complications.

2.7 Review of Literature

The application of radiation therapy for benign conditions has evolved significantly over the decades, with numerous retrospective studies, case series, and select randomized controlled trials (RCTs) contributing to the evidence base.

Shen et al. reviewed over 70 studies and concluded that postoperative radiation reduced keloid recurrence by over 60%, especially when delivered within 24 h of excision [2]. Electron therapy and brachytherapy both showed effective outcomes, with minimal adverse effects.

Seegenschmiedt et al. have established the efficacy of single-fraction RT (7–8 Gy) for HO prevention following hip arthroplasty, with outcomes comparable to NSAIDs and fewer complications [3]. A Cochrane review confirmed that both RT and indomethacin were effective, but RT had the advantage in patients at high GI risk [7].

The University of Pittsburgh and Karolinska Institute have demonstrated obliteration rates of 60–90% after SRS for cerebral AVMs, depending on lesion size and dose [4]. Delayed occlusion (1–3 years) is expected, and risk of hemorrhage significantly declines post-RT.

Leksell Gamma Knife studies involving over 500 patients report pain relief in 75–85% with doses of 80–90 Gy, with minimal facial numbness [5]. Randomized data is limited, but outcomes are consistent across institutions.

Seegenschmiedt and Micke published extensive German experience using low-dose RT for painful osteoarthritis and inflammatory disorders, reporting improvement in pain and function in over 70% of cases [6]. Grave's ophthalmopathy has shown response rates of 60–80% in randomized trials comparing RT with corticosteroids [9].

Cuttler et al. reported no significant increase in malignancy rates in patients treated with RT for benign diseases, particularly with doses <10 Gy and small fields [8]. This supports its safety when applied judiciously. More high-quality, multicentric trials are needed to better define indications, optimal doses, and long-term outcomes.

2.8 Future Directions

Future developments in radiation therapy for non-malignant diseases will likely focus on personalized treatment planning, improved safety, and broader evidence through prospective studies.

1. Prospective Clinical Trials
   While retrospective data are abundant, there is a pressing need for randomized controlled trials to establish standard protocols, especially for less common indications. Comparative studies with pharmacologic and surgical alternatives would help solidify RT's role in clinical algorithms.
2. Molecular and Radiobiological Insights
   Understanding the molecular underpinnings of conditions like keloids, AVMs, and neurogenic pain can help identify specific radiation-sensitive targets. Advances in biomarkers may allow better prediction of treatment response and risk of toxicity.
3. Technological Advancements
   Emerging modalities such as proton therapy and FLASH RT may further reduce normal tissue exposure, making RT even safer for benign applications. These are particularly useful in pediatric or younger patients.
4. Expanding Indications
   As evidence builds, newer indications such as refractory autoimmune diseases (e.g., rheumatoid arthritis, Crohn's disease) and chronic degenerative conditions could be explored. Low-dose radiation's immune-modulating potential opens doors to innovative treatments.
5. Policy and Education
   In many regions, reluctance to use RT for benign disease persists due to fear of secondary malignancy and lack of training. Educational programs, guideline development, and inclusion in radiation oncology curricula could promote appropriate use.

Radiation therapy for non-malignant conditions holds immense potential. Continued research, technological refinement, and clinical integration will help unlock its full benefits while minimizing risks.

2.9 Conclusion

It means that now with proper radiobiologic proof and evidence based studies available now radiation is being used in benign conditions frequently. With its ability to modulate inflammatory, fibroproliferative, and vascular processes, RT offers durable relief in a range of conditions including keloids, heterotopic ossification, arteriovenous malformations, and trigeminal neuralgia. With the development in modern radiation techniques, precise delivery with minimal side effects and long-term benefits can be achieved. Patient selection, timing, dose optimization, and interdisciplinary coordination are key to maximizing outcomes. Despite the historical concerns about long-term toxicity, contemporary evidence suggests that when applied judiciously, RT is both safe and effective.

References

1. Loeffler JS, Kooy HM. Clinical indications for radiation therapy. In: Radiation oncology: technology and biology. Springer; 2013.
2. Shen J, et al. Efficacy of adjuvant radiotherapy for keloids: a meta-analysis. Int J Radiat Oncol Biol Phys. 2015;91(3):543–50.
3. Seegenschmiedt MH, et al. Prevention of heterotopic ossification with radiation therapy: a review. Int J Radiat Oncol Biol Phys. 2001;50(3):597–604.
4. Kondziolka D, et al. The role of radiosurgery for cerebral arteriovenous malformations. Neurosurg Clin N Am. 2013;24(4):605–18.
5. Régis J, et al. Gamma Knife radiosurgery for trigeminal neuralgia: a review of 497 patients. Neurosurgery. 2010;66(6):1026–32.
6. Seegenschmiedt MH, Micke O, et al. Radiotherapy for benign diseases. clinical guidelines and evidence-based practice. Strahlenther Onkol. 2015;191(5):377–94.
7. Pakos EE, et al. Radiotherapy vs NSAIDs for the prevention of heterotopic ossification: a meta-analysis. Clin Orthop Relat Res. 2009;467(3):718–27.
8. Cuttler JM, et al. Can low-dose radiation prevent cancer? J Radiat Res. 2013;54(6):943–4.
9. Bartalena L, et al. Randomized trial of low-dose RT versus steroids for Graves' ophthalmopathy. J Clin Endocrinol Metab. 2010;95(6):2407–15.

Ethical Considerations for Treatment of Benign Diseases with Radiation Therapy

3

Kanika Sood Sharma

3.1 Introduction

Radiation therapy is primarily employed in cancer care; however, its application in benign diseases such as keloids, heterotopic ossification, and Graves' orbitopathy remains relevant in modern medicine. The use of RT in oncology often involves decisions under urgent or life-threatening circumstances and mostly offers survival benefits; benign disease scenarios, on the other hand, typically unfold in a more elective context. Thereby the ethical considerations in setting are distinct and nuanced.

The principle imperative to "do no harm" becomes critical in benign cases, since these patients usually have normal life expectancy and may experience relatively mild disease burdens [1]. The decision to utilize radiotherapy for benign conditions transcends clinical considerations and demands a more thorough ethical evaluation. Considerations of long-term risks, especially radiation-induced malignancy, have to be weighed against short-term functional or symptomatic gains. International Commission on Radiological Protection (IRCP) Publication establishes the core guidelines for safeguarding individuals from the risks associated with ionizing radiation in medical settings. These principles are essential to ensure that the advantages of medical radiation use outweigh potential risks for both patients and healthcare professionals [2].

Moreover, in these situations, informed consent is not merely a routine legal formality but serves as the foundation of ethical practice. It has to be ensured that patients are fully aware of their options, fully understand the potential benefits and harms, and are supported in making a decision consistent with their values and preferences. Before embarking on radiation therapy for benign diseases, a comprehensive ethical

K. Sood Sharma (✉)
Department of Radiation Oncology, Dharamshila Narayana Superspeciality Hospital, New Delhi, Delhi, India

K. Sood Sharma (ed.), *Radiation Therapy for Benign Disorders*, https://doi.org/10.1007/978-981-95-6635-8_3

analysis of the use of RT for benign diseases, with a special emphasis on the centrality of the informed consent process is imperative.

3.2 Ethical Principles in the Management of Benign Diseases

3.2.1 Autonomy

Respect for patient autonomy is foundational to the ethical medical practice landscape. With respect to benign diseases, this principle mandates that all patients be fully informed and empowered to make decisions about their care. Studies reveal that patients frequently overestimate the benefits and underestimate the risks of RT. Structured communication protocols significantly improve understanding, and standardized consent forms and visual tools enhance patient recall and comprehension [3].

Unlike cancer treatments, where the urgency of treatment might compress decision timelines, benign disease management allows for more deliberate, thoughtful patient participation. Hence, multiple counseling and consultation sessions may be required to permit the patient to understand the plan of care and its implications, thereby exercising the power of autonomy.

The well-informed consent process becomes the means by which autonomy is realized. It should include a balanced presentation of the expected outcomes, uncertainties, risks, and available alternatives. Wherever available, the relevant clinical evidence may be shared to bring in objectivity into the facts presented. Autonomy also demands a non-directive approach from clinicians, ensuring that patients do not feel pressured to accept a particular treatment merely because it is offered.

3.2.2 Beneficence and Non-maleficence

Beneficence requires that clinicians act to benefit the patient, while non-maleficence obligates them to avoid harm. These so-called twin principles are in constant play in the treatment of benign disease with RT. The benefits of RT in this context are often symptomatic relief or improved function, not survival. In contrast, the harms may sometimes include serious long-term consequences such as secondary malignancies, tissue damage, or infertility. There may be certain predictable accompaniments of the treatment that should be listed with the percentage of likelihood. However, some consequences are not predicted by any threshold values but need to be informed and documented. As per Gigerenzer et al., a key foundation of statistical literacy is clear and transparent communication of risks. To enhance understanding, they suggest presenting information using frequency statements rather than single-event probabilities, absolute risks instead of relative risks, and mortality rates rather than survival rates. Additionally, natural frequencies should be used in place of conditional probabilities. There is a need for further psychological research into effective visual and numerical methods for conveying risk, as well as for training healthcare professionals in these communication strategies [4]. Stacey et al. found individuals who use decision aids tend to feel more knowledgeable, better informed, and have greater clarity about their personal values. They are also more likely to take an active role in decision-making and to have a more accurate understanding of risks. Increasing evidence suggests that decision aids support choices that align with individuals' values. Importantly, the use of decision aids does not negatively impact health outcomes or patient satisfaction. Recent updates show that decision aids, whether used during or before consultations, further enhance knowledge and improve the accuracy of risk perception [5].

These risk-benefit estimates must be more conservative than those employed in oncologic care. For instance, while the risk of inducing cancer may be acceptable in treating a life-threatening tumor, it may be ethically unjustifiable when addressing a non-debilitating keloid. Consequently, RT should typically be reserved for benign conditions that are refractory to standard therapies and cause significant morbidity or distress.

3.2.3 Justice

The principle of justice in healthcare involves fair distribution of resources and equitable access to treatment. In the case of RT for benign conditions, justice raises several questions, particularly in the public sector, where the patients awaiting access to oncologic therapy may be higher:

- Should expensive and resource-intensive treatments be allocated to non-malignant conditions when cancer patients may be awaiting access?
- Are there disparities in access to RT for benign disease based on socioeconomic status, geography, or insurance coverage?
- Are patients being selected appropriately based on clinical indications, or is treatment availability influencing clinical decisions?

Justice also requires that ethical guidelines and indications for RT in benign diseases be standardized and transparent, minimizing variability in practice.

3.3 Clinical Rationale and Indications for RT in Benign Diseases

3.3.1 Historical Perspective

In the early to mid-twentieth century, when the long-term risk estimates for RT were not available, RT was used for numerous benign conditions, including acne, tonsillitis, and tinea capitis. Over time, as the long-term risks of ionizing radiation became better understood and many other effective treatment modalities evolved in benign conditions, the practice declined. The late twentieth century has witnessed tremendous progress in radiation therapy planning and delivery. Therefore, recent decades have witnessed a cautious re-evaluation of radiation in benign conditions, primarily driven by technological advancements and improved understanding of dose-response relationships.

Current interest has focused on precise, low-dose RT applications with highly conformal techniques. These advancements have revived interest in RT for select benign diseases, especially in countries with robust radiation oncology infrastructure such as Germany and the Netherlands.

3.3.2 Current Indications

RT is considered for benign diseases where conventional treatments are inadequate, contraindicated, or associated with high morbidity. Common indications have expanded over the years and include:

- *Heterotopic Ossification*: Postoperative prophylaxis, particularly in hip arthroplasty.
- *Keloids*: Particularly recurrent keloids post-excision.
- *Plantar Fasciitis*: For patients with chronic pain refractory to other modalities.
- *Dupuytren's Contracture*: In early proliferative stages.
- *Graves' Orbitopathy*: Moderate to severe active disease unresponsive to steroids.
- *Arteriovenous Malformations and Hemangiomas*: In select refractory cases.

To offer radiation therapy in any of the above indications, a multidisciplinary discussion and individualized risk-benefit analysis are essential prior to recommending RT for these indications.

3.4 The Consent Process: An Ethical Imperative

Qualitative studies suggest that patients value honest, empathetic communication and prefer clinicians who take the time to explain risks clearly. Engaging patients as partners in decision-making is associated with higher satisfaction and improved outcomes. The consent-taking process is also a part of this communication and documentation of the facts discussed. Informed consent is also a legal obligation. Failure to adequately document consent can expose providers to litigation. Regulatory bodies may require specific protocols and quality checks before RT can be offered for benign conditions. ASTRO (2021) and DEGRO (2020) guidelines highlight the importance of explicit risk disclosure and emphasize the need for tailored, indication-specific consent processes. These organizations recommend standardized consent templates and documentation protocols [6–8]. The consensus guidelines for the radiotherapy of non-malignant diseases have been collaboratively developed by all participating institutions of the German Working Group on

Radiotherapy. These guidelines provide a foundation for quality assessment, prospective clinical trials, and outcomes research [9, 10].

3.4.1 Elements of Informed Consent

The consent process should be thorough, patient-centered, and well documented. Key elements include:

- *Capacity*: Determining the patient's ability to understand and reason. In most countries, 18 years is considered the age of giving valid consent.
- *Disclosure*: Comprehensive explanation of the medical condition, rationale for utilization of RT as a treatment modality, expected benefits, possible side effects (both immediate and delayed), uncertainties, and available alternatives.
- *Comprehension*: Clinicians should verify that patients have understood the information, and the consent is documented in the language of the patients' understanding.
- *Voluntariness*: Ensuring the decision is free from coercion.
- *Documentation*: Detailed records of discussions and patient preferences. Video documentation on a case-by-case basis may be required.

3.4.2 Risk Communication

Patients must be given realistic, understandable information about potential harms. For example:

- "There is a 0.5% (5 in 1000) chance of developing a radiation-induced malignancy over the next 20–30 years."
- Visual aids, analogies (e.g., comparing risks to common life events), and decision aids can facilitate better understanding.
- Discussing uncertainties in current knowledge is essential for trust-building.

3.4.3 Alternatives and Shared Decision-Making

Ethical consent demands full disclosure of alternatives, including:

- Watchful waiting or no treatment.
- Surgical options.
- Pharmacological therapies.
- Physical or rehabilitative interventions.

Shared decision-making acknowledges that risk tolerance and quality of life expectations vary among individuals. It enhances patient satisfaction and aligns treatment with patient values.

3.4.4 Special Populations and Vulnerabilities

- *Children*: Require both parental consent and, where appropriate, child assent. Greater sensitivity to long-term risks is necessary.
- *Cognitively Impaired Adults*: Legal guardians must be involved. Ethical practice demands that even cognitively impaired individuals be engaged in decisions to the extent possible.
- *Cultural and Language Barriers*: Utilize trained interpreters and culturally tailored educational materials to ensure understanding.

3.4.5 Ongoing Consent

Consent should be seen as a dynamic, continuous process. Follow-up conversations are crucial, especially if new information arises or treatment plans evolve.

3.5 Recommendations for Ethical Practice

- Develop and implement standardized consent protocols for benign indications.
- Use multimodal educational approaches: verbal explanations, printed materials, and digital aids.
- Integrate shared decision-making tools into clinical workflows.
- Provide training in risk communication and ethical reasoning for radiation oncologists.
- Encourage patient feedback to refine and improve consent practices.
- Establish institutional review mechanisms for the use of RT in benign diseases.

3.6 Conclusion

Treating benign diseases with radiation therapy presents unique ethical challenges. While the technology enables highly targeted treatment, the ethical responsibility to minimize harm and ensure informed, voluntary patient participation remains paramount. Clinicians must rigorously apply the principles of autonomy, beneficence, non-maleficence, and justice. The informed consent process, when properly conducted, serves as the ethical cornerstone of care in these scenarios.

As the field evolves, ongoing attention to patient-centered communication, risk assessment, and equitable resource allocation will ensure that RT for benign diseases is used judiciously, safely, and ethically. This approach not only upholds the dignity and rights of patients but also reinforces the integrity of the radiation oncology profession.

References

1. World Medical Association. World Medical Association Declaration of Helsinki: ethical principles for medical research involving human subjects. JAMA. 2013;310(20):2191–4. https://doi.org/10.1001/jama.2013.281053.
2. Do KH. General principles of radiation protection in fields of diagnostic medical exposure. J Korean Med Sci. 2016;31(Suppl 1):S6–9. https://doi.org/10.3346/jkms.2016.31.S1.S6. Epub 2016 Jan 29. PMID: 26908991; PMCID: PMC4756345.
3. Olejarczyk JP, Young M. Patient rights and ethics. [Updated 2024 May 6]. In: StatPearls [Internet]. Treasure Island (FL): StatPearls Publishing; 2025. Available from: https://www.ncbi.nlm.nih.gov/books/NBK538279/.
4. Gigerenzer G, Gaissmaier W, Kurz-Milcke E, Schwartz LM, Woloshin S. Helping doctors and patients make sense of health statistics. Psychol Sci Public Interest. 2007;8(2):53–96. https://doi.org/10.1111/j.1539-6053.2008.00033.x. Epub 2007 Nov 1.
5. Stacey D, Légaré F, Lewis K, Barry MJ, Bennett CL, Eden KB, Holmes-Rovner M, Llewellyn-Thomas H, Lyddiatt A, Thomson R, Trevena L. Decision aids for people facing health treatment or screening decisions. Cochrane Database Syst Rev. 2017;4(4):CD001431. https://doi.org/10.1002/14651858.CD001431.pub5. Update in: Cochrane Database Syst Rev. 2024;1:CD001431. 10.1002/14651858.CD001431.pub6. PMID: 28402085; PMCID: PMC6478132.
6. Gutiontov SI. Informed consent in radiation oncology. Int J Radiat Oncol Biol Phys. 2021;109(1):29–35. https://doi.org/10.1016/j.ijrobp.2020.08.064.
7. Seegenschmiedt M-H, Micke O, Niewald M, Mücke R, Eich H, Kriz J, Heyd R. DEGRO guidelines for the radiotherapy of non-malignant disorders: part III: hyperproliferative disorders. Strahlenther Onkol. 2015;191(7):541–8. https://doi.org/10.1007/s00066-015-0818-2.
8. Ott OJ, Niewald M, Weitmann HD, Jacob I, Adamietz IA, Schaefer U, Keilholz L, Heyd R, Muecke R, German Cooperative Group on Radiotherapy for Benign Diseases (GCG-BD). DEGRO guidelines for the radiotherapy of non-malignant disorders. Part II: painful degenerative skeletal disorders. Strahlenther Onkol. 2015;191(1):1–6. https://doi.org/10.1007/s00066-014-0757-3. Epub 2014 Sep 20.
9. Micke O, Seegenschmiedt MH, German Working Group on Radiotherapy in Germany. Consensus guidelines for radiation therapy of benign diseases: a multicenter approach in Germany. Int J Radiat Oncol Biol Phys. 2002;52(2):496–513. https://doi.org/10.1016/s0360-3016(01)01814-4.
10. Tzoulaki I, ANOVA Study Group. Risk of cancer after radiation therapy for benign disease: a systematic review and meta-analysis. Cancer Epidemiol Biomarkers Prev. 2016;25(1):21–31.

Future Directions and Innovations: Role of Low-Dose Radiation Therapy (LDRT) in Alveolitis and Related Pulmonary Inflammatory Conditions

4

Kanika Sood Sharma and Ritvik Agarwal

4.1 Introduction: Context and Rationale for LDRT in Alveolitis

Alveolitis, characterized by inflammation of the alveoli, is a frequent pathological finding in a range of pulmonary disorders which includes idiopathic interstitial pneumonias, autoimmune-related lung diseases, and viral pneumonias [1]. The inflammation disrupts alveolar architecture, impairs gas exchange, and can lead to respiratory failure. Conventional treatments such as corticosteroids and immunosuppressants have variable efficacy and can cause systemic side effects. Inflammatory and degenerative diseases have been managed for many years by low-dose radiotherapy (LDRTs), usually running at less than 1 Gy; however, the matter is less well explored or extrapolated, and nothing is yet statistically definitive.

Its anti-inflammatory and immunomodulatory effects have been recognized since the early twentieth century, but modern radiation oncology has focused mainly on cancer treatment. Amid the COVID-19 pandemic, there has been a resurgence of interest in using LDRT as a therapeutic approach, motivated by its potential to enhance patient outcomes during this period of heightened clinical urgency.

In its historical use in managing pneumonia and its known anti-inflammatory properties, radiation therapy was revisited as a potential therapeutic option during the COVID-19 pandemic, with the aim of improving patient outcomes [2, 3].

K. Sood Sharma (✉) · R. Agarwal
Dharamshila Narayana Superspeciality Hospital, Delhi, India

K. Sood Sharma (ed.), *Radiation Therapy for Benign Disorders*,
https://doi.org/10.1007/978-981-95-6635-8_4

4.2 Immunological and Molecular Mechanisms of LDRT in Alveolitis and Viral Pneumonia

COVID-19-associated pneumonia generally progresses through two distinct stages. In the early phase, an intensified immune response is triggered to reduce and control the initial viral burden. As the disease advances, this response may become exaggerated, resulting in excessive secretion of cytokines and chemokines by immune and endothelial cells. This overproduction drives a hyperinflammatory state known as the cytokine storm (CS) [4–6].

The resulting inflammation leads to severe impairment of alveolar gas exchange, thereby reducing blood oxygenation levels. Additionally, proteinaceous exudates tend to accumulate in the alveoli, and the formation of hyaline membranes contributes to mucous plug development, further obstructing gas exchange. Proinflammatory cytokines also activate coagulation pathways—particularly the extrinsic pathway—through the induction of tissue factor and factor VIIa. Consequently, coagulopathy becomes a common clinical feature in advanced-stage COVID-19, often linked with widespread systemic inflammation [7, 8].

Radiation therapy, specifically low-dose radiation therapy (LDRT), has been explored as a treatment modality in such cases due to its anti-inflammatory and immunomodulatory capabilities. Both immune and endothelial cells—major sources of cytokines—exhibit similar radiosensitivity profiles. LDRT targets these cells, helping to temporarily suppress the cytokine storm. Lung epithelial cells, being relatively resistant to radiation, sustain less damage, thereby preserving alveolar gas exchange.

Moreover, radiation promotes apoptosis, which assists in clearing alveolar mucous and enhances absorption. It also induces beneficial changes in the microvasculature that lead to endothelial cell renewal, further improving oxygen exchange [9, 10]. Macrophages, another critical component of the immune response, exist in two major phenotypes: M1 (proinflammatory) and M2 (anti-inflammatory). LDRT supports a shift toward the M2 phenotype, thereby contributing to an overall anti-inflammatory milieu [11, 12]. The radiation dose of <1 Gy leads to an anti-inflammatory state due to polarization of M2 macrophages. Whereas a dose >1 Gy causes polarization of M1 macrophages, creating a proinflammatory microenvironment [13]. Low-dose lung irradiation can potentially mitigate the severity of pneumonitis, thereby reducing the risk of death. Table 4.1 showcases the mechanism of action of LDRT.

4.3 Radiation Planning

The aim of the treatment is to deliver radiation to bilateral lungs in a single sitting using 6 MV photon beams. Treatment methods that reduce exposure risk to healthcare personnel during both planning and administration are highly preferred. If target matching radiotherapy is being considered, existing diagnostic CT imaging can be used for planning purposes.

Table 4.1 Mechanism of action of LDRT

Mechanism	Key process	Outcome
Immune cell modulation	Reduces pro-inflammatory neutrophils/leukocytes Increases regulatory B cells and M2 macrophages	Balances immune response Monocytic cells as therapy biomarkers
Cytokine regulation	Induces TGF-β within 24 h Suppresses IL-6, IL-1β, and TNF-α Modulates chemokine levels	Mitigates cytokine storm Controls immune cell trafficking
M2 polarization	Promotes M2 macrophage phenotype Secretes anti-inflammatory factors	Reduces edema Restores alveolar integrity Enhances tissue repair

The planning target volume (PTV) should consist of the entire lung volume with an additional 1.2 cm margin. The radiation field should then incorporate this PTV, with a further 8 mm margin which ensures adequate coverage [14].

Patients are positioned in supine position such that their hands are extended above the head. For improved comfort and positioning, a breast board can be used to create a semi-Fowler's position, elevating head and shoulders.

Radiation is typically administered using an anteroposterior/posteroanterior (AP/PA) beam configuration. The dose is calculated at the mid-plane level, ideally using a source-to-surface distance (SSD) of 100 cm, and the depth should be determined by the diagnostic scan or inter-parietal chest measurement.

For critically ill patients who cannot be shifted onto a treatment couch, a single posterior or anterior field using 6 MV photons may be applied while the patient is on a trolley. This may be done using an open field, manually set up, and delivered with twice the usual monitor units (MUs). Both conventional jaw-defined or MLC-defined open fields can be employed.

To streamline the process, manual dose calculation is recommended. If available, treatment delivery through the emergency module of the linear accelerator can be used, but a thorough "time-out" verification must be implemented to prevent significant treatment errors.

Since lung density may vary, especially in patients with COVID-19-related pneumonia, dose calculations must be adjusted accordingly, following the guidelines laid out in TG-17.

4.4 Treatment Portals

The patient is positioned in the supine orientation with both arms raised above the head. To identify the appropriate dose prescription point, the linear accelerator's gantry is first rotated to 90°, allowing for the acquisition of a lateral chest X-ray portal image. Once this imaging is complete, the gantry is returned to the 0-degree position, and the radiation field is adjusted to adequately encompass both lungs.

- *Superior field border*: Positioned just above the lateral end of the clavicle and extended 1 cm beyond the lung apex, as confirmed on portal imaging.
- *Inferior field border*: Extended down to the level of the L1 vertebra (transpyloric plane) to ensure inclusion of the costophrenic angles.
- *Lateral borders*: Positioned to extend into air margins beyond both sides of the thoracic cavity, ensuring full lung coverage.

Radiation Dosage A single fraction dose of 75 cGy is prescribed at the midpoint of the anterior-posterior chest separation, using 6 MV X-ray photon beams.

During the entire procedure, the patient's oxygen saturation is to be continuously monitored via a pulse oximeter. The monitor is oriented toward a CCTV camera to allow real-time observation from the control area. Upon completion of the radiation delivery, the patient is transported back to the inpatient unit along the same designated corridor. The linear accelerator room must then be thoroughly sanitized in accordance with the vendor's established protocols for cleaning and disinfection.

4.5 Clinical Trials of LDRT in COVID Pneumonia

Animal studies have provided robust evidence that LDRT improves survival and reduces lung inflammation in models of viral pneumonia. For instance, mice infected with influenza A virus and treated with whole-lung LDRT exhibited markedly increased survival rates, reduced lung edema, and decreased airway and vascular inflammation compared to untreated controls. Importantly, LDRT did not affect viral titers, indicating that its therapeutic effect is mediated through modulation of host inflammatory responses rather than direct antiviral activity. Initial pilot studies demonstrated that a single fraction of 0.5–0.7 Gy delivered to both lungs was safe and associated with rapid improvement in oxygenation and clinical symptoms in patients with moderate to severe COVID-19 pneumonia. These studies reported no acute radiation toxicity and suggested potential to reduce ICU admissions and ventilator dependence.

Long-term safety studies in murine models have demonstrated that low-dose radiation therapy (LDRT), when administered at doses up to 1.8 Gy, does not lead to significant adverse effects such as radiation pneumonitis or pulmonary fibrosis. This contrasts sharply with high-dose radiation (e.g., 10 Gy), which has been associated with severe lung damage. These findings affirm the safety profile of LDRT and support its potential utility in managing pulmonary inflammatory diseases. In the context of COVID-19, where specific and consistently effective medical treatments remain lacking, supportive hospital-based care—especially in intensive care units (ICUs)—has been the primary recourse for approximately 5% of patients who progress to advanced disease stages [4].

Historically, low-dose radiotherapy was used to manage infectious respiratory conditions before the widespread availability of pharmacologic treatments. The resurgence of interest in LDRT stems from the pathophysiological features of COVID-19 pneumonitis, particularly the cytokine storm characterized by excessive levels of proinflammatory mediators such as interleukin-6 (IL-6) and tumor necrosis factor-alpha (TNF-α), which often precipitate respiratory failure. LDRT, particularly at doses below 100 cGy, exerts an anti-inflammatory effect by downregulating proinflammatory macrophages while promoting the activity of anti-inflammatory macrophages and immune cells—such as those producing interleukin-10 and transforming growth factor-β1—as well as natural killer (NK) T cells. This modulation of immune activity may help counteract the dysregulated immune response in COVID-19. Prior to the 1940s, LDRT was commonly employed to treat viral pneumonias, and historical data suggest that whole-lung irradiation may prevent the onset of cytokine storm and acute respiratory distress syndrome (ARDS).

More recent investigations, though limited by small sample sizes and short-term follow-up, have reported promising outcomes using LDRT doses ranging from 0.5 to 1.5 Gy [3, 15]. Both preclinical and clinical evidence point to a favorable safety profile. One of the earliest peer-reviewed trials conducted in the United States involved a safety evaluation of 1.5 Gy LDRT in elderly patients (median age: 90 years) with bilateral pulmonary infiltrates, oxygen dependency (without mechanical ventilation), and high comorbidity burdens—conditions that are typically associated with poor prognosis. This Phase I safety study (ClinicalTrials.gov Identifier: NCT04366791) enrolled seven patients; however, one was transferred to the ICU and another died prior to receiving LDRT, resulting in five patients receiving the treatment. No acute exacerbation of the cytokine storm or treatment-related adverse events were observed. Four of the five treated patients showed clinical improvement within 3–96 h post-irradiation. The trial successfully met its primary safety endpoint, demonstrating 7-day survival in all irradiated participants [16].

In India, a pilot study conducted at AIIMS IRCH yielded a 90% clinical response rate, reinforcing the feasibility and potential effectiveness of LDRT for patients with moderate to severe COVID-19 pneumonia. Nine patients experienced complete recovery, most within 3–7 days. One patient with a history of hypertension experienced clinical deterioration and died 24 days after treatment. Importantly, no participants in the study developed acute radiation toxicity [17]. Additional data from unpublished studies conducted at centers in Trichy and AIIMS Patna further support the viability of this approach in Indian clinical settings.

Ongoing trials include a Phase 2, single-arm study (NCT04427566), designed to assess 30-day mortality in patients requiring mechanical ventilation. Participants in this study receive 0.8 Gy of LDRT along with possible investigational treatments. Another key study is a randomized, multi-institutional clinical trial (NCT04466683) enrolling hospitalized patients who present with hypoxemia, fever, or pulmonary compromise, but who are not yet intubated. In the initial phase, participants are randomized to receive LDRT at either 0.35 Gy or 1 Gy. Based on pre-specified interim analysis, the trial will continue with randomization between standard of care (SOC) alone and SOC plus the more efficacious and safer of the two LDRT doses.

To achieve the full therapeutic potential of LDRT, precise optimization of the dose, timing, and patient selection are essential. The immunomodulatory benefit of LDRT is maximized when delivered during the early respiratory phase, where the intervention window is relatively narrow. The PRE-VENT trial [18] is currently enrolling patients with fever, cough, or dyspnea lasting fewer than 9 days, aiming to reduce the need for mechanical ventilation. Patients with advanced disease already requiring mechanical ventilation or exhibiting established pulmonary fibrosis are less likely to benefit. However, those who do not respond to standard therapies such as steroids or remdesivir may be ideal candidates for LDRT. Given the recent surge in steroid-induced mucormycosis among COVID-19 survivors, LDRT offers a compelling steroid-sparing alternative worth serious consideration.

Most current studies have prioritized enrolling patients aged 60 and older to minimize the risk of radiation-induced secondary malignancies. Nevertheless, emerging data—including from IRCH and the PRE-VENT trial—show that LDRT can be safely delivered to patients as old as 50 years of age.

Before initiating low-dose radiation therapy (LDRT), several technical and logistical factors must be carefully addressed. Foremost among these is ensuring the safety of healthcare personnel involved in administering the treatment. Adequate personal protective equipment (PPE) should be provided to all staff members to mitigate exposure risks. Additionally, the linear accelerator (LINAC) vault should be maintained under negative pressure—meaning the air pressure within the treatment room must be lower than that outside—to reduce the risk of airborne transmission.

To further enhance infection control, it is advisable to schedule the treatment of COVID-19 patients at the end of the day. This timing allows for thorough disinfection of the treatment room by the infection control team, in accordance with institutional sanitation protocols.

Various dose schedules have been explored in the literature, with single-fraction doses ranging from 3 Gy to 15 Gy. Among these, a 7 Gy dose has been most frequently employed. The PRE-VENT trial specifically examined two lower dose regimens: 0.35 Gy and 1.0 Gy. Notably, doses approaching or exceeding 1 Gy are considered to carry a higher risk of promoting proinflammatory responses and may also increase the likelihood of secondary malignancies. Therefore, a dose of up to 1 Gy is generally considered reasonable for achieving immunomodulatory benefits without incurring undue risk [19–21].

Although the theoretical risk of long-term stochastic effects—such as premature aging and radiation-induced malignancies—cannot be entirely ruled out, the very low doses used in LDRT for pneumonia make the likelihood of such outcomes highly implausible.

4.6 Radiation Dose Considerations

The radiation doses employed in the treatment of pneumonia using LDRT are typically less than 1% of those administered in conventional cancer radiotherapy, generally remaining well below 1 Gy. These low doses fall far beneath the established tolerance thresholds for critical organs such as the heart and stay cumulatively within safe exposure limits for other sensitive organs—for instance, 15–20 Gy for the thyroid, 45 Gy for the stomach, and 23–28 Gy for the kidneys. According to long-term epidemiological risk models, the estimated excess lifetime cancer risk in adjacent organs is minimal, with a latency period of approximately 10 years for any potential manifestation. Given the acute and potentially fatal nature of severe pneumonia, the risk–benefit ratio strongly favors therapeutic intervention, particularly when weighed against these rare and theoretical late effects [20].

Dose optimization strategies, including precise planning and organ shielding, play a crucial role in minimizing exposure to surrounding tissues. Among organs contributing most to potential radiation-related risk are the lungs and breasts. However, the likelihood of damage to out-of-field organs remains very low—estimated at less than 0.06 excess cases per 10,000 for lifetime attributable risk (LAR) in females, a figure approximately 22 times higher than that for males of the same age group. Even so, these risks remain modest. For a 60-year-old male, the effective doses from LDRT are comparable to those used in high-dose interventional radiology procedures, and the associated LAR is estimated to be about 8 times that of a standard cardiac CT scan when the prescription dose is 50 cGy [22].

Therefore, in clinically deteriorating patients with limited or no alternative treatment options, LDRT may be reasonably considered as a viable therapeutic modality.

4.7 Future Directions

Future directions and innovations in LDRT for alveolitis and pulmonary inflammation focus on optimizing efficacy, expanding applications, and integrating advanced technologies. Personalized treatment strategies using biomarkers such as immune cell profiles and cytokine levels aim to predict patient responses and tailor therapy. Combining LDRT with antiviral agents, corticosteroids, or immunomodulators may enhance outcomes while reducing systemic drug doses. Beyond COVID-19, LDCT shows potential for idiopathic pulmonary fibrosis, autoimmune lung diseases, and other pneumonias, warranting systematic evaluation. Technological advancements like image-guided and intensity-modulated radiotherapy could refine precision targeting of inflamed areas while sparing healthy tissue. Mechanistic research into pathways involving TGF-β, IL-10, and macrophage polarization will inform clinical trial design and biomarker development. Ultimately, large-scale randomized trials are critical to establish LDRT's safety, optimal dosing, and role alongside existing therapies, solidifying its position as a standard treatment for inflammatory lung conditions.

References

1. Bourke SC, Clague H. Review of cryptogenic fibrosing alveolitis, including current treatment guidelines. Postgrad Med J. 2000;76(900):618–24.
2. Rödel F, Frey B, Gaipl U, et al. Modulation of inflammatory immune reactions by low-dose ionizing radiation: molecular mechanisms and clinical application. Curr Med Chem. 2012;19(12):1741–50.
3. Calabrese EJ, Dhawan G. How radiotherapy was historically used to treat pneumonia: could it be useful today? Yale J Biol Med. 2013;86(4):555–70.
4. Thomas-Ruddel D, Winning J, Dickmann P, et al. Coronavirus disease 2019 (COVID-19): update for anesthesiologists and intensivists March 2020. Anaesthesist. 2020;70(Suppl 1):1–10. https://doi.org/10.1007/s00101-020-00760-3.
5. Fajgenbaum DC, June CH. Cytokine storm. N Engl J Med. 2020;383(23):2255–73.
6. Tay MZ, Poh CM, Rénia L, MacAry PA, Ng LFP. The trinity of COVID-19: immunity, inflammation and intervention. Nat Rev Immunol. 2020;20(6):363–74.
7. Connors JM, Levy JH. COVID-19 and its implications for thrombosis and anticoagulation. Blood. 2020;135(23):2033–40.
8. Iba T, Levy JH, Levi M, Thachil J. Coagulopathy in COVID-19. J Thromb Haemost. 2020;18(9):2103–9.
9. Rödel F, Frey B, Gaipl U, Keilholz L, Fournier C, Manda K, et al. Modulation of inflammatory immune reactions by low-dose ionizing radiation: molecular mechanisms and clinical application. Curr Med Chem. 2012;19(12):1741–50.
10. Arenas M, Sabater S, Hernández V, et al. Anti-inflammatory effects of low-dose radiotherapy. Strahlenther Onkol. 2012;188(1):975–81.
11. Meziani L, Mondini M, Petit B, et al. Low doses of radiation increase the immunosuppressive profile of lung macrophages during viral pneumonia. Int J Radiat Oncol Biol Phys. 2021;109(1):195–206.
12. Rödel F, Keilholz L, Herrmann M, et al. Radiobiological mechanisms in inflammatory diseases of low-dose radiation therapy. Int J Radiat Biol. 2007;83(6):357–66.
13. Rödel F, Hofmann D, Auer J, et al. The anti-inflammatory effect of low-dose radiation therapy: induction of TGF-β1 and suppression of E-selectin expression. Radiat Res. 2002;158(2):543–50.
14. Yuan L, Kim S, Palta J, Hagan MP. An efficient planning technique for low dose whole lung radiation therapy for covid-19 pandemic patients. Phys Imaging Radiat Oncol. 2020;16:85–8. https://doi.org/10.1016/j.phro.2020.10.004. Epub 2020 Oct 12. PMID: 33072896; PMCID: PMC7550039.
15. Kumar R, Haresh KP, Sharma DN, Gupta A, Gupta S, Vellaiyan S, et al. Low-dose radiotherapy for COVID 19: a radioimmunological perspective. J Cancer Res Ther. 2021;17(2):295–302.
16. Hess CB, Buchwald ZS, Stokes W, Nasti TH, Switchenko JM, Weinberg BD, et al. Low-dose whole-lung radiation for COVID-19 pneumonia: planned day 7 interim analysis of a registered clinical trial. Cancer. 2020;126(23):5109–13.
17. Sharma DN, Guleria R, Wig N, et al. Low dose radiation therapy for COVID-19 pneumonia: a pilot study. Br J Radiol. 2021;94(1126):20210187. https://doi.org/10.1101/2020.11.16.20231514.
18. George DW, Minesh PM, James SW, Arnab C, C. LR, James F. Investigating low-dose thoracic radiation as a treatment for COVID-19 patients to prevent respiratory failure. Radiat Res. 2020;194(1):1–8. https://doi.org/10.1667/RADE-20-00108.1.
19. Mitigating coronavirus-induced acute respiratory distress syndrome by radiotherapy. TrinitatGarcía,Hernándeza Maite Romero, Expósitob Beatriz Sánchez- Volume 153, December 2020, Pages 289–295.
20. Venkatraman P, Sahay JJ, Maidili T, Rajan R, Pooja S. Breakthrough of COVID-19 using radiotherapy treatment modalities. Radiother Oncol. 2020;148:225–6.

21. Dhawan G, Kapoor R, Dhawan R, Singh R, Monga B, Giordano J, et al. Low dose radiation therapy as a potential life saving treatment for COVID-19- induced acute respiratory distress syndrome (ARDS). Radiother Oncol. 2020;147:212–6.
22. Low dose radiation therapy for COVID-19: Effective dose and estimation of cancer risk Trinitat García-Hernández, Maite Romero-Expósito,Beatriz Sánchez-Nieto Volume 153, December 2020, Pages 289–295.

Stereotactic Radiosurgery in Benign Brain Tumours: Overview

5

Shyam Singh Bisht, Rishabh Arora, Ayushee Saini, Tapan Kapoor, and Deepak Gupta

5.1 Meningioma

5.1.1 Background

Meningiomas are the commonest primary intracranial tumors arising from the meninges and account for roughly one-third of all primary central nervous system (CNS) tumors [1]. They are typically slow-growing and benign (WHO grade 1 in ~80% of cases), though a minority can be atypical or malignant (grade 2:15–18%; grade 3:1–3%) [1].While complete resection can be curative in low grade, it is not always feasible—approximately 20–30% of meningiomas are in locations where total removal is impossible or carries high morbidity (e.g., skull base sites like cavernous sinus, clival, or optic nerve sheath meningiomas) [2]. There remains a 5% 5-year recurrence rate for grade 1 meningiomas that increases to 40% for grade 2 meningiomas and higher for grade 3. Radiation therapy (fractionated radiation therapy and radiosurgery) has emerged as the reliable second pillar: used as adjuvant after subtotal resection or definitively when surgery is not possible. SRS provides durable control (~90% at 5–10 years in modern series) with functional preservation [2]. Contemporary practice tailors observation, surgery, and SRS/RT to tumor biology, location, and patient priorities [3].

S. S. Bisht (✉) · R. Arora · A. Saini · D. Gupta
Division of Radiation Oncology, Medanta—The Medicity, Gurugram, India

T. Kapoor
Bhagwan Mahavir Cancer Hospital and Research Center, Jaipur, India

K. Sood Sharma (ed.), *Radiation Therapy for Benign Disorders*,
https://doi.org/10.1007/978-981-95-6635-8_5

5.1.2 Pathogenesis

Meningiomas arise from arachnoid cap cells, usually manifesting as slow-growing, dural-based tumors. Their biology is shaped by distinct molecular drivers. Roughly 40–60% harbor sporadic NF2 gene mutations on chromosome 22, disrupting the tumor-suppressor merlin and predisposing to multiple lesions in neurofibromatosis type 2, and 50–75% of patients with germline mutations develop meningiomas [4]. Higher-grade (atypical or anaplastic) meningiomas often show alterations such as TERT promoter mutations and homozygous deletions of CDKN2A/B, which confer the capacity for limitless replication and are strongly associated with more aggressive, rapidly recurring tumors, and presence of TERT promoter mutation or CDKN2A/B loss now qualifies a meningioma as WHO grade 3 in the 2021 WHO classification due to their adverse prognostic significance. Many grade 1 meningiomas express abundant progesterone receptors, and their growth can sometimes be influenced by hormonal changes. Meningiomas uniformly express somatostatin receptors (particularly SSTR2), which not only allows diagnostic imaging with radiolabeled somatostatin analogs but also provides a therapeutic avenue via peptide receptor radionuclide therapy. Importantly, benign meningiomas usually have low mitotic activity (hence their slow growth), but they can still be controlled by radiation due to their intrinsic radiosensitivity. In benign meningiomas, which proliferate slowly, radiation may not shrink the tumor immediately but can halt its growth and gradually cause tumor cells to lose reproductive capacity.

5.1.3 Role of Radiosurgery/Radiation Therapy

Radiation therapy plays a vital role in the multidisciplinary management of meningiomas, either as a primary treatment or as an adjuvant to surgery. Current consensus guidelines and clinical practice indicate RT in several scenarios:

- Inoperable or high-risk cases: Definitive RT (radiosurgery/fractionated radiosurgery) is recommended for patients who have symptomatic, growing, or life-threatening meningiomas that cannot be safely resected due to location or medical comorbidities [5].
- Incompletely resected tumors: For a benign (grade I) meningioma that was subtotally resected (STR) or has residual tumor, adjuvant SRS is often considered to reduce recurrence risk. Retrospective series have reported 5-year progression-free survival (PFS) rates as low as 40–60% after subtotal resection alone [2]. In the NRG Oncology RTOG 0539 study (Phase II trial), patients with residual or recurrent benign meningiomas (classified as "intermediate-risk") who received adjuvant RT had an excellent 3-year PFS of 94%, significantly better than historical controls (3-year PFS ~70%) with surgery alone [6]. A recent prospective "observation-only" cohort for low-risk meningiomas (newly diagnosed grade I with gross-total resection) showed 5- and 10-year PFS rates of 89% and 85%, respectively, but among those with STR the 5-year PFS was only ~73% [7].

- Adjuvant RT for higher-grade meningiomas: For atypical (WHO grade II) and anaplastic (grade III) meningiomas, the risk of recurrence after surgery is high, so adjuvant RT is generally recommended even after gross total excision [5, 8].
- Recurrent disease: Radiation is commonly used for recurrent meningiomas of any grade, especially if a second surgery is not feasible. Stereotactic radiosurgery has been particularly effective for small recurrent nodules, achieving high local control with minimal treatment time. For multiple recurrences or previously irradiated tumors, re-irradiation can be considered on a case-by-case basis (sometimes with advanced techniques like proton therapy to spare already irradiated tissues).

Patient selection is based on tumor size, location, presence of symptoms and comorbidities (Table 5.1). Small (<3 cm), well-circumscribed tumors not compressing the optic apparatus are ideal for single-fraction SRS. Larger or critically located lesions are managed with fractionated RT to protect adjacent structures. Older or medically fragile patients often benefit from primary RT, while younger patients with resectable disease may still undergo surgery to avoid long-term radiation exposure.

5.1.4 Radiation Technique

- Fractionated external beam RT (EBRT): Standard for large, residual, or surgically inaccessible tumors. Typical dose is 50–54 Gy in 1.8–2 Gy fractions for grade I, and up to 59–60 Gy for grade II/III [2, 5]. IMRT and VMAT allow sharp dose fall-off, limiting exposure to optic nerves, brainstem, and cochlea and should be used.

Table 5.1 Suggested Radiation, dose and fractionations schedule for different WHO grades of meningioma. (GTR: Gross total resection; STR: Subtotal resection; SRS: Stereotactic Radiosurgery; FSRS: Fractionated Radiosurgery; cFRT: Conventionally fractionated Radiotherapy; Fx:Fractions)

Grade/extent of excision	RT	Dose: SRS	Dose: F SRS	Dose: cFRT
WHO Grade1, GTR	Observation			
WHO Grade 1, STR/recurrent	SRS/FSRS/ cFRT	13–14 Gy	24 Gy/3Fx---30 Gy/5Fx	50–54 Gy/25–30 Fx
WHO Grade 2, GTR	SRS/FSRS/ cFRT	15-18Gy	24Gy/3Fx--30Gy/5Fx	54Gy-59.4Gy/27-33Fx
WHO Grade 2, STR/recurrent	SRS/ FSRS/ cFRT	15–18 Gy	27Gy/3Fx--35Gy/5Fx	59.4Gy/33Fx
WHO Grade 3, any	cFRT(SRS/ FSRS- evidence lacking)	18–24 Gy	30Gy/3Fx–40Gy/5Fx	60Gy/30Fx ± GTV Boost
Radiological low grade (non-operated)	SRS/ FSRS/ cFRT	13–14 Gy	24 Gy/3 Fx–30 Gy/5	50–54 Gy/25–30 Fx

- Stereotactic radiosurgery (SRS): Ideal for small (<3 cm), well-circumscribed tumors not abutting the optic apparatus. Single-session Gamma Knife or linac-based SRS delivers 12–16 Gy, achieving ~90–95% 5-year control [2]. When tumors lie close to sensitive structures, fractionated stereotactic radiosurgery (FSRS; e.g., 24–30 Gy in 3–5 fractions) reduces toxicity risk while maintaining high control which is comparable to SRS [9]. The choice between single vs. multi-fraction radiosurgery depends on OAR constraints and tumor size—if OAR dose would exceed safe limits with single-fraction, hypofractionation is chosen (Figs. 5.1, 5.2).
- Proton therapy: Exploits the Bragg peak to reduce exit dose, useful for skull base tumors or younger patients where long-term toxicity is a concern. There are case series that report 5- to 10-year control rates of 85–95%, comparable to photons but with potentially less integral brain dose.

5.1.5 Toxicity

Acute effects include fatigue, localized alopecia, and occasional skin erythema during fractionated RT; SRS may cause transient headache or nausea. Steroids are sometimes prescribed to counter early edema. Subacute toxicities (weeks–months post-RT) largely stem from peritumoral edema, which can transiently worsen neurological symptoms. Symptomatic edema is more common after single-fraction SRS in larger tumors; fractionated schedules reduce this risk. Late toxicities are the main concern given long survival. With modern dosing, serious complications are uncommon:

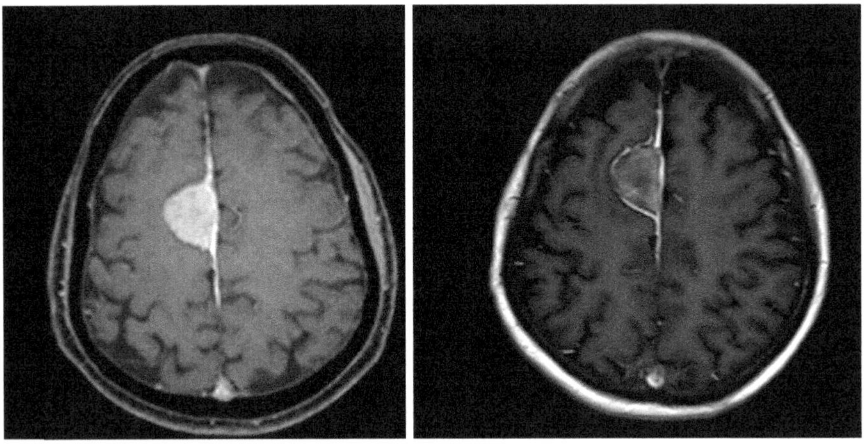

Fig. 5.1 Pattern of response in Meningioma after SRS: Pre–SRS(left panel) image displays a well defined rounded dural based T1-weighted contrast enhancing lesion, and 1 year post-SRS(right panel) image displays heterogenous loss of contrast enhancement with development of patchy necrosis suggestive of response. SRS dose delivered was 24Gy in 3 sessions on Cyberknife VSI platform. (Courtesy-Radiation Oncology, Medanta The Medicity)

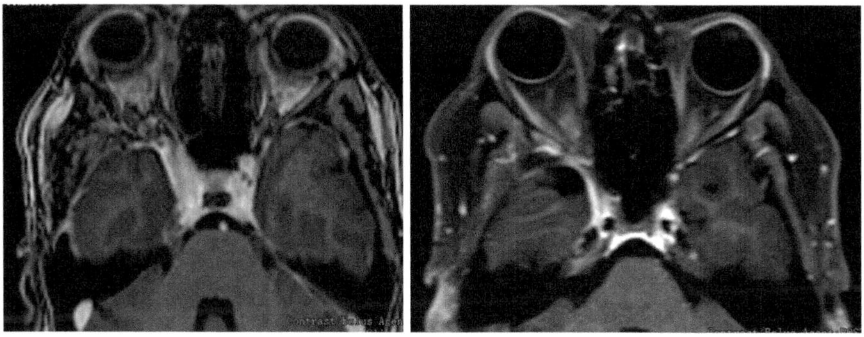

Fig. 5.2 Cavernous sinus meningioma: Pre-SRS (left panel) image displays T1-weighted contrast enhancing lesion in right cavernous sinus and right panel image(5 years post SRS) displays near complete resolution of the dural thickening. (Courtesy-Radiation Oncology, Medanta The Medicity)

- Radiation necrosis occurs in <5% and is usually manageable with steroids; rare severe cases may require surgery.
- Cranial neuropathies are rare when dose constraints are respected. The optic nerves/chiasm should remain ≤54 Gy (fractionated) or ≤8–10 Gy (SRS) to avoid optic neuropathy.
- Endocrine dysfunction may arise when the pituitary/hypothalamus lies in-field, warranting long-term hormonal follow-up [3].
- Hearing loss can occur if cochlear dose exceeds ~45 Gy mean.
- Secondary malignancy is rare (<2% at 20 years) and risk is lower with conformal techniques and protons.

When to consider for SRS/fractionated SRS in meningioma

- Radiologically non-G2/3.
- Size: Small (<2 cm); 2–4 cm (Fx SRS).
- Symptoms: asymptomatic or minimally symptomatic.
- Compression: no/minimal compressive symptoms.
- Edema: nil or minimal edema.
- Distance from serial OAR: At least 2–3 mm.
- Residual post-surgery: grade I residual.
- Recurrent: grades II, III (selected).

5.2 Vestibular Schwannoma

5.2.1 Background

Vestibular schwannoma (VS) is a benign Schwann cell tumor of the vestibulocochlear nerve, accounting for 8–10% of intracranial tumors and the most common cerebellopontine angle neoplasm [10]. Most cases are unilateral and sporadic, while about 5–7% occur with the genetic syndrome neurofibromatosis type 2 (NF2) that causes bilateral VS. Although benign and slow-growing, VS can lead to significant morbidity. Patients typically present with unilateral sensorineural hearing loss (in ~90% of cases), tinnitus, and balance difficulties [10]. Historically, the management of VS has evolved considerably. In the early twentieth century, attempted surgical removal carried high risks—operative mortality was on the order of 20–40%, and permanent facial paralysis was common. In parallel, stereotactic radiosurgery (SRS) emerged as a less invasive treatment option. The Gamma Knife was first used to treat a VS in 1969, and through the 1980s–1990s, SRS gained acceptance as an effective modality for small-to moderate-sized VS. Today, management of vestibular schwannoma is highly individualized. The main options include initial observation ("watch and wait" with serial MRI) for small asymptomatic tumors, microsurgical resection, and SRS (either single-fraction SRS or fractionated stereotactic radiosurgery, FSRS) [11].

5.2.2 Pathogenesis

Vestibular schwannomas arise from Schwann cells due to inactivation of the NF2 tumor-suppressor gene on chromosome 22q. Loss of NF2 function leads to a deficiency of the merlin protein (schwannomin), which normally regulates contact inhibition in cells. Merlin inactivation removes these growth restraints, resulting in unregulated Schwann cell proliferation and tumor formation. VS are benign encapsulated neoplasms (WHO grade I) composed of Schwann cells; they typically exhibit a low mitotic index but can still gradually expand. The natural growth rate is variable (on average ~2 mm per year in diameter). As a VS enlarges beyond the internal auditory canal into the cerebellopontine angle, it can compress and displace the brainstem and cranial nerves, producing progressive neurological deficits (hearing loss, facial nerve palsy, trigeminal nerve impairment, etc.) and potentially life-threatening brainstem compression if the tumor grows large enough [10]. Koos grading system is used for VS (Table 5.2).

5.2.3 Role of Radiosurgery/Radiation Therapy

Radiosurgery is a key modality for vestibular schwannoma, especially for small-to-moderate tumors (<3 cm), and residual or recurrent disease. SRS/FSRS achieves long-term tumor control rates of 90–95%, comparable to microsurgery but with lower morbidity. SRS is particularly advantageous for preserving facial and trigeminal nerve function, with permanent facial paralysis occurring in <2% of modern series [12]. Hearing preservation is possible in ~50–70% at 5 years, though rates decline over time [12].

Management is individualized according to tumor size (Koos grade), tumor growth, presence of symptoms, and patient comorbidities (Fig. 5.3):

Table 5.2 Koos grading system for Vestibular Schwannoma

Grade	Tumor extent
1	Intracanalicular tumor
2	Tumor extends into cistern but not reaching to brainstem
3	Reaching the brainstem surface
4	Deforming the brainstem surface and shifting the fourth ventricle

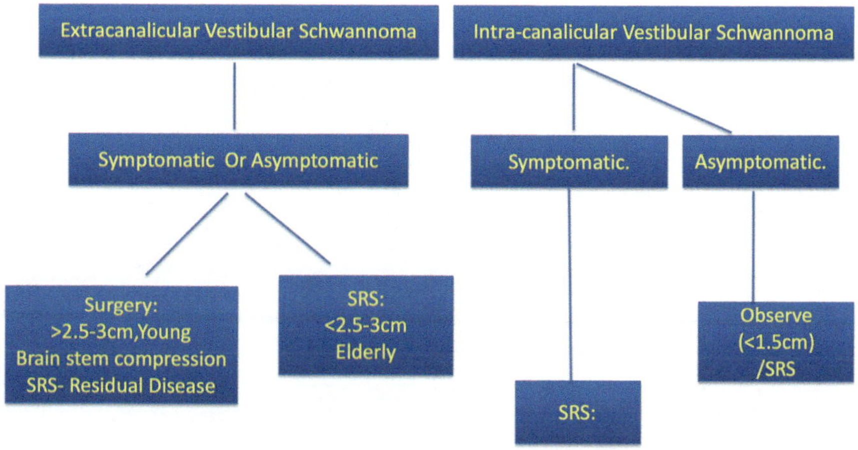

Fig. 5.3 Simplified Treatment algorithm for vestibular schwannoma

- *Observation*: Preferred for small, asymptomatic lesions (Koos I) or elderly/comorbid patients due to the slow growth rate (average 0.7 ± 1.4 mm/year; 82% grow less than 1 mm/year). Of late the role of observation in small acoustic schwannoma has come into question as delivering SRS in observation failure cases may further lead to poor hearing preservation.
  A large tumor and tinnitus at diagnosis increase the odds of higher growth rate.
- *Single-fraction RS*: Standard for small-to moderate-sized tumors (Koos I–III; volume <15 cc) without significant brainstem compression or fourth ventricle deviation; strong consensus for marginal doses of 12–13 Gy [13].
  For every 1 cc increase in median tumor volume, 5-year PFS fell by 1.5% [14].
- *Fractionated SRS*: Option for small to moderate tumors (<30 mm or approx.30 cc (Koos grade II-III)), especially when close to critical structures. No statistically significant difference in 5-year tumor control rates, hearing, trigeminal and facial nerve preservation rates between single-dose RS and FSRS, as per many retrospective series comparing treatment of patients with RS v/s FSRS [15].
- *Surgery*: Recommended for large tumors with mass effect (Koos IV), tumors causing significant brainstem compression or fourth ventricle deviation or with features of facial nerve involvement, or when rapid decompression is necessary.

5.2.4 Radiosurgery Doses and Fractionation Regimens for Vestibular Schwannoma

The International Stereotactic Radiosurgery Society (ISRS) Practice Guideline provides a detailed systematic review of radiation therapy (RT) doses, techniques, and outcomes for vestibular schwannoma patients. The two primary RT modalities discussed are single-fraction radiosurgery (RS, including Gamma Knife and linear accelerator-based RS) and fractionated stereotactic radiation therapy (FSRT, both conventional and hypofractionated). Typical post-SRS response is shown in Fig. 5.4.

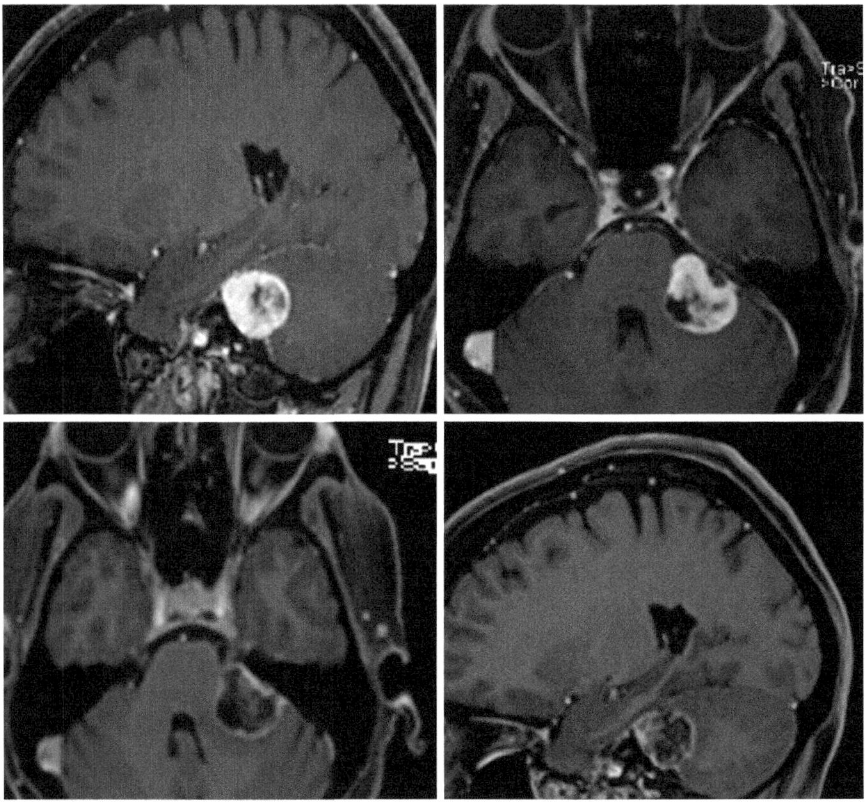

Fig. 5.4 MRI images of patient with vestibular schwannoma Pre-SRS (upper 2 panels) and 1-year post-SRS images(lower 2 panels). PreSRS images in sagittal and axial sections displays contrast enhancing lesion in left CP angle and post SRS images displays loss os enhancement with development of necrosis within the tumor. Dose delivered was 19.5Gy in 3 sessions at 80% prescription isodose on Cyberknife VSI platform. (Courtesy-Radiation Oncology, Medanta The Medicity)

5.2.4.1 Modalities

Stereotactic Radiosurgery (SRS)

- Gamma Knife/Cyberknife: Single session, typically 12–13 Gy prescribed for tumor margin at present (started with 18–20 Gy in 1980s→ reduced to 14–16 Gy in 1990s due to high complications).
- 5-year tumor control rates of 91–99%; hearing preservation rates of 41–79%; facial nerve preservation 95–100%; trigeminal nerve preservation 79–99% [17].
- Linear accelerator: Similar marginal doses yield ~90% 5-year control; facial and trigeminal preservation rates 96% (hearing function not assessed) [18].

Fractionated Stereotactic Radiotherapy (FSRT)

- Hypofractionated regimens: Prescribed at tumor margin or to the PTV 5 Gy × 5 sessions, 6 Gy × 3 sessions.
- Tumor control ranges, 96–100%; hearing preservation, 70–76%; facial and trigeminal nerve preservation, 99–100% [19].

5.2.5 Toxicity Profile

Radiosurgery for vestibular schwannoma is generally well tolerated. *Acute effects* are mild, including transient headache, imbalance, or nausea, usually resolving with conservative care or short steroid courses. *Late toxicities* are more relevant. Progressive hearing loss remains the most common, with serviceable hearing preserved in ~50–70% at 5 years and ~25–50% at 10 years [10, 16]. Recommended cochlear doses are shown in Table 5.3. Facial and trigeminal nerve dysfunctions are uncommon (<2–5%), with most cases being mild sensory changes. Symptomatic brainstem injury or radionecrosis is exceedingly rare (<1%) when modern dose constraints are respected [12]. Hydrocephalus can occur in ~1–2% due to pseudoprogression or CSF pathway obstruction (Fig. 5.5).

Table 5.3 Suggested dose constraints for Cochlea in Vestibular Schwannoma SRS/FSRS

	SRS	Fractionated SRS
Mean dose	<4 Gy	17 Gy(3 fractions) 25 Gy(5 fractions)
Maximum dose	4 Gy to modiolus of cochlea	

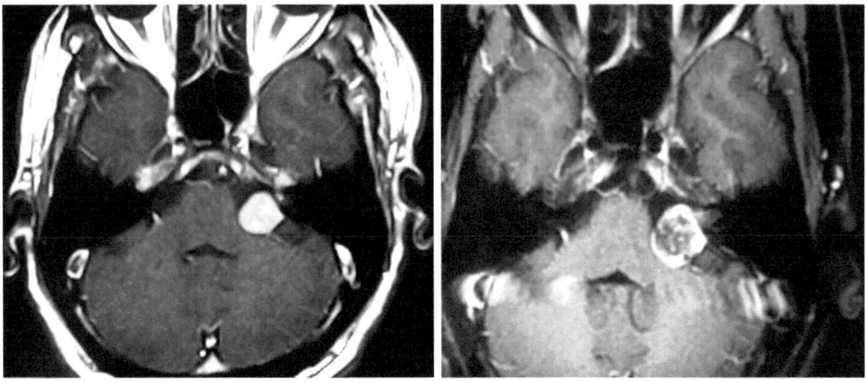

Fig. 5.5 Pseudo progression after SRS in Vestibular Schwannoma. Left panel image displays well defined enhancing lesion before SRS and right panel image, 12 months after SRS demonstrate increase in size of lesion with heterogenous contrast enhancement and areas of necrosis suggestive of pseudo progression. (Courtesy-Radiation Oncology, Medanta The Medicity)

5.3 Pituitary Adenomas

5.3.1 Background

Pituitary adenomas (PA) are benign neoplasms of the anterior pituitary that account for approximately 10–15% of primary intracranial tumors. The annual incidence is around 4 per 100,000 population, with increasingly frequent detection due to widespread MRI use [20]. Clinically, they are classified based on size (microadenomas <10 mm, macroadenomas ≥10 mm) (Fig. 5.6) and hormone secretion: functioning (hormone-secreting), such as prolactinomas, somatotroph adenomas causing acromegaly, corticotroph adenomas causing Cushing's disease, and thyrotroph adenomas; and non-functioning, which typically manifests through mass effect producing headaches, visual field loss (classically bitemporal hemianopsia from optic chiasm compression), or cranial nerve palsies. Most are sporadic, though a minority arise in familial syndromes (e.g., MEN1, Carney complex). Most common pituitary adenomas are prolactinomas. Pituitary adenomas historically were managed with transcranial surgery until the transsphenoidal surgical approach (pioneered in the mid-twentieth century) greatly reduced morbidity. Conventional radiotherapy for pituitary tumors was introduced in the 1960s as an adjunct for residual or unresectable disease [21].

5.3.2 Pathogenesis

Pituitary adenomas (recently termed pituitary neuroendocrine tumors, PiNETs) arise from monoclonal expansion of adenohypophyseal cells. The exact molecular pathogenesis is complex and not fully understood. Most cases are sporadic; only

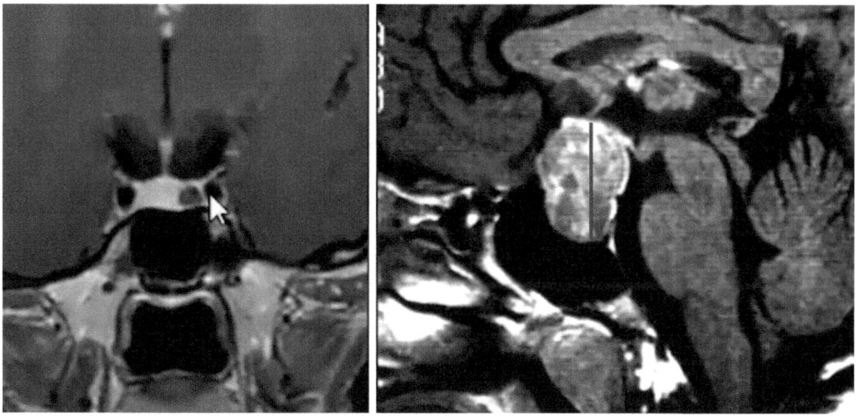

Fig. 5.6 Pituitary Microadenoma (Left panel coronal section image) versus Pituitary macroadenoma (Right panel sagittal section image), more than 1 cm cranio-caudal extent. (Courtesy-Radiation Oncology, Medanta-The Medicity)

~5% are familial. These tumors are typically slow-growing and histologically benign, but they can exhibit locally invasive behavior, extending into the cavernous sinus, suprasellar region, or bone [21] Functional adenomas secrete excess hormones (e.g., prolactin, growth hormone, ACTH), leading to clinical syndromes (acromegaly, gigantism, Cushing's disease, etc.), whereas nonfunctioning adenomas cause symptoms via mass effect (most critically, optic chiasm compression causing visual field defects).

5.3.3 Role of Radiation Therapy/Radiosurgery

Radiation therapy in PA achieves long-term local control while minimizing treatment-related morbidity. Although "benign," pituitary adenomas can cause serious neurologic or endocrine dysfunction via mass effect or hormone hypersecretion. Complete surgical removal may be infeasible. In functional pituitary adenomas, radiation not only inhibits cell proliferation but also curtails hormone overproduction—as hyperfunctioning adenoma cells are damaged, hormone levels fall over time. This process is protracted; hormone normalization may take months to years post-RT, depending on baseline levels [22]. Surgery is the first-line treatment for most pituitary adenomas, but RT plays a crucial role in a number of scenarios. Adjuvant RT is indicated for residual adenomatous tissue after surgery, especially if there is tumor invasion into areas not safely resectable (such as cavernous sinus) or if postoperative imaging shows significant remnant. In cases of recurrent adenomas after prior surgery, RT is often the treatment of choice to achieve long-term control. For functional (hormone-secreting) adenomas, RT is typically reserved for patients whose disease is not cured by surgery [23]. In acromegaly or Cushing's disease, if surgical resection fails to normalize hormonal levels, radiosurgery is followed by medical therapies (like somatostatin analogs, or adrenal-blocking drugs) to gradually reduce hormone hypersecretion [23]. Prolactinomas are a special case—medical therapy with dopamine agonists is first line and very effective followed by surgery if medical therapy fails. SRS is needed if the tumor is refractory to medication or the patient cannot tolerate lifelong medical management [24]. Primary radiation (without surgery) for pituitary adenoma is less common but may be considered in patients unfit for surgery or who decline surgery, particularly if the tumor is small and well away from the optic chiasm [20]. Nonfunctioning adenomas that demonstrate growth on serial imaging or threaten vision can also be treated with RT if surgery is contraindicated. Overall, pituitary RT is indicated for residual or recurrent adenomas, persistent hormone excess after surgery/medications, inoperable tumors (due to medical comorbidities or skull base invasion), and occasionally as primary therapy for progressive tumors in patients who are poor surgical candidates [25, 26]. RT is noninvasive, making it particularly valuable for lesions in surgically inaccessible locations such as the cavernous sinus (Fig. 5.7).

5.3.4 Dose and Fractionation Regimens

SRS dosing for pituitary tumors depends on tumor type and proximity to the optic apparatus. Common practice is a single-fraction dose of 15–16 Gy to the tumor margin for nonfunctioning adenomas and 18–25 Gy for functional adenomas. Higher doses yield better hormone normalization rates, especially in acromegaly and Cushing's, but the optic chiasm should generally receive <8–10 Gy in one fraction to avoid neuropathy; therefore, if the adenoma is too close to the chiasm, the SRS dose is lowered or fractionation is used. Hypofractionated stereotactic

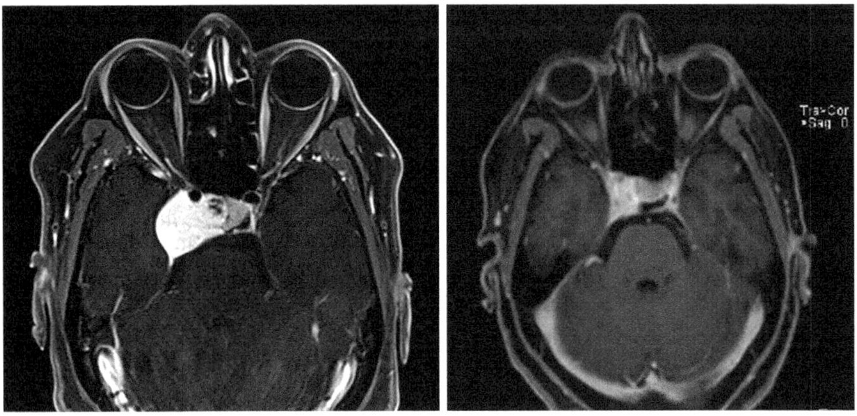

Fig. 5.7 SRS in pituitary adenoma invading cavernous sinus. PreSRS (left panel) image displays nonfunctional pituitary adenoma invading right cavernous sinus which has demonstrated good regression, at 2 years post SRS (right image panel). Dose delivered was 24Gy in 3 sessions at 70% prescription isodose on Cyberknife VSI platform. (Courtesy-Radiation Oncology, Medanta-The Medicity)

schedules (e.g., 21 Gy in 3 fractions, 25 Gy in 5 fractions, or 35 Gy in 7 fractions) have also been employed for adenomas that are adjacent to optic nerves, as a compromise that allows a higher total dose than single-fraction SRS while splitting the dose to protect the optic apparatus. Thus, the aim should be to maintain cumulative biologically effective dose (BED) around 80 Gy(a/b^3). Conventional fractionated regimens historically ranged from 45 to 54 Gy delivered in 1.8–2 Gy per fraction over 5–6 weeks [20]. In modern practice, a typical prescription is about 45–50.4 Gy in 25–28 fractions for both nonfunctioning and functioning adenomas. This dose achieves ~90 % tumor control at 10 years in multiple series [22, 24]. For secreting adenomas, some centers treat toward the upper end (50–54 Gy) to maximize the chance of hormonal remission [23].

Important organs at risk are optic chiasma, optic nerves, stalk of pituitary, remaining pituitary gland, hypothalamus. During SRS, aim should be to keep optic chiasma dose maximum and 0.2 cc below 10Gy and 8 Gy, 17.4Gy and 15.4 Gy, 25Gy and 23 Gy in 1, 3 and 5fractions respectively. Studies have suggested to keep mean stalk dose below 7 Gy. Constraints for hypothalamus are not well known.

5.3.5 Toxicity

Acute toxicities from pituitary RT are generally mild—transient headache, fatigue, nausea, or temporary hormonal fluctuations that resolve quickly. Sometime pseudoprogression is also seen after SRS, usually within 6 month to year. The most frequent long-term effect is hypopituitarism, which can develop gradually over years and requires lifelong endocrine monitoring and replacement. With modern stereotactic or conformal techniques, the risk of radiation-induced optic neuropathy is very low (<1% rate when maximum dose to chiasma is kept less than 8 Gy). Rare late effects include cranial nerve deficits, neurocognitive changes, or secondary intracranial tumors. Careful target delineation, strict adherence to optic/brainstem dose limits, and use of highly conformal or fractionated regimens have markedly reduced the incidence and severity of these complications.

5.4 Glomus Tumor

5.4.1 Background

Glomus jugulare tumors (jugular paragangliomas) are rare benign skull base tumors arising from neural crest-derived paraganglia in the jugular foramen. They comprise <1% of intracranial tumors. Glomus tumors typically present in middle age (median ~55–60 years) with a strong female predominance [27]. Patients often report pulsatile tinnitus, hearing loss, and lower cranial nerve deficits due to local invasion. Tumors are hypervascular and have proximity to critical structures like the carotid artery, jugular vein, and brainstem which poses significant risks, including cranial nerve damage and excessive bleeding [28]. In the late twentieth century, stereotactic radiosurgery (SRS) emerged as a noninvasive alternative for glomus tumors, given their radiosensitivity and difficult surgical anatomy. Today, modern radiation techniques (including SRS and highly conformal external beam RT) play a key role in the multidisciplinary management of these benign intracranial tumors.

5.4.2 Pathogenesis

Glomus jugulare tumors are parasympathetic paragangliomas that originate from paraganglionic chief cells in the adventitia of the jugular bulb. These cells, derived from the neural crest, normally act as chemoreceptors [29]. Glomus tumors are highly vascular lesions (classically exhibiting a "salt-and-pepper" MRI appearance due to flow voids). They typically remain benign, with only ~1–5% undergoing malignant transformation or metastasis. Pathophysiologically, even benign glomus tumors can be locally aggressive: they infiltrate the temporal bone and skull base, erode bone, and encase cranial nerves IX–XI and vessels. A small subset (estimated 1–3%) of head/neck paragangliomas are functional, secreting catecholamines that cause systemic symptoms (e.g., hypertension, tachycardia) [30].

5.4.3 Role of Radiosurgery/Radiation Therapy

Radiation induces endothelial damage and fibrosis within the tumor's extensive vasculature, reduces blood flow, and starves the tumor of nutrients. Over time, treated glomus tumors often show sclerosis and shrinkage, relieving pressure on cranial nerves. Importantly, because these tumors are not malignant, SRS doesn't eradicate but rather durable control is achieved—turning an active growing lesion into an inert one. Given the high surgical morbidity for these tumors, SRS is frequently used as definitive primary treatment for glomus jugulare tumors. SRS is indicated for small-to medium-sized glomus tumors that cause symptoms or demonstrate growth, especially when they are confined to the skull base without extensive neck extension. In many contemporary series, asymptomatic or minimally symptomatic glomus tumors may be managed with an initial observation ("wait-and-scan") approach, but if there is clear growth or notable symptoms (e.g., worsening tinnitus, cranial nerve palsies), radiation is recommended to prevent further progression [31]. Adjunctive RT is also used postoperatively in cases of subtotal resection. In fact, a combined approach is common: surgical debulking of large tumors to relieve brainstem or nerve compression, followed by radiation to treat residual disease, yields good control with lower overall morbidity. Thus, indications include inoperable or unresectable glomus tumors (due to difficult location or patient factors), residual tumor after partial resection, recurrent tumors after prior surgery, and bilateral/multiple paragangliomas where a conservative strategy is needed. For younger patients with intact lower cranial nerve function, some experts still favor primary surgery (with careful nerve monitoring) to achieve debulking [28]; however, even in those cases, adjuvant radiation might be added to address microscopic disease.

A meta-analysis [32] found that radiosurgery achieved ~97% tumor control with no procedure-related mortality and low permanent complication rates. Many patients even experience improvement of preexisting neurological symptoms after RT as the tumor shrinks or at least stops compressing nerves. Thus, for glomus tumors, the benefit of RT lies in its favorable risk-benefit profile: high efficacy in tumor control and symptom stabilization, with far fewer cranial neuropathies than surgery. Radiosurgery is also cost-effective and usually done outpatient, avoiding the prolonged hospital stay and recovery of open skull base surgery [33].

5.4.4 Radiation Dose

The recommended SRS dose is in the range of 12–18 Gy to the tumor margin. Many series have used a median of ~15 Gy, which has proven quite successful—a systematic review found that marginal doses ≥15 Gy are associated with local control rates >90% [34]. Doses up to 20–25 Gy in one fraction have been reported for larger tumors or partial brainstem contact, sometimes with staging of the treatment, but the risk of cranial neuropathy rises with higher doses. As such, if the glomus tumor is large or encases nerves, practitioners often choose hypofractionated SRS (for example, 3–5 fractions of ~5–7 Gy each). Hypofractionation allows a higher biological dose to the tumor (e.g., total ~30–35 Gy in 5 fractions) while allowing normal tissue sub-lethal damage repair between fractions, thus reducing cranial nerve injury risk [35]. Proton therapy can be used for glomus tumors as well, typically with similar total doses (e.g., 50.4 Gy[RBE] in 28 fractions); the advantage is reduced dose to off-target tissues like the contralateral ear or brain, but outcomes are comparable to photon RT in terms of tumor control [36].

For glomus tumors, special considerations include the tumor's vascularity and potential secretory nature. While RT is effective, a highly vascular glomus may bleed or swell transiently post-RT, so patients are observed for any acute cranial nerve swelling symptoms; significant post-SRS swelling is uncommon, but peritumoral edema can occur. In functioning paragangliomas (secreting catecholamines), patients should be on appropriate alpha-/beta-blockade medications before undergoing RT because radiation could (theoretically) provoke catecholamine release. Another unique factor for head and neck paragangliomas is the possibility of multiple tumors (e.g., synchronous carotid body tumor and glomus). In such cases, RT can be targeted to each tumor sequentially or within the same plan if nearby, avoiding multiple morbid surgeries.

Acute effects are usually mild and self-limited—transient headache, fatigue, localized skin erythema, or temporary ear fullness/tinnitus. Occasionally patients may experience transient cranial nerve irritation but serious acute toxicity is rare. Late effects include the risk of sensorineural hearing loss, especially if cochlear doses are high, as well as very rare lower cranial-nerve palsies or vestibular dysfunction. With modern SRS/FSRS, the incidence of significant new cranial-nerve deficits is <5%, and radionecrosis or secondary malignancy is extremely uncommon. Careful cochlear/brainstem sparing and dose constraint adherence have markedly reduced these risks.

5.5 Chordoma of the Skull Base

5.5.1 Background

Chordomas are rare, slow-growing malignant tumors derived from remnants of the notochord. They primarily arise along the axial skeleton, with the skull base (clivus) and sacrococcygeal regions being the most common sites. At the skull base, chordomas account for approximately *35–40% of cases* [37]. Although histologically low to intermediate grade, their locally invasive behaviour and proximity to critical neurovascular structures make management challenging. Historically, surgery was the cornerstone of treatment, with limited success due to incomplete removal and high recurrence rates. The advent of microsurgical and endoscopic endonasal techniques improved resection outcomes, yet gross total excision remains difficult [38]. Currently radiation therapy/radiosurgery has emerged as an essential adjunct [39].

5.5.2 Pathogenesis

These tumors are characterized by the presence of *physaliferous cells*, which are vacuolated cells embedded in a myxoid stroma. Immunohistochemically, chordomas typically express *brachyury*, a transcription factor that is a highly specific marker of notochordal differentiation, as well as cytokeratins, S100, and epithelial membrane antigen (EMA) [41]. Pathophysiologically, chordomas are locally invasive, eroding bone and infiltrating dura, cranial nerves, and vasculature, but they metastasize infrequently (5–10%) [42].

5.5.3 Role of Radiation Therapy/Radiosurgery

It has the ability to sterilize residual microscopic disease and control tumors in surgically inaccessible regions. Consequently, RT is considered indispensable in long-term disease control, particularly where radical surgery is unachievable [40]. Although chordomas are relatively radioresistant compared to other malignancies, high-precision and escalated doses ($\geq$70 Gy in photon-equivalent dosing) achieve durable local control [43]. Proton and carbon ion therapies, with their superior dose distributions, enhance tumoricidal effects while sparing adjacent structures such as the optic apparatus and brainstem [44].

5.5.3.1 Indications

- *Adjuvant RT* following subtotal or gross total resection (standard of care).
- *Definitive RT* in unresectable cases or patients unfit for surgery.
- *Salvage RT* for recurrences after surgery.
- *Boost therapy* with SRS in selected cases.

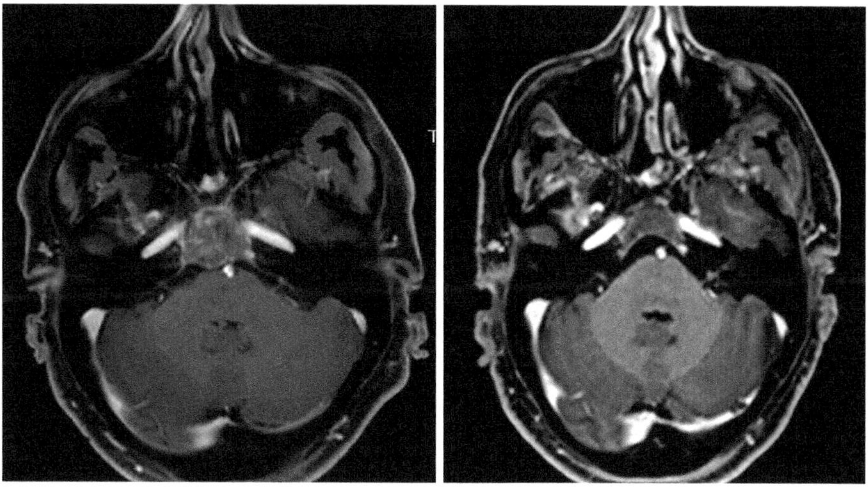

Fig. 5.8 MRI Image displays Clival chordoma, preSRS (left panel image) and 1-year, post SRS (right panel image) showing good regression after dose of 40Gy in 5 fractions on Cyberknife VSI platform. Maximum dose received by brainstem was limited to 29.9Gy by accepting lower coverage of target posteriorly without compromising overall dose to tumor. (Courtesy-Radiation Oncology, Medanta-The Medicity)

Chordomas are inherently radioresistant, necessitating *high doses* for effective control (Fig. 5.8). However, dose escalation is limited by proximity to optic nerves, chiasm, and brainstem. SRS, proton beam therapy, and carbon ion therapy overcome these limitations with superior dose distributions.

In conclusion, RT is indispensable in chordoma care. Its role is complementary to surgery and, in select cases, definitive. Despite inherent radioresistance, technological advances have transformed RT into the most effective tool for durable disease control at the skull base.

References

1. Yarabarla V, Mylarapu A, Han TJ, McGovern SL, Raza SM, Beckham TH. Intracranial meningiomas: an update of the 2021 World Health Organization classifications and review of management with a focus on radiation therapy. Front Oncol [Internet] 2023 Aug 22 [cited 2025 Sep 15];13. Available from: https://www.frontiersin.org/journals/oncology/articles/10.3389/fonc.2023.1137849/full.
2. Radiation therapy for WHO grade I meningioma - Day - Chinese Clinical Oncology [Internet]. [cited 2025 Sep 21]. Available from: https://cco.amegroups.org/article/view/15325/html.
3. EANO guideline on the diagnosis and management of meningiomas - PubMed [Internet]. [cited 2025 Sep 21]. Available from: https://pubmed.ncbi.nlm.nih.gov/34181733/.
4. Clark VE, Erson-Omay EZ, Serin A, Yin J, Cotney J, Ozduman K, et al. Genomic analysis of non-NF2 meningiomas reveals mutations in TRAF7, KLF4, AKT1, and SMO. Science. 2013;339(6123):1077–80.

5. Target volume delineation for radiotherapy of meningiomas: an ANOCEF consensus guideline | Radiation Oncology | Full Text [Internet]. [cited 2025 Sep 21]. Available from: https://ro-journal.biomedcentral.com/articles/10.1186/s13014-023-02300-w.
6. Intermediate-risk meningioma: initial outcomes from NRG Oncology RTOG 0539 - PubMed [Internet]. [cited 2025 Sep 21]. Available from: https://pubmed.ncbi.nlm.nih.gov/28984517/.
7. Low-risk meningioma: initial outcomes from NRG Oncology/RTOG 0539 - PubMed [Internet]. [cited 2025 Sep 21]. Available from: https://pubmed.ncbi.nlm.nih.gov/35657335/.
8. High-risk Meningioma: Initial Outcomes From NRG Oncology/RTOG 0539 - PubMed [Internet]. [cited 2025 Sep 21]. Available from: https://pubmed.ncbi.nlm.nih.gov/31786276/.
9. Stereotactic radiosurgery versus stereotactic radiotherapy in the management of intracranial meningiomas: a systematic review and meta-analysis - PubMed [Internet]. [cited 2025 Sep 21]. Available from: https://pubmed.ncbi.nlm.nih.gov/31153149/.
10. Thielhelm T, Goncalves S, Welford S, Mellon E, Cohen E, Nourbakhsh A, et al. Understanding the radiobiology of vestibular schwannomas to overcome radiation resistance. Cancer. 2021;13:4575.
11. Brun L, Mom T, Guillemin F, Puechmaille M, Khalil T, Biau J. The recent management of vestibular schwannoma radiotherapy: a narrative review of the literature. J Clin Med. 2024;13(6):1611.
12. Germano IM, Sheehan J, Parish J, Atkins T, Asher A, Hadjipanayis CG, et al. Congress of neurological surgeons systematic review and evidence-based guidelines on the role of radiosurgery and radiation therapy in the management of patients with vestibular schwannomas. Neurosurgery. 2018;82(2):E49–51.
13. Stereotactic radiosurgery for vestibular schwannomas: analysis of 317 patients followed more than 5 years - PubMed [Internet]. [cited 2025 Sept 23]. Available from: https://pubmed.ncbi.nlm.nih.gov/16094154/.
14. Weil RS, Cohen JM, Portarena I, Brada M. Optimal dose of stereotactic radiosurgery for acoustic neuromas: a systematic review. Br J Neurosurg. 2006;20(4):195–202.
15. Combs SE, Engelhard C, Kopp C, Wiedenmann N, Schramm O, Prokic V, et al. Long-term outcome after highly advanced single-dose or fractionated radiotherapy in patients with vestibular schwannomas - pooled results from 3 large German centers. Radiother Oncol. 2015;114(3):378–83.
16. Tuleasca C, Kotecha R, Sahgal A, de Salles A, Fariselli L, Paddick I, et al. Large vestibular schwannoma treated using a cranial nerve sparing approach with planned subtotal microsurgical resection and stereotactic radiosurgery: meta-analysis and International Stereotactic Radiosurgery Society (ISRS) practice guidelines. J Neuro-Oncol. 2025;173(2):245–62.
17. Timmer FCA, Hanssens PEJ, van Haren AE, van Overbeeke JJ, Mulder JJS, Cremers CWRJ, et al. Follow-up after gamma knife radiosurgery for vestibular schwannomas: volumetric and axial control rates. Laryngoscope. 2011;121(7):1359–66.
18. Friedman WA, Bradshaw P, Myers A, Bova FJ. Linear accelerator radiosurgery for vestibular schwannomas. J Neurosurg. 2006;105(5):657–61.
19. Hansasuta A, Choi CYH, Gibbs IC, Soltys SG, Tse VCK, Lieberson RE, et al. Multisession stereotactic radiosurgery for vestibular schwannomas: single-institution experience with 383 cases. Neurosurgery. 2011;69(6):1200–9.
20. Gupta T, Chatterjee A. Modern radiation therapy for pituitary adenoma: review of techniques and outcomes. Neurol India. 2020;68(Suppl 1):S113.
21. Hemaidia RM, Cebula H, Goichot B, Noel G. Radiation therapy in functioning and no functioning pituitary neuroendocrine tumor: systematic review of the recent literature after 2011. Front Endocrinol [Internet]. 2024 Nov 12 [cited 2025 Sept 27]; 15. Available from: https://www.frontiersin.org/journals/endocrinology/articles/10.3389/fendo.2024.1468724/full.
22. Minniti G, Gilbert DC, Brada M. Modern techniques for pituitary radiotherapy. Rev Endocr Metab Disord. 2009;10(2):135–44.
23. Green S, Lehrer EJ, Cifarelli CP, Recinos PF, Sheehan JP, Ziu M, et al. Congress of neurological surgeons systematic review and evidence-based guidelines for the role of radiosurgery for patients with functioning pituitary adenomas. Neurosurgery. 2025;97(3S):S36.

24. Almeldin D, Fersht N, Kosmin M. Radiotherapy for pituitary tumors. In: Feingold KR, Ahmed SF, Anawalt B, Blackman MR, Boyce A, Chrousos G, et al., editors. Endotext [Internet]. South Dartmouth (MA): MDText.com, Inc.; 2000 [cited 2025 Sept 27]. Available from: http://www.ncbi.nlm.nih.gov/books/NBK278955/.
25. Sasaki R, Murakami M, Okamoto Y, Kono K, Yoden E, Nakajima T, et al. The efficacy of conventional radiation therapy in the management of pituitary adenoma. Int J Radiat Oncol Biol Phys. 2000;47(5):1337–45.
26. Sheehan JP, Starke RM, Mathieu D, Young B, Sneed PK, Chiang VL, et al. Gamma Knife radiosurgery for the management of nonfunctioning pituitary adenomas: a multicenter study. J Neurosurg. 2013;119(2):446–56.
27. Wanna GB, Sweeney AD, Haynes DS, Carlson ML. Contemporary management of jugular paragangliomas. Otolaryngol Clin N Am. 2015;48(2):331–41.
28. Tomasello F, Conti A. Judicious management of jugular foramen tumors. World Neurosurg. 2015;83(5):756–7.
29. Semaan MT, Megerian CA. Current assessment and management of glomus tumors. Curr Opin Otolaryngol Head Neck Surg. 2008;16(5):420–6.
30. Fussey JM, Kemeny AA, Sankar S, Rejali D. Successful management of a catecholamine-secreting glomus jugulare tumor with radiosurgery alone. J Neurol Surg B Skull Base. 2013;74(6):399–402.
31. Prasad SC, Mimoune HA, D'Orazio F, Medina M, Bacciu A, Mariani-Costantini R, et al. The role of wait-and-scan and the efficacy of radiotherapy in the treatment of temporal bone paragangliomas. Otol Neurotol. 2014;35(5):922–31.
32. Radiosurgery of glomus jugulare tumors: a meta-analysis - International Journal of Radiation Oncology, Biology, Physics [Internet]. [cited 2025 Sept 27]. Available from: https://www.redjournal.org/article/S0360-3016(11)00666-3/fulltext.
33. Shakeri A, Portanova A, Sakano H, Singh DP. Glomus jugulotympanicum tumor treated with radiation therapy: a case report with review of literature. J Clin Imaging Sci. 2024;14:14.
34. Fatima N, Pollom E, Soltys S, Chang SD, Meola A. Stereotactic radiosurgery for head and neck paragangliomas: a systematic review and meta-analysis. Neurosurg Rev. 2021;44(2):741–52.
35. Paulissen JMJ, Zegers CML, Houben RM, Hofstede D, Kars M, van Santen HM, et al. Radiotherapy-induced hypothalamic-pituitary axis dysfunction in adult brain, head and neck and skull base tumor patients—a systematic review and meta-analysis. Clin Transl Radiat Oncol. 2025;51:100900.
36. Pencil-beam scanning proton therapy for the treatment of glomus jugulare tumours - Kubeš - 2022 - Journal of Medical Radiation Sciences - Wiley Online Library [Internet]. [cited 2025 Sept 27]. Available from: https://onlinelibrary.wiley.com/doi/full/10.1002/jmrs.612.
37. McMaster ML, Goldstein AM, Bromley CM, Ishibe N, Parry DM. Chordoma: incidence and survival patterns in the United States, 1973–1995. Cancer Causes Control. 2001;12:1.
38. Cavallo LM, Cappabianca P, Galzio R, et al. Endoscopic endonasal transclival approach to chordomas of the craniovertebral junction. Neurosurg Focus 19(1):E2, 2005.
39. Castro JR, Linstadt DE, Bahary JP, et al. Experience in charged particle irradiation of tumors of the skull base: 1977–1992. Int J Radiat Oncol Biol Phys. 1994;29:647.
40. Weber DC, Rutz HP, Pedroni ES, et al. Results of spot-scanning proton radiation therapy for chordoma and chondrosarcoma of the skull base: the Paul Scherrer Institute experience. Int J Radiat Oncol Biol Phys. 2005;63:401.
41. Vujovic S, Henderson S, Presneau N, et al. Brachyury, a crucial regulator of notochordal development, is a novel biomarker for chordomas. J Pathol. 2006;209:157.
42. Walcott BP, Nahed BV, Mohyeldin A, et al. Chordoma: current concepts, management, and future directions. Lancet Oncol. 2012;13:e69.
43. DeLaney TF, Liebsch NJ, Pedlow FX, et al. Long-term results of Phase II study of high-dose photon/proton radiotherapy in chordoma. Surg Oncol. 2014 Aug;110(2):115-22.
44. Schulz-Ertner D, Karger CP, Feuerhake A, et al. Carbon ion radiotherapy for chordomas and low-grade chondrosarcomas of the skull base. Int J Radiat Oncol Biol Phys.2002 May 1;53(1):36-42

Unraveling the Mystery of Meningiomas 6

Indu Bansal, Sonali Karnwal, and Meenakshi Sanwaria

6.1 Background

Among the primary central nervous system tumors, meningioma arising from the meningeal layers of brain or spinal cord is the most commonly occurring tumor [1]. It comprises about 37.6% of all CNS tumors and around 50% of benign brain tumors [2]. As per the World Health Organization (WHO) 2021 grading, CNS WHO grade 1 tumor constitutes 80.1% of cases, grade 2 18.3%, and grade 3 around 1.5% [3]. Most of the grade 1 tumors are benign and grow very slowly. Aggressive behavior, high chances of recurrence, poor clinical outcomes with high chances of mortality are seen with atypical and anaplastic varieties [4]. A total of 1–3% of meningiomas may show malignant transformation with 5-year overall survival of 32–64% [1]. These tumors decrease the quality of life due to neurological deficits, and in 20% cases, they may show malignant behavior [5].

The incidence is more in older people with the average age of presentation being around 66 years, and the incidence in children is 1.5%. Although intraventricular location is rare overall but is commonly seen in children mainly in lateral ventricle followed by third and 4th ventricle [5]. The overall 5-year survival is better for non-malignant cases ranging from 97% to 87% and is worse for malignant meningiomas ranging from 50% to 85% [6].

6.2 Aetiology, Epidemiology, and Risk Factors

Harvey Cushing hypothesized in 1922 that meningiomas originates from the meninges of the brain and spinal cord and from the arachnoid cap cells [4]. The peak incidence is around the sixth and seventh decades and age itself is a risk factor for

I. Bansal (✉) · S. Karnwal · M. Sanwaria
Department of Radiation Oncology, Paras Hospital, Gurugram, Haryana, India

K. Sood Sharma (ed.), *Radiation Therapy for Benign Disorders*,
https://doi.org/10.1007/978-981-95-6635-8_6

its development [4]. Exposure of brain to ionizing radiation puts the patient at 6–10 times more risk of developing meningiomas [4]. The risk is more after some dental procedures, cranial radiation for ALL, radiation for tinea capitis, or for atomic bomb survivors [1, 4, 5, 7]. Patients with a positive family history of meningiomas or those with family history of Von Hippel Lindau syndrome (VHL), neurofibromatosis type 2 (NF2), multiple endocrine neoplasia (MEN) have a high risk of developing higher grade tumor or may develop multiple meningiomas [1, 5, 7].

Usually females present with benign meningiomas, while males are twice at risk of atypical or anaplastic meningiomas. The progesterone receptor expressing tumors seen in 70–80% cases have favorable prognosis and less chances of recurrence, and estrogen receptor expression is seen rarely [4]. Increased risk of meningiomas has been seen in smokers, after methotrexate exposure, with high body mass index, in women of reproductive age, and in women with breast cancer, and it has been observed that the size of meningioma may change during menstrual cycle, during pregnancy, or during menopause [7].

6.3 Genomics and Biology

The meningiomas have usually been classified as per the grade of tumor but now many molecular bimarkers are being used for stratification and prognostication of meningiomas [5]. The first gene thought to be responsible for meningioma development is neurofibromatosis-2 (*NF2*) on chromosome 22q12.2 [8]. It has inhibitory effect on PI3K/Akt, Raf/MEK/ERK, and mTOR signaling pathways in non-meningioma cells which leads to overexpression of yes-associated protein 1 (YAP1), and Hippo signaling pathway is also deregulated [8]. Hence, meningiomas with NF2 alterations are usually higher grade and more aggressive, although benign NF2-mutant cases may also be seen. The NF2 mutation is seen in 37% of grade 1, 60% of grade 2, and 69% of grade 3 tumors [8].

Meningiomas without any NF2 alterations may have other mutations such as TRAF7/KLF4, SUFU, AKT1, SMO, and POLR2 [8]. Meningiomas with these "non-NF2" mutations have better prognosis due to low-grade presentation and fewer chromosomal alterations which leads to better outcomes with conventional treatment [8]. The location of NF2-altered meningiomas is usually along the cerebral hemisphere or in the posterior or lateral skull base. But non-NF2 altered meningiomas are usually located in the anterior skull base [8]. The anterior falx location is seen with meningiomas associated with combined NF2/SMARCB1 mutations [8]. SMARCE 1 loss is usually seen in clear cell type and BAP1 loss is seen with rhabdoid and papillary variants [8].

TERT mutation and H3K27me3 loss are usually associated with worse survival. The association of ARID1A, PTEN, and PBRM1 mutations leads to a higher grade of meningioma [8]. The homozygous deletion of CDKN2A/B is also associated with significantly shorter PFS. Other meningiomas associated syndromes include Werner syndrome, Gorlin syndrome, and Cowden syndrome [8]. Additional genomic regions which are recurrently lost in meningiomas include 14q, 1p, 6q, and 18q [9].

TERT mutation and H3K27me3 loss are usually associated with worse survival. Presence of mutations such as PTEN, PBRM1, or ARID1A or homozygous deletion of CDKN2A/B indicates a higher-grade meningiomas and a short PFS [8]. Association of meningioma has also been seen with Werner syndrome, Gorlin syndrome, and Cowden syndrome [8]. A number of other genomic alterations seen in meningiomas are loss of 14q, 1p, 6q, and 18q [9].

6.4 Location and Symptoms

Most of the meningiomas have supratentorial location. Meningioma is usually located in para-sagittal area, convexities of brain, sphenoid ridges, olfactory areas, and anterior and posterior para-falcine region [1]. But they may also be seen in suprasellar, cerebello-pontine angle, intraorbital, intraventricular, and spinal locations [1].

Meningiomas are slow-growing tumors and may progress slowly over months or years. Some patients may have no symptoms, but few patients may present with neurological deterioration. Occasionally, meningiomas may grow to a very large size before becoming symptomatic [1]. The symptoms depend on the location and size of the tumor and include headache, dizziness, visual impairments, papilledema, behavioral changes, and anosmia as shown in Table 6.1. If it is a very large tumor, it may cause obstructive hydrocephalus which may lead to increase in intracranial pressure (ICP) and may cause papilledema; patient may feel nauseous and may have vomiting episodes [1].

6.5 Spinal Meningiomas

Out of all primary intradural spinal tumors, spinal meningiomas constitute around 30–38% and are seen more commonly in 80.3% of females [1]. The most common location is in the thoracic spine in posterior, postero-lateral, or lateral segments and is also seen in the anterior part of cervical spine or in lumbosacral region [10]. The most common varieties are meningothelial, fibroblastic, and transitional types of meningiomas. Androgen receptors (AR+) and estrogen receptors (ER+) are more commonly expressed in spinal than in intracranial meningiomas. They usually present with gradually progressive myelopathy or radiculopathy [10]. The symptoms include limb weakness, paraesthesia, gait disturbances, and bowel/bladder dysfunction [10]. Depending on the location of the tumor and pressure on nerve roots, patient may present with upper or lower motor neuron deficits [10]. Weakness, muscle pain, and loss of reflexes may be the signs of lower motor neuron involvement [10].

Most spinal meningiomas are well circumscribed with strong homogenous enhancement on T2w and may show hypo-intensity on T1-weighted images. Occasionally dural tail may be appreciated on T2w images [10]. They are divided into 4 types based on MRI findings [11]:

Table 6.1 Location and symptoms of meningioma

Location	Features	Symptoms	Molecular alteration
Convexity	May be silent	Seizures, headache, hemiparesis	Chromosome 22q deletions and/or NF2 mutations
Parasagittal/falx	Involve motor cortex usually leg)	C/L limb weakness or paraplegia, urinary incontinence or seizures	
Sphenoid wing	Involve cranial nerves, optic apparatus and cavernous sinus	Visual disturbances, proptosis or orbital symptoms, facial numbness and weakness, multiple cranial n. palsies (III, IV, V1, V2, VI)	Mutations in AKT1, TRAF7, SMO, and/or PIK3CA
Olfactory groove		Anosmia or frontal lobe symptoms as apathy, personality change, executive dysfunction, Foster Kennedy syndrome	Mutations in AKT1, TRAF7, SMO, and/or PIK3CA
Tuberculum sellae/ suprasellar		Bitemporal hemianopia or may mimic pituitary adenomas	Mutations in AKT1, TRAF7, SMO, and/or PIK3CA
Posterior fossa (petrous ridge, foramen magnum)		Ataxia, dysarthria, nystagmus, cranial n. palsies, hydrocephalus	Mutations in AKT1, TRAF7, SMO, and/or PIK3CA.
Intraventricular	Arise in trigone of lateral ventricle	Can cause hydrocephalus, headache, and mental status changes	
Spinal	Thoracic spine MC	Myelopathy, radiculopathy, limb weakness, paresthesias, gait disturbances, bowel, bladder dysfunction	Chromosome 22q deletions and/or NF2 mutations

1. Type A: tumors with homogenous enhancement after contrast administration and may be attached to dura (may or may not have a dural tail).
2. Type B: oval-shaped tumors which show hypo-intensity on T2w images.
3. Type C: "en plaque" meningioma, which have a diffuse sheet-like growth along the dura.
4. Type D: spinal meningiomas which do not fall into type A, B, or C categories.

Ginko leaf sign helps to differtiate spinal meningiomas from schwannomas [12]. It is best seen on contrast-enhanced T1W images. The distorted spinal cord which is pushed to one side by the tumor is represented as leaf and the strap represents stretched denticulate ligament [9]. The chances of recurrence are very high ranging from 1.3% to 14.7%, so maximal safe resection should be attempted [7]. The atypical and anaplastic varieties may in 0.1% cases metastasize extracranially to lungs and pleura, but occasionally intraspinal and vertebral spread may also occur [10] (Fig. 6.1).

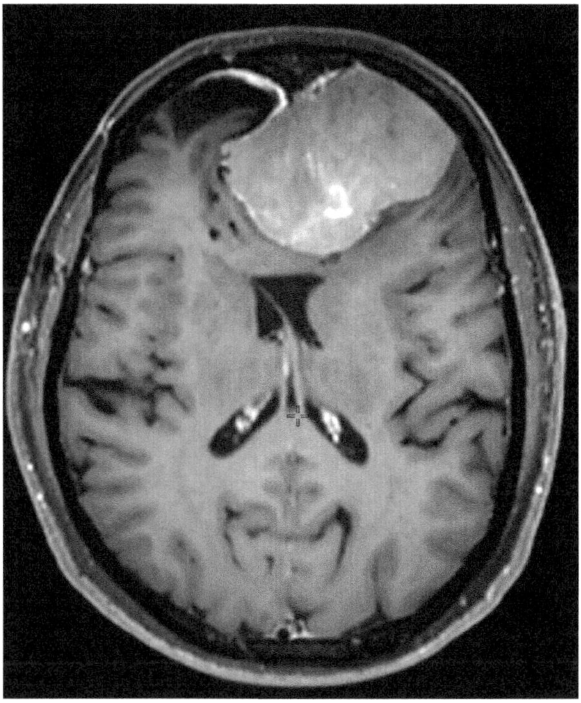

Fig. 6.1 Axial T1 w contrast image: showing homogenously enhancing large solitary lesion at bifrontal region. (Source: Paras Hospital)

The surgery for spinal meningioma should be attempted if the benefit of tumor removal outweighs the risks involved. No adjuvant treatment is needed for WHO grade 1 meningiomas [10]. For WHO grade 3 and WHO grade 2 with recurrence, adjuvant radiation is recommended [10]. Upfront radiosurgery is not usually recommended for grade 2 or 3 meningiomas, but if we get a margin of 2–3 mm between the meningioma and the spinal cord, it may be offered in inoperable patients. The FSRS dose is 21 Gy/3F. Chemotherapy may be used in recurrent and aggressive meningiomas [10].

6.6 Pediatric Meningiomas

Meningiomas account for only 2.2–3.6% of all brain tumors in pediatric age group and is seen in 0.4–2.5% of all meningioma cases [8]. The incidence is equal in males and females with a higher predilection for intraventricular location and spinal cord [8]. NF2 mutations and loss of chromosome 22 are very common and seen in 47–72% of cases [8]. Other mutations such as AKT1, SMO, KLF4, and TRAF7 (non-NF2 driver mutations) are rarely seen but YAP1-fusions may occasionally be seen in certain cases [3]. All pediatric patients should be screened for NF2 mutations and other genetic conditions should also be ruled out at the time of diagnosis [3]. As spinal meningiomas are common in children, it is preferable to do a full craniospinal imaging at the time of diagnosis. Surgery is the preferred treatment, and gross total resection (GTR) leads to better progression-free survival (PFS) and overall survival (OS). There is insufficient evidence for advantage of adjuvant radiation and the treatment decision should be individualized [3].

6.7 Grading of Meningiomas

As per WHO 2021 classification, depending on the number of mitosis and other histopathological and molecular features, 3 grades for meningiomas are described as shown in Table 6.2 [1]. Grade 1 or typical meningiomas constitute 80–81% cases, atypical or grade 2 lesions are seen in 17–18% cases, and anaplastic or

Table 6.2 Grading of meningiomas

	Grade 1	Grade 2	Grade 3
Nomenclature	Typical	Atypical	Anaplastic
Incidence	80%	17–18%	1.7%
Mitotic rate Ki-67	<4 mitosis /10HPF	4–19 mitosis/10HPF (at least 2.5/mm^2) 2–7.5%-25%	> 20 or more mitoses/ 10 HPF >25%
Histology	9 histologic variants Meningothelial. Fibrous. Transitional. Psammomatous. Secretory. Angiomatous. Microcystic. Lymphoplasmacytic. Metaplastic absence of atypical, anaplastic, or rhabdoid features histologically.	3 histologic variants: atypical, clear cell, chordoid Or Unequal brain invasion(not only perivascular spread or indentation of brain without pial breach) Or At least 3 of the following Increased cellularity Small cells with high N:C ratio Prominent nuceloli Sheeting Foci of spontaneous necrosis	3 histologic variants: anaplastic, rhabdoid, papillary Or Franka anaplasia (sarcoma, carcinoma, or melanoma like appearance) Or TERT promoter mutation Or homozygous deletion of CDKN2A and /or CDKN2B Papillary and rhabdoid features alone no longer qualify for WHO grade 3
Recurrence rate	7–25%	29–52%	50–94%
Special features	>70% of meningiomas PR+, hyperostosis of bone can be seen		Similar to high-grade sarcomas, carcinoma, or melanomas with a high rate of DM

grade 3 meningiomas are seen in 1.7% patients [1]. Grade 1 and grade 2 are considered non-malignant meningiomas with 10-year OS rates of 83%, whereas grade 3, 20% of grade 1, and 15% of grade 2 can show malignant behavior with 10-year OS of only 65%. Malignant cell types include hemangiopericytoma, malignant fibrous histiocytoma, papillary meningioma, and benign metastasizing meningioma [13].

The 10-year recurrence rate of meningiomas can reach 20% [1]. In grade 1, the recurrence rate (RR) is low ranging from 7% to 25%; in grade 2, it is 29–52%, while high recurrence rates of about 50–94% have been seen in higher-grade meningiomas [1, 3].

If there is gross residual tumor after surgery, the chances of recurrence are very high, while the growth rate of tumor indicates about the chances of detection of a recurrence early [14] It's important to understand the difference between mitotic index, ki-67, and Mib-1. Mitotic index gives information about cellular proliferation, whereas Ki-67 indicates about time to recurrence and is a cellular marker for proliferation [14]. It is the ratio between the number of population of cells undergoing mitosis to its total number of cells, measured on fresh tissue sample or on frozen section. MIB-1-monoclonal antibody targeted against different epitopes of same proliferation-related antigen can be measured on paraffin block. MIB-1 index is more sensitive than mitotic rate [14]. A higher MIB-1 index is associated with worse prognosis. Benign meningioma may have a MIB-1 index of 1.9%, while atypical and anaplastic meningiomas may have Mib index of 4.5% and 11.7%, respectively [4].

Brain invasion is seen in only 9.4% of grade 1 while 41% of WHO grade 2 and 100% of WHO grade 3 meningiomas may habe brain invasion [8]. The presence of brain invasion is sufficient to call a meningioma as grade 2 tumor; however, the association of only brain invasion with adverse outcomes in the absence of other poor prognostic features is still unclear [8]. If the tumor cells infiltrate the adjacent brain parenchyma and there is no connective tissue layer or well-defined plane between the tumor and brain and there is reactive astrocytosis in surrounding brain, it indicates brain invasion [8]. There are three types of brain invasion—tongue-like protrusion, clustered or clustered nests, and diffuse growth [8]. Males usually show finger-like invasions while females have clustered type invasion [8]. Radiologic features such as loss of CSF cleft, indistinct brain-tumor interface, or peritumoral edema may indicate brain invasion [8].

Usually, it is recommended not to remove the grossly normal adjacent brain during meningioma surgery [8]. It has been noted that the gross impression of brain invasion during surgery may not be reliable, as invasion may not be evident grossly always and even leptomeningeal adhesion may be misinterpreted as brain invasion [8]. There is no clarity if we should include extra brain parenchymal margin during radiation in all cases, or margin should only be added in recurrent tumors, in patients with documented evidence of brain invasion, or in patients with high risk of brain involvment depending on high grade tumor, anatomic location and in patients with high risk features on imaging or molecular reports [8]. So, it is recommended to give extra margin to brain parenchyma as per case to case basis.

6.8 Radiological Features of Meningiomas

Meningiomas are commonly seen as well-delineated, extra-axial tumors, which may displace the adjacent brain and are usually diagnosed when they become symptomatic [15]. CT head with bone window setting is a useful tool for patients who are unfit for MRI. Hyperostosis and calcified meningiomas are also easy to see on a CT scan [7]. Contrast CT head shows meningiomas as a homogenous, dense, enhanced dural-based lesions with or without brain edema. Non-contrast head CT scan helps in hyperdense or iso-dense dural-based lesions. MRI brain with contrast should always be done whenever possible as it is the gold standard radiological tool for diagnosis and for monitoring response to treatment [7, 8].

Usually, meningiomas are single lesions but sometimes they may be multiple if associated with genetic syndromes as NF2 [5]. Mostly, meningiomas show strong isointense enhancement on T1W after contrast administration and are hyperintense on T2W and FLAIR MRI sequences [7]. MRI spectroscopy with its capability to differentiate metabolic and chemical contents of healthy normal brain from the tumor is a useful tool to detect malignant meningiomas [7]. Some meningiomas (25%) may show calcification, 50% may have perilesional edema, and 72% may have dural tail [8].

Bone infiltration has been reported in 7–18% of meningiomas and may be visualized even if there is no radiologic bone abnormality [16]. Some tumors may show hyperostosis due to reactive changes or due to tumor infiltration and it may be seen in calvarial or skull base bones adjacent to meningiomas as shown in Figs. 6.2 and 6.3 [16]. Hyperostosis may present as homogenous, periosteal, three-layered, or diploic patterns and is seen in 23–90% of cases histologically. Hyperostosis may lead to more chances of recurrence, but there is no clarity if the infiltrated bone is a nidus for recurrence, or due to bone infiltration, tumor shows aggressive behavior [16]. So, till further research is available, the clinician should take an individualized decision regarding the inclusion of suspicious areas of bone invasion or hyperostosis when planning radiotherapy for meningioma [16].

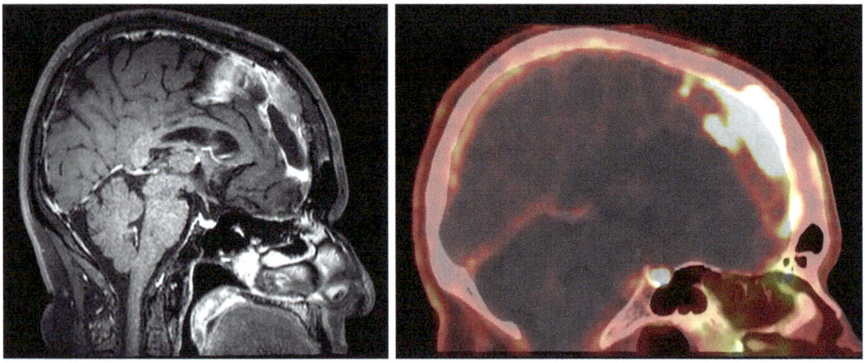

Fig. 6.2 Comparison of MRI and NOTANOC scan. Sagittal view comparing the extent of meningioma on MRI versus NOTANOC scan. (Source: Paras Hospital, Gurugram)

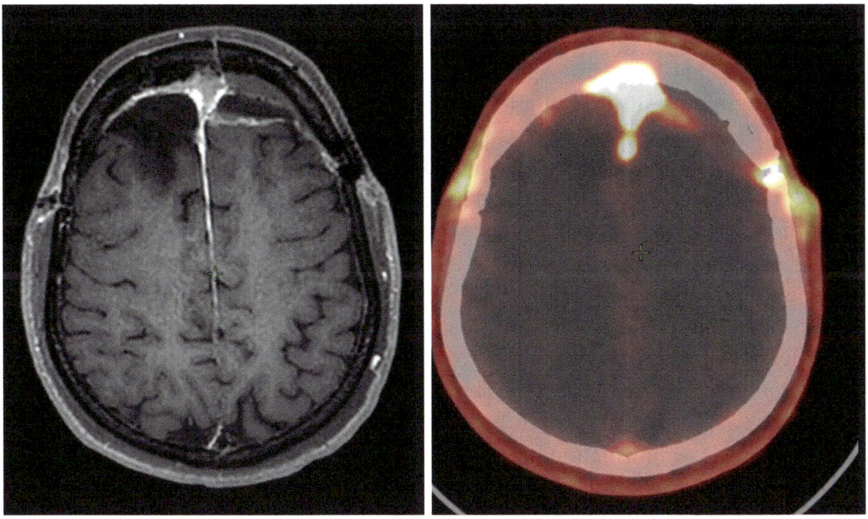

Fig. 6.3 Comparison of MRI and NOTANOC scan. MRI scan: axial view showing bone infiltration. NOTANOC scan showing intense uptake in recurrence setting, thus helping in proper delineation of the lesion. (Source: Paras Hospital, Gurugram)

Dural tail involvement is seen on MRI as a gradually tapering, hyper-intense, thickened dura adjacent to a meningioma and may be seen in other dural-based tumors as well [17]. If dural tail is seen, pleomorphic xantho-astrocytoma should also be ruled out as differential diagnosis [17]. The dural invasion may be seen in approximately 88% cases, and 95% of the involvement is within 2.5 cm of the tumor base. It may be seen as smooth and tapering enhancement and may be nodular, or have mixed smooth and nodular patterns [17]. It has been seen that 44% of "smooth" dural pattern may have tumor cells up to 1.5 cm, while in nodular and mixed patterns dural invasion may be seen in up to 3 cm. So, during radiation planning, 2 cm margins may cover 82% of tumors, and 2.5 cm margin is enough to cover 95% of cases of dural tail invasion [16].

Around 60% of meningiomas may show peritumoral brain edema and it may not always correlate to the size of tumor [17]. If peritumoral edema increases by 1 centimeter, the chances of brain invasion go up by 20%. It is hyperintense on T2 W images. As the blood–brain barrier is disrupted, the extracerebral protein-rich fluid accumulates in the brain which appears as vasogenic edema. The most common reasons for brain edema are no visible arachnoid plane on MRI, high levels of ki-67 index, presence of irregular tumor margins, and the release of vascular tumor cells [17]. Secretory, microcystic, angiomatous, and lympho-plasmacyte-rich meningiomas commonly cause disproportionately large degree of edema [8].

Cerebral venous sinuses are seen as duplicated dura mater and have a vascular endothelium. They show contrast with the surrounding venous and arterial structures [17]. During radiation planning, the wall of the sinus should be included in the CTV in grade 2/3 meningiomas if it is in contact with the GTV but there is no macroscopic invasion [17]. As the risk of thrombosis is high, high-dose radiation should be used safely on the venous sinuses [17].

Mushroom-like appearance may be seen at times in cystic lesions due to tumor invagination in the brain parenchyma. Due to the entrapment of CSF or cerebral cortical vessels between the lesion and cortex, CSF vascular cleft may be seen in certain tumors. It helps in differentiating extra-axial lesion from an intra-axial meningioma [18]. Water buckling sign is seen when the gray-white junction is preserved even in the presence of brain edema which leads to buckling or inward compression of the white matter [19]. It is due to extracerebral fluid collection in extra-axial lesions. Sun-burst features and mother-in-law sign are other features of meningiomas. In mother-in-law sign, there is early enhancement in arterial phase and is persistently opacified during the venous phase [19].

Conventional angiography may be useful if there is suspicion of invasion of a major sinus as superior sagittal or lateral sinus by the tumor and MRI angiography is not giving clear information [7]. In such situations, 3D venous angiography may help in knowing about the patency of the sinus and its collateral venous drainage. Digital subtraction angiography (DSA) helps in differetiating between pial and dural blood supply and also tells about the feeding arteries of meningioma [7]. It's a very useful tool for giant meningiomas (>5 cm) [7]. Currently, the role of preoperative embolization is declining due to the perceived risk of postoperative cardiovascular complications [7]. But in petroclical meningiomas, if feeding arteries are not accessible to surgeons, preoperative embolization may help occlude the meningeal branch of ascending pharyngeal artery or the tentorial branch of the internal carotid artery [7].

The radiological signs which predict malignancy are rapid growth, extensive brain or bone invasion, or lesions which are bright on T2W (such as meningothelial, angioblastic, or with hemangiopericytic elements). Increase in perfusion, increase in T2W signal, and decreased apparent diffusion coefficient of the tumor also point toward aggressive meningioma.

6.9 Is There Any Role of PET Scans for Meningioma?

Traditionally, CT scan and MRI brain have been used for evluation of meningiomas. They help to identify the extent of meningioma, its bony infiltration and are also used for initial treatment planning, for delineation of treatment volumes, for monitoring the response and for follow up evaluation [15]. But unfortunately, it is difficult with these modalities alone to delineate meningiomas correctly, especially for meningiomas with complex geometry, which are close to skull base, in orbital or para-falcine areas, with sagittal sinus or cavernous sinus involvement, and also in ascertaining degree of infiltration of trans-osseous growth [15]. Also, sometimes it's very difficult to differentiate residual/recurrent tumor and scar tissue, especially if patient has undergone surgery or radiation. In addition, artifacts and calcifications may give false findings on MRI. The role of PET scan for such situations is emerging [15].

18-FDG PET has not found to be very sensitive for meningiomas as these are slow-growing tumors with moderately elevated glucose metabolism [15]. Moreover, because of normal high physiological uptake of glucose in cerebral cortex, the sensitivity to detect meningioma from normal brain parenchyma is low [15]. As the 18F-PET does not show any accumulation in the pituitary, it may help detect intrasellar invasion of meningioma or to differentiate grade 1 from grade 2/3 meningiomas [15]. A threshold of 1.05 of the tumor-to-gray matter ratios of FDG uptake has been recommended in differentiating grade 1 meningiomas from grade 2/3 and a ratio of 0.85 in tumor relapses [15].

As somatostatin receptors subtype 2 is expressed in 100% of meningiomas, various radiolabeled somatostatin receptor ligands (SSTR ligands) such as DOTATOC, DOTATATE, and DOTANOC/ NOTANOC have been used to diagnose meningiomas [15]. Recent data is emerging for the role of SSTR2 ligands for diagnostic (e.g. Ga68 scan) as well as for therapeutic purposes (e.g. use of 177Lu or Y90). The concept of theragnostics is also gaining value in meningiomas [15]. These tracers provide improved lesion contrast relative to background as they are not taken up by bones or unaffected brain parenchyma [15]. But note that as pituitary gland has normal physiological uptake, it might be difficult to evaluate lesions close to sella [15]. In addition, 68 Ga-DOTATATE PET/CT may be used to differentiate optic nerve sheath lesions from meningiomas of the optic nerve [15].

6.10 Special Situations

6.10.1 Incidental/Asymptomatic Meningiomas

Incidental meningiomas may be seen in 20% cases. They have a slow rate of growth (average <5% increase in volume per year), but around 5–8% of patients may develop new lesions in 4.1 years [8]. More than 60% have self-limiting growth, so they may be observed by serial imaging without any treatment [7]. But most of the lesions progress within 5 years [8].

The imaging features which predict higher risk of progression are large size, no calcification, hyperintense enhancement on T2-W MRI, peritumoral edema, large tumor at diagnosis (>10 cm^3), non-skull base location, and lesion sitting close to dural venous sinus or neurovascular structures [7, 8]. It is recommended to do an annual MRI at least for 5 years for suspected or WHO grade 1 meningioma after which the imaging interval may be doubled [7, 8].

IMPASSE study (Incidental Meningioma Progression During Active Surveillance or After Stereotactic Radiosurgery) included small meningiomas without any symptoms or incidental meningiomas. It showed a tumor control rate of 99.4% in meningioma cohort that received SRS compared to 62.1% in the observation cohort. These patients were matched for patient age, volume, and location of tumor and had similar follow-up imaging [8].

6.10.2 Meningioma En-Plaque (MEP)

Meningioma en-plaque (MEP) is a WHO grade 1 meningioma, constitutes 2–10% of all meningiomas, mainly occurs intracranially, and is less often seen in the spine [1]. These are carpet- or sheet-like lesions which can invade medullary spaces and grow along dural surface and cause significant intra-osseous infiltration in 13–49% of cases and can extensively infiltrate in the bones, dural surfaces, or soft tissues (as seen in sphenoid ridge and calvarial bones) [1]. On histopathological examination, whorls and syncytia of meningothelial cells may be seen in the hyperostosis in MEP. It may have different patterns—homogenous, periosteal, three-layer, and diploic [1].

6.10.3 Radiation-Induced Meningiomas (RIM)

RIM may develop due to iatrogenic or environmental exposure to radiation treatment. It usually has a latent occurrence with a period ranging from 2 to 63 years, following radiation exposure [1]. Its location depends on the site of the radiation exposure such as in the cranium or in the spinal location [1]. In comparison with spontaneous meningiomas, RIM may be multiple and show fast growth rate. Some of the tumors may have pathological malignant features, for example, high MIB-1 labeling index >10%, and may have high risk of tumor recurrence within 1 year of surgery [14]. They may also show high vascular endothelial growth factor (VEGF) levels and show mRNA expression [14].

6.10.4 Cystic Meningiomas

The meningiomas with intratumoral or peritumoral cysts are known as cystic meningiomas and account for about 4–7% of meningiomas [1, 18]. It is difficult to diagnose them from intra-axial glial tumor or metastasis [1, 18]. There are several hypotheses about their formation. Some people believe it is due to necrosis or degeneration of tumor cells. It may also happen due to arteriolar hyalinization inside the tumor known as oasis phenomenon, due to secretions from the tumor or due to a peripheral CSF containing arachnoid cyst [1, 18]. The classification of intracranial cystic meningiomas is given in Table 6.3 [1, 18].

6.10.5 Ossified Meningiomas

WHO classification defines ossified meningiomas as grade 1 metaplastic meningiomas [1]. They can have intracranial or spinal location and constitute about 1–5% of all spinal meningiomas [1]. These are not seen commonly, have a slow growth rate, and may show extensive ossification or calcification but this is different than that seen in psammomatous meningiomas [1]. The clear mechanism of ossification is not understood but seems to be associated with metaplasia of arachnoid and interstitial cells [1].

Table 6.3 Classification of cystic meningiomas

	Nauta classification
Type 1	Represents a single or multiple intratumoral cysts, mainly within a tumor
Type II	Represents a single or multiple intratumoral cysts located peripherally to meningiomas and surrounded by the tumor cells
Type III	Represents single or multiple peritumoral cysts located peripherally to the meningioma lying adjacent to the parenchyma
Type IV	Represents a single or multiple peritumoral cysts with walls formed by the arachnoid located between the meningioma and adjacent brain parenchyma
	EL-FILKI classification: explains the association between the cyst contents and location
Type A	Containing CSF or clear fluid divided into two locations, A1 and A2
A1	Extra-tumoral cystic meningioma containing CSF and surrounded by the arachnoid membrane
A2	Extra-tumoral containing clear fluid not surrounded by an arachnoid membrane
Type B	Containing a xanthochromic fluid divided into two locations, B1 and B2
B1	Extra-tumoral cystic meningioma not surrounded by a wall
B2	Surrounded by a thin rim of an enhancing tumor
Type C	Containing a yellowish or dark brown fluid located intratumorally
Type D	Both clear fluids of peritumoral or extra-tumoral cysts and small intratumoral dark brown cysts

6.10.6 Treatment

The management of meningioma involves observation, surgery, radiation, somatostatin analogues, and other systemic agents in relapsed or refractory meningiomas. For asymptomatic incidental meningiomas, radiological surveillance may be done, but for patients who have large and symptomatic tumors, maximal safe surgery is the standard of care.

6.10.7 Surgery

Surgery is the standard treatment for meningiomas. The goal of surgery is not just to minimise the neurological symptoms but it also helps to get a tissue diagnosis and to reduce the mass effect [7]. Every attempt should be made for maximal safe resection of the lesion with the involved dura with low morbidity and preservation of function [7]. This is possible only if exact delineation of tumor including bony involvement and dural infiltration is possible before surgery [7]. But sometimes it's not possible to exactly know tumor infiltration, especially in certain areas as skull base, orbit, and para-falcine locations, or whether sagittal sinus or cavernous sinus is involved, or in cases of trans-osseous growth [7]. For radiation-induced meningiomas, complete surgical resection is better if safer to do [7].

It is very critical to ensure that in order to achieve clear margins, no injury to critical structures occurs and various patient- and tumor-specific factors must be taken into account, such as grade of tumor, location and accessibility of resection of tumor, radiologic imaging features, symptoms of patient, and options of salvage treatment such as SRS or salvage RT [16]. Various prognostic factors for severe complications after surgery include long surgery >4 hrs, age >70 years, KPS <70 [16].

Extent of resection (EOR) has been defined by EORTC and RTOG as either gross total resection (GTR) or subtotal resection (STR) [20]. Another classification is Simpson grading system which was established in 1957 by Dr. Donald Simpson. It is an excellent tool which calculates local recurrence risk after correlation with the degree of tumor resection, associated dural resection, and the involvement of hyperostotic bone. It has been divided into 6 grades, which tell about rates of recurrence as shown in Table 6.4 [20].

Vinding et al., found that radiological assessment alone is not enough to rule out residual tumor disease as even with finest resolution of MRI, residual disease up to 1,000,000 cells can be left undetectable [14]. Vinding et al., proposed a novel Copenhagen grading system that combines the extent of resection after surgery with immuno-histochemistry and imaging findings on MRI or DOTATOC-PET scan after 3 months. It was done specifically for WHO grade 1 tumor [14]. After surgery, biopsy is taken from four different quadrants of the surgical margin, or a complete strip of dura surrounding the lesion is sent separately for histopathology (labeled as "complete resection margin") [14]. In addition, biopsies are also obtained from resection margins of the choroid plexus in case of intra-ventricular and posterior third ventricular meningiomas. "Area of Doubt (AOD)" is the area outside the

Table 6.4 Simpson grading scale for extent of resection

Grade	Extent of resection	Recurrence risk
Grade 0	Complete tumor removal plus an additional 2–3 cm from tumor insertion site	
Grade 1	Complete macroscopic or gross total resection (GTR) with the attached dura and involved abnormal bone, dural sinus	9%
Grade 2	Complete macroscopic or GTR with coagulation of the dural attachment	19%
Grade 3	Complete macroscopic or GTR without resection or coagulation of the attached dura or any extradural extensions, such as the involved abnormal bone, invaded dural sinus	29%
Grade 4	Partial resection of the tumor	40%
Grade 5	Simple decompression of the tumor with or without a biopsy	

surgical margin where the surgeon might have left residual tumor, i.e., along the dura or bony structures [14].

The Copenhagen Grade is thus a combination of histopathology (0 or 1) and radiological imaging (0 or 1) [14]. It is expressed as 0/0, 1/0, 0/1, or 1/1 depending on the empirical observations [14]. Histopathology is reported as "1" if at least one of resection margin—or AOD biopsies—is found to be positive for tumor by routine histology plus IHC for EMA and SSTR2 or there is brain invasion [14]. At 3 months after surgery, routine MRI or CT is done along with 68Ga-DOTATOC-PET CT. If no tumor is detected, it's classified as grade 0 and if a specific 68Ga-signal is seen, it is labeled as grade 1 [14]. This grading system might help in giving more information about aggressiveness of tumor and in deciding further treatment [14].

Tumors located in certain locations such as sphenoid wing, olfactory groove, cerebello-pontine angle, petro-clival region, saddle tubercle, or those involving venous sinuses, blood vessels, or cranial nerves or with brain invasion have increased risk of complications during surgery and require more advanced surgical techniques [5]. With the availability of micro-tools, better operating microscopes, advancements in neuroimaging, surgical neuro-navigation and intra-operative neuromonitoring, ultrasonic aspiration devices, and endovascular embolization techniques, it is now possible to finely dissect the tumor from the nerves, vessels, and eloquent areas [4, 5].

Some studies report a 5-year OS of 78–91% and 41–65% for atypical and anaplastic meningiomas, respectively, but the 10-year survival is only 53% in atypical and only 0% in anaplastic varieties [4]. Even after complete resection, the 5-year recurrence rate is 29–58% for grade 2 and 72–94% for grade 3 meningiomas. Depending on the extent of resection, residual meningiomas may be observed or treated with conformal radiotherapy or stereotactic radiosurgery [4]. As the 5-year risk of progression for incompletely resected meningiomas is 83–100%, they should be treated with radiation [4].

6.11 Radiation Treatment Planning

Standard management of meningiomas includes safe maximal surgical resection. Radiation therapy is a very important tool in the armamentarium to control meningiomas [4]. The goal of radiation is to decrease the rate of proliferation and growth rate of meningiomas [4]. Radiation after surgery is usually advised for anaplastic meningiomas regardless of the amount of resection, for partially resected atypical meningiomas, and for recurrent meningiomas; however, the role of radiotherapy for completely resected atypical meningiomas is a point of discussion [4]. It is also considered a first-line treatment for some meningiomas in critical locations as that of optic nerve sheath or the cavernous sinus [5]. The indications for definitive radiotherapy (RT) include symptomatic, progressive, or life-threatening inoperable meningiomas [17].

While deciding radiation therapy for any patient, it is important to take into consideration the size, location and grade of tumor, extent of resection, the surrounding critical organs at risk, any history of prior radiation, and the dose and technique of prior radiation [17]. Accurate target volume delineation is a very critical step for planning radiation fields for meningiomas. It is important to accurately fuse the CT and MRI images as sometimes in skull base meningiomas and sphenoid wing meningiomas, it is difficult to make a differentiation between normal dura and bone [17].

6.11.1 Radiation Treatment Planning Procedure

Informed written consent should be obtained before the procedure from every patient. Thermoplastic brain cast/SRS brain cast is preferred for conventional and conformal techniques. A radiation planning CT without contrast with 1 mm slice thickness is mandatory for SRS-/FSRS-based treatments [17, 21]. This RT planning scan should be properly fused with post-contrast enhanced 3D T1-W MRI and T2 W images for proper delineation of target volume. It is also advisable to fuse with a preoperative MRI scan for IMRT planning for assessing the preoperative GTV [17, 21]. The MRI used for delineation should ideally be within 4 weeks of RT or less if the tumor is of rapidly progressive variety [17, 21].

Some studies have shown that PET imaging with DOTATOC or DOTANOC tracers helps in improving GTV delineation in certain cases, especially in post-radiation or recurrent cases. The contouring guidelines as per ANOCEF group are shown in Table 6.5 [17, 21]. The comparison of different guidelines as recommended by the

Table 6.5 Anocef contouring guidelines

	Grade 1	Grade 2	Grade 3
GTV (IMRT/SRT)	Whole tumor or postop residue including nodular dural enhancement, contrast-enhanced thickened meninges, directly invaded bone	Whole tumor or postop residue including nodular dural enhancement, contrast-enhanced thickened meninges, directly invaded bone	Whole tumor or postop residue including nodular dural enhancement, contrast-enhanced thickened meninges, directly invaded bone
CTV (IMRT)	Same as GTV	Add 5 mm to GTV, hyperostosis, around invaded bone and along normal meninges and venous sinuses; include drill holes and osteostomy areas	Add 10 mm margins to GTV in normal bone, hyperostosis, invaded bone, normal meninges, venous sinuses, optic or cranial n. contacting GTV; include drill holes and osteotomy areas and 10 mm of peri-tumoral edema; exclude arteries, cortical bone, cranial flap
CTV (SRT)	Same as GTV In post op setting include only the residual enhancement and not the excision cavity	SRT is not recommended	SRT is not recommended

European Society for Radiation and Oncology Advisory Committee on Radiation Oncology Practice (ESTRO-ACROP), National Comprehensive Cancer Network (NCCN), and Association of French-speaking Neuro-oncologists (ANOCEF) for proper targeting of the gross lesion and additional margins is shown in Table 6.6 [22].

Conventional fractionation radiation therapy with intensity-modulated radiation therapy (IMRT) and single-fraction or multiple-fraction stereotactic

Table 6.6 Different consensus guidelines

	RTOG 0539	ROAM/ EORTC 1308	ANOCEF	ESTRO-ACROP	NCCN
GTV	Nodular enhancement, post op cavity, hyperostosis, directly invaded bone	Nodular enhancement and postop cavity, including hyperostosis and directly invaded bone, dural tail	Whole tumor or post op residue including nodular dural enhancement, contrast enhanced thickened meninges, directly invaded bone	Visible tumor with only thickened proximal dural tail, not linearly enhancing or unenhanced dura	Gross tumor if present, surgical bed
CTV	Gr 1-GTV = CTV Gr 2- GTV to CTV expansion 1 cm, 0.5 cm around natural barriers Gr 3- 1 cm GTV to CTV expansion SRS- no margin to GTV	Gr 1-GTV=CTV Gr 2- 1 cm GTV to CTV expansion Gr 3- 1 cm GTV to CTV expansion	Gr 1-GTV=CTV Gr-2- 0.5 cm GTV to CTV expansion Gr3- 1 cm GTV to CTV expansion, escalate dose if possible	Gr 2- 1–2 cm GTV to CTV expansion Gr 3- 1–2 cm GTV to CTV expansion include pre-op tumor bed	Gr 2- 0.5–2 cm margin to GTV Gr 3- 2–3 cm margin,
Venous sinus			Include in Gr 2/3 if in contact with GTV, avoid high dose		
Cortical bone			Do not include if not invaded, whole bone flap not included but include 1 cm if bone invaded in Gr 2/3. Include drill holes, osteotomy areas, cranioplasty	Include	

(continued)

Table 6.6 (continued)

	RTOG 0539	ROAM/ EORTC 1308	ANOCEF	ESTRO-ACROP	NCCN
Hyperostosis	Include in GTV	Include in GTV	Do not include in Gr 1 but include in gr 2/3	Include in Gr 2/3	
Peritumoral edema		Include whole in CTV for Gr 3	Include 5 mm for Gr 2 and 1 cm for grade 3 but not whole edema	Include in Gr 2/3	
Cranial or optic nerves			Include in Gr 3 if they are in contact with GTV, optic n., margin of 0–5 mm along sheath		

radiosurgery have been shown to be effective for patients with high tumor control rates ranging from 85% to 100% at 5 years [5]. While both have been associated with high rates of tumor control, fractionated RT may be preferred for larger tumors (>2–3 cm) or tumors close to brainstem or optic nerves [8]. Small cavernous sinus meningiomas and optic nerve sheath meningiomas are better controlled with conventional fractionated RT and have similar rates of symptomatic improvement after treatment [8].

Stereotactic radiosurgery (SRS) can be used for grade 1 meningiomas, for patients who are unfit for surgery, skull base meningiomas, or recurrent or incompletely resected meningiomas [8]. Single-fraction SRS is used in meningiomas with <3 cm maximum diameter or tumors located more than 3 mm from critical structures [5]. Primary or recurrent multiple intracranial meningiomas treated with stereotactic radiosurgery have an OS of 95% and a 5-year OS of 90% [5].

The evidence on SRS for meningiomas with grade 2 and 3 is limited and tumor control even with a marginal dose of 13 Gy is poor and ranges from 50% and 17% at 2–2.5 years, respectively [8] The European Association of Neuro-Oncology (EANO) does not approve the use of SRS for grade 2 and 3 tumors, outside of recurrent settings; however, some studies have described similar results for smaller tumors [23].

The prescription doses for SRS are 12-18 Gy to the 50% isodose line for Gamma knife and the dose is prescribed at 60-70% isodose line for cyberknife and to 80% isodose line for Linac- based treatments [8]. The dose prescription for SRS is 13–15 Gy given in a single fraction and 21–25 Gy given in three to five fractions [21]. For tumors larger than 3 cm in diameter or that involve critical brain regions such as brainstem or optic apparatus, dose fractionation of 50–55 Gy in 25–33 daily fractions or 54 Gy/27 fractions at 1.8 Gy per fraction is employed while single-fraction SRS can be used for smaller lesions away from the optic structures [21].

The factors which lead to improved local control after SRS are higher marginal dose, size of tumor (<10 cc), grade 1 tumor, primary SRS in place of adjuvant radiation, treatment in <1 year after onset of symptoms, female gender, and young age [8]. The risk factors for recurrence after SRS include male sex, grade 2/3 disease, tumor volume >6 ml [25] or >10 cc [8] [24], dose <12 Gy, parasagittal/para-falcine location, venous sinus invasion, multifocal disease, recurrent disease, or RT-induced tumors [8, 25]. So, it is preferable not to use SRS in certain situations such as primary grade 2/3 tumors, presence of peritumoral edema, venous sinus occlusion or involvement, large-sized meningiomas, or tumors that are adjacent to brainstem or cranial nerves [8, 25].

The patients may have very high rate of perilesional edema ranging from 2.5% to 50% post-SRS [4]. The risk factors which lead to increased risk of perilesional edema are previous radiation, larger tumor, high grade of tumor, and para-sagittally located tumors [4]. It is advisable to treat larger meningiomas with FSRS [4]. With fractionated radiosurgery (FSRS) with RT dose of 15–35 Gy over 3–6 fractions, similar local control to SRS has been noted but there is less perilesional edema (around 2.7–26%) [4]. One study has shown that as the dose per fraction increases, the rate of perilesional edema also increases—t is 2.7% with 6 Gy per fraction or less but 8.8 and 11.9% with 7–14 Gy and 15 Gy or higher [4].

There is still no clarity about offering adjuvant RT after complete resection of grade 2 meningiomas [26, 27]. It is important to do proper tumor and risk stratification to identify patients at risk for recurrence and then tailor subsequent management [26, 27]. This issue was addressed by two important trials—RTOG 0539 and EORTC trials. These trials categorized meningiomas into low-, intermediate-, and high-risk groups as shown in Table 6.7 [26, 27]. A risk scoring system for meningioma was also developed by Fioravanzo et al. It is a scoring system based on five features: male sex, parasagittal location, Simpson grade 3, mitotic index >6/10 HPF, and presence of sheeting. Each is given 1 score. If the score >2, it is associated with 4.7 times increased risk of recurrence [26, 27].

The NRG Oncology/RTOG 0539 is a phase II trial that investigated the results of adjuvant RT in patients with recurrent grade 1 and completely resected meningiomas [28]. In a first report, results of 49 patients of intermediate-risk meningiomas

Table 6.7 Risk stratification of meningiomas

Risk category	Grade	Adjuvant treatment	Results
Low risk	Grade 1 whether GTR or STR	No adjuvant RT	3-year PFS 91.8% 5-year PFS-86.1% 3-year OS 92.5%
Intermediate risk	Newly diagnosed grade 2 after GTR, recurrent grade 1 after any resection	RT 54 Gy/30 F	3-year PFS-93.8%
High risk	New or recurrent grade 3 regardless of resection, recurrent grade 2, grade 2 after subtotal resection	60 Gy/30 F with SIB (RTOG 0539)	3-year PFS-59.2% OS 78.6%

who were treated with IMRT or 3DCRT at a dose of 54 Gy/30 fractions were reported [28]. Of the evaluable patients, 44 (84.6%) received IMRT, and 50 (96.2%) were treated per protocol or with acceptable variation [28]. 3-year PFS was 93.8%, local failure rates were only 4.1%, and 3-year overall survival rate was 96% [28]. The clinical outcomes between atypical meningiomas after GTR or recurrent benign meningiomas were same and only grade 1 or 2 adverse reactions were seen [28].

In a second report from the same RTOG 0539 trial, results of 53 patients with high-risk meningiomas, who were treated with IMRT at a dose of 54 Gy/30 F with simultaneous integrated boost to GTV up to 60 Gy/30 F, were presented [29]. At 4 years FU, 3-year progression-free survival was 58.8%, overall survival was 78.6%, and local control was 68.9% [29]. Combined acute and late adverse events were seen in 40% of patients, but these were limited to grades 1-3 toxicity and one grade 5 event was seen [29]. Per central review, 92.9% of recurrences were within the RT planning target volume [29]. The authors concluded that higher RT doses, such as highly conformal, radiosurgery, or brachytherapy boost, are beneficial but require more validation [29].

In the EORTC 22042-26042 phase II study, 56 newly diagnosed patients with grade 2 atypical menigiomas who had gross total resection were included. The patients received adjuvant RT 60 Gy/30 F and the results were reported [30]. Five patients did not receive the planned dose of radiation, three did not complete RT due to grade 3 CSF leakage, nausea, vomiting or radiation dermatitis on scar and 2 patients received a higher dose of 70 Gy [30]. 3-year PFS was 88.7%, overall survival was 98.2%, and local failure was seen in 14.3% [30]. Late grade 3 toxicity was seen in 14%. This trial showed benefit of radiation in 70% patients of atypical meningiomas even after complete resection [30].

EORTC 22942 study demonstrated that patients with WHO grade 2 meningiomas treated with postop radiation at a dose of 60 Gy have a 3-year PFS of 70% [20]. Overall, 2- and 5-year progression-free survival of 65.0% and 38.4% and 2- and 5-year overall survival of 84.8% and 67.9%, respectively, were seen [30]. Among the patients who received adjuvant RT, the 2- and 5-year PFS of 81.6% and 57.7% and the 2- and 5-year OS were 89.3% and 71.2%, respectively [20].

There is still a lot of controversy regarding the advantage of postoperative radiation in patients with complete resection of WHO grade 2 meningiomas. This important question is being investigated with two phase III randomized trials NRG BN-003 (NCT03180268) and ROAM/EORTC-1308 (ISRCTN71502099), but the results are awaited.

ROAM/EORTC 1308 trial is an international, multicentric, randomized phase III controlled trial randomizing the patients to receive adjuvant RT or observation after surgery of atypical meningioma. The dose of radiation will be 60 Gy/30F [31]. The results are expected soon and it might help clarify the controversy regarding adjuvant radiation [31].

Alliance/NCI trial A071401 is a phase II trial of targeted therapy in recurrent or progressing Grade 1-3 meningiomas with somatic NF2 mutations [32]. The role and efficacy of FAK inhibitor, GSK2256098, in patients with NF2 loss was demonstrated [32]. The eligible cohort was treated with GSK2256098, 750 mg twice daily till the progression of disease [32]. The 6-month PFS and response rate were assessed using McDonald response criteria [30]. In patients with grade 1 meningioma, the observed progression-free survival was 83%, while in grade 2/3 meningiomas, it was 33% [32]. This trial showed the efficacy of GSK2256098 in recurrent or progressive setting but it requires further evaluation [32].

Some people have tried dose escalation in higher-grade meningiomas [8]. The phase II MARCIE trial treated incompletely resected WHO grade 2 meningiomas, with intensity-modulated radiation or fractionated stereotactic radiation at a dose of 50.4 Gy/28 fractions followed by a carbon-ion (C12) boost dose of 18 Gy/6 fractions [33]. The 3-year PFS and local control were 80.3% and 86.7%, but a large number of patients had contrast enhancement post-treatment and one treatment-associated death occurred, so the study was prematurely terminated [33].

6.11.2 Response Assessment After Treatment

Meningiomas show a slow response to radiation and only 20–30% of meningiomas show a decrease in the size of tumor over many months [8]. It is unclear if reduction in size of lesion or size stabilization should be assessed as response and if any suspicion of tumor progression warrants a change in management [8]. As per the RANO working group, 6-month PFS could be a viable endpoint, and if there is 25% increase in the tumors bi-dimensional size, it may be considered as definite progression. As per ICON definition, tumor progression is when a radiologic progression warrants a change in management of patient [8]. DOTATOC-PET scan may show a decrease in the uptake value as a marker of response [8].

MRI is considered to be the standard imaging modality for response assessment [7]. It is recommended that surveillance should be done on gadolinium-enhanced T1W sequence and size should be measured on T2W sequence but small meningiomas may be observed on T2 sequence as well [7].

6.11.3 Complications of Treatment

The non-surgical complications are increase in the size of tumor, chances of disease recurrence, and rapid growth of tumor [34]. Some meningiomas may progress to grade 2 or 3, get calcified, invade the brain invasion, or rarely show metastasis. The complications of surgery include risk of hematoma formation, infection, CSF leakage, injury to neighboring structures, risk of aspiration pneumonia, deep vein thrombosis, risk of stroke, myocardial ischemia, etc [34]. Cranial radiosurgery leads to risk of cranial nerve deficits, radio-necrosis, and post-radiation edema [34]. The side effects of conventional radiation with doses of 54–60 Gy range from 0% to 17% and may include mild skin reactions, fatigue, headache, cognitive changes, incoherent thinking, gradual memory disturbances, altered hormone levels (if pituitary receives radiation), loss of appetite, etc [34]. Most of these side effects are temporary and gradually decrease sometime after treatment. These can be managed easily with lifestyle modifications and medications, but cognitive changes may be permanent [34].

6.12 Conclusion

Meningiomas represent the most common primary intracranial tumors, arising predominantly from arachnoid cap cells. While the majority of meningiomas are non-malignant and grow slowly, their clinical presentation, behavior, and prognosis can vary significantly depending on histological grade, location, and extent of involvement with critical neurovascular structures. Advances in neuroimaging have enhanced early detection and accurate diagnosis, while surgical resection remains the cornerstone of treatment, often supplemented by radiotherapy in higher-grade or recurrent tumors. Recent insights into the molecular and genetic characteristics of meningiomas have opened new avenues for classification, prognostication, and the development of targeted therapies. The 2021 WHO classification now integrates molecular characteristics alongside histological features, signifying a shift toward precision medicine in neuro-oncology. Despite these advances, challenges remain, particularly in the management of high-grade, recurrent, and surgically inaccessible tumors. Future research must focus on improving risk stratification, identifying novel biomarkers, and refining therapeutic approaches, including immunotherapy and molecularly targeted agents. Ultimately, a multidisciplinary approach that combines clinical expertise, surgical innovation, and personalized medicine is essential for best outcomes and maintaining the quality of life for patients with meningioma.

References

1. Alruwaili AA, De Jesus O. Meningioma. [Updated 2023 Aug 23]. In: Stat Pearls [Internet]. Treasure Island (FL): Stat Pearls Publishing; 2025.
2. Ostrom QT, Gittleman H, Xu J, Kromer C, Wolinsky Y, Kruchko C, Barnholtz-Sloan JS. CBTRUS statistical report: primary brain and other central nervous system tumors diagnosed in the United States in 2009–2013. Neuro Oncol. 2016;18(Suppl 5):v1–75.
3. Louis DN, Perry A, Wesseling P, Brat DJ, Cree IA, Figarella-Branger D, et al. The 2021 WHO classification of tumors of the central nervous system: a summary. Neuro Oncol. 2021;23(8):1231–51.
4. Wilson MW, Youngblood DF, Miyagishima D, Jin L, Gupte T, Li C, et al. Associations of meningioma molecular subgroup and tumor recurrence. Neuro Oncol. 2021;23(5):783–94.
5. Caruso G, Ferrarotto R, Curcio A, Metro L, Pasqualetti F, Gaviani P, et al. Novel advances in treatment of meningiomas: prognostic and therapeutic implications. Cancers (Basel). 2023;15(18):4521.
6. Ostrom QT, Truitt G, Gittleman H, Brat DJ, Kruchko C, Wilson R, Barnholtz-Sloan JS. Relative survival after diagnosis with a primary brain or other central nervous system tumor in the National Program of cancer registries, 2004 to 2014. Neurooncol Pract. 2020;7(3):306–12.
7. Goldbrunner R, Minniti G, Preusser M, et al. EANO guidelines for the diagnosis and treatment of meningiomas. Lancet Oncol. 2016;17(9):e383–91.

8. Wang JZ, Landry AP, Raleigh DR, Sahm F, Walsh KM, Goldbrunner R, et al. Meningioma: International Consortium on Meningiomas consensus review on scientific advances and treatment paradigms for clinicians, researchers, and patients. Neuro Oncol. 2024;26(10):1742–80.
9. Wiemels J, Wrensch M, Claus EB. Epidemiology and aetiology of meningioma. J Neurooncol. 2010;99(3):307–14.
10. Saraf SS, McCarthy BJ, Villano JL. Update on meningiomas. Oncologist. 2011;16(11):1604–13.
11. Yeo JM, MacArthur D, Davis J, Scott I, Gran B. An unusual cause of cranial dural thickening. Case Rep Neurol Med. 2020;2020:8877738.
12. Krishnan P. Gingko leaf sign: a classical imaging finding in spinal meningiomas. Asian J Neurosurg. 2023;18(1):228–9.
13. Meningioma Grading [Internet]. www.hopkinsmedicine.org. Available from: https://www.hopkinsmedicine.org/health/conditions-and-diseases/meningioma-grading.
14. Corniola MV. Why we need new classification models in meningioma management. Acta Neurochir. 2022;164:1381–3.
15. Galldiks N, Albert NL, Sommerauer M, Grosu AL, Ganswindt U, Law I, et al. PET imaging in patients with meningioma: report of the RANO/PET group. Neuro-Oncology. 2017;19(12):1576–87.
16. Chen WC, Choudhury A, Youngblood MW, Polley MC, Lucas CG, Mirchia K, et al. Targeted gene expression profiling predicts meningioma outcomes and radiotherapy responses. Nat Med. 2023;29(12):3067–76.
17. Martz N, Salleron J, Dhermain F, Vogin G, Daisne JF, Mouttet-Audouard R, et al. Target volume delineation for radiotherapy of meningiomas: an ANOCEF consensus guideline. Radiat Oncol. 2023;18(1):113.
18. Nauta HJ, Tucker WS, Horsey WJ, Bilbao JM, Gonsalves C. Xanthochromic cysts associated with meningioma. J Neurol Neurosurg Psychiatry. 1979;42(6):529–35.
19. Jacobi-Postma L, Duyndam D. Enhancement patterns in CNS disease [Internet]. The Radiology Assistant; 2023.
20. Rogers L, Zhang P, Vogelbaum MA, Perry A, Ashby LS, Modi JM, et al. Intermediate-risk meningioma: initial outcomes from NRG Oncology RTOG 0539. J Neurosurg. 2017;129(1):35–47.
21. Combs SE, Baumert BG, Bendszus M, Bozzao A, Brada M, Fariselli L, et al. ESTRO ACROP guideline for target volume delineation of skull base tumors. Radiother Oncol. 2021;156:80–94.
22. Horbinski C, Nabors LB, Portnow J, Baehring J, Bhatia A, Bloch O, et al. NCCN guidelines® insights: central nervous system cancers, version 2.2022: featured updates to the NCCN guidelines. J Natl Compr Canc Netw. 2023;21(1):12–20.
23. Goldbrunner R, Stavrinou P, Jenkinson MD, Sahm F, Mawrin C, Weber DC, et al. EANO guideline on the diagnosis and management of meningiomas. Neuro-Oncology. 2021;23(11):1821–34.
24. Kuhn EN, Chan MD, Tatter SB, Ellis TL. Stereotactic radiosurgery for meningiomas. Stereotact Funct Neurosurg. 2012;90(6):365–9.
25. Yarabarla V, Mylarapu A, Han TJ, McGovern SL, Raza SM, Beckham TH. Intracranial meningiomas: an update of the 2021 World Health Organization classifications and review of management with a focus on radiation therapy. Front Oncol. 2023;13:1137849.
26. Fioravanzo A, Caffo M, Bonaventura R, Gardiman MP, Ghimenton C, Lus T, et al. A risk score based on 5 clinico-pathological variables predicts recurrence of atypical meningiomas. J Neuropathol Exp Neurol. 2020;79(5):500–7.
27. Rogers L, Barani I, Chamberlain M, Kaley T, McDermott M, Raizer J, et al. Meningiomas: knowledge base, treatment outcomes, and uncertainties. A RANO Review. J Neurosurg. 2015;122(1):4–23.
28. Rogers CL, Pugh SL, Vogelbaum MA, Perry A, Ashby LS, Modi JM, et al. Low-risk meningioma: initial outcomes from NRG Oncology/RTOG 0539. Neuro Oncol. 2023;25(1):137–45.
29. Rogers CL, Won M, Vogelbaum MA, Perry A, Ashby LS, Modi JM, et al. High-risk meningioma: initial outcomes from NRG Oncology/RTOG 0539. Int J Radiat Oncol Biol Phys. 2020;106(4):790–9.

30. Weber DC, Ares C, Villa S, Peerdeman SM, Renard L, Baumert BG, et al. Adjuvant postoperative high-dose radiotherapy for atypical and malignant meningioma: a phase-II parallel non-randomized and observation study (EORTC 22042-26042). Radiother Oncol. 2018;128(2):260–5.
31. Jenkinson MD, Javadpour M, Haylock BJ, Young B, Gillard H, Vinten J, etal. The ROAM/EORTC-1308 trial: Radiation versus Observation following surgical resection of Atypical Meningioma: study protocol for a randomised controlled trial. Trials. 2015;16:519. https://doi.org/10.1186/s13063-015-1040-3. PMID: 26576533; PMCID: PMC4650615.
32. Brastianos PK, Twohy EL, Gerstner ER, Kaufmann TJ, Iafrate AJ, Lennerz J, etal. A071401: Phase II Trial of Focal Adhesion Kinase Inhibition in Meningiomas with Somatic NF2 Mutations. J Clin Oncol. 2023;41(3):618–628. https://doi.org/10.1200/JCO.21.02371. Epub 2022 Oct 26. PMID: 36288512; PMCID: PMC9870228.
33. Deng MY, Maas SLN, Hinz F, Karger CP, Sievers P, Eichkorn T, Meixner E, etal. Efficacy and toxicity of bimodal radiotherapy in WHO grade 2 meningiomas following subtotal resection with carbon ion boost: Prospective phase 2 MARCIE trial. Neuro Oncol. 2024;26(4):701–712. https://doi.org/10.1093/neuonc/noad244. PMID: 38079455; PMCID: PMC10995516.
34. Dawley T, Rana Z, Abou-Al-Shaar H, et al. Major complications from radiotherapy following treatment for atypical meningiomas. Neurosurg Focus. 2019;46(6):E5.

Pituitary Adenoma

7

Arnav Sharma, Jishnu Prem, and Jhanja Mohapatra

7.1 Background

Pituitary adenomas are benign, slow-growing intracranial tumors that account for approximately 10–20% of all primary brain tumors [1, 9]. They are classified as functioning (hormone-secreting) or non-functioning (NFPA) and are further divided by size into microadenomas (<1 cm) and macroadenomas (>1 cm) [9]. Functioning adenomas present with hormonal syndromes such as Cushing's disease, acromegaly, or prolactinomas, while NFPAs typically present at a larger size due to compressive symptoms like visual disturbances, headache, or hypopituitarism [1, 9].

Transsphenoidal surgery remains the first-line treatment for most pituitary adenomas, aiming for maximal safe resection [1]. However, complete excision is often limited by cavernous sinus invasion or proximity to critical neurovascular structures. Medical management is primarily reserved for functioning tumors: dopamine agonists for prolactinomas, and somatostatin analogues, growth hormone receptor antagonists, or steroidogenesis inhibitors for acromegaly and Cushing's disease, especially when surgery is not curative or feasible [2, 3]. Medical therapy is generally ineffective for NFPAs.

Radiation therapy (RT) is indicated for residual, recurrent, or inoperable tumors, or when hormonal remission is not achieved with surgery or medical therapy [1, 9]. Historically, conventional external beam radiotherapy (CRT) was used, but was associated with significant long-term morbidity, particularly hypopituitarism and cerebrovascular risks [4]. The advent of stereotactic radiosurgery (SRS) and fractionated stereotactic radiotherapy (FSRT) has enabled more precise delivery of radiation, minimizing exposure to critical structures such as the optic chiasm and

A. Sharma (✉) · J. Prem · J. Mohapatra
Department of Radiation Oncology, Dharamshila Narayana Superspeciality Hospital, New Delhi, India

K. Sood Sharma (ed.), *Radiation Therapy for Benign Disorders*,
https://doi.org/10.1007/978-981-95-6635-8_7

temporal lobes [5]. These advances have expanded the role of RT from a salvage option to a key component of multimodal therapy.

Despite their benign nature, untreated or progressive pituitary adenomas can cause significant endocrine and neurologic morbidity. RT offers a durable, non-invasive means of tumor control and hormonal regulation, especially when surgery or medications are ineffective [1, 4, 5, 9].

7.2 Pathogenesis

Pituitary adenomas arise from the anterior pituitary (adenohypophysis) and are generally benign, slow-growing tumors. Their pathogenesis involves a complex interplay of genetic mutations, epigenetic alterations, and hormonal influences [4, 5, 8, 10].

7.3 Molecular Pathways and Genetic Drivers

Somatic mutations play a significant role in functional adenomas:

- *GNAS mutations* are frequently identified in somatotroph adenomas, contributing to excess growth hormone secretion [8, 10].
- *USP8 mutations* are commonly seen in corticotroph adenomas causing Cushing's disease [10, 11].
- *MEN1, AIP, and CDKN1B mutations* are implicated in familial syndromes like *MEN1, FIPA* (familial isolated pituitary adenomas), and *MEN4* [4, 11, 12].
- Disruptions in cell cycle regulation, such as *cyclin D1 overexpression* and *p27kip1 loss*, promote unchecked cellular proliferation [4, 8, 11].

Epigenetic modifications, altered microRNA expression, and dysregulated signaling pathways (e.g., MAPK, PI3K/AKT) further contribute to tumorigenesis [10, 11]. Hormonal factors, particularly estrogen, are linked to prolactinoma development [4, 8, 11].

7.4 WHO CNS 2021 Classification

The *WHO Classification of Tumors of the Central Nervous System (CNS), fifth edition (2021)*, replaced the term *"pituitary adenoma"* with *"pituitary neuroendocrine tumor (PitNET)"* to better reflect their neuroendocrine origin and biological behavior [13]. This shift emphasizes:

- Lineage-based classification: Tumors are categorized by transcription factor expression (e.g., *PIT1, SF1, TPIT*), guiding their differentiation into lactotroph, somatotroph, corticotroph, gonadotroph, or thyrotroph tumors [12, 13].

- Recognition of *high-risk histological subtypes* (e.g., sparsely granulated somatotroph tumors, Crooke's cell tumors, silent corticotroph tumors), which are associated with more aggressive behavior and higher recurrence rates [12–14].
- Integration of molecular pathology to predict prognosis and tailor treatment [12, 14].

This updated classification enhances the understanding of tumor behavior and guides treatment decisions, particularly regarding the use of targeted therapies and radiation modalities [12–14].

Despite their benign nature, PitNETs can exhibit local invasiveness (especially into the cavernous sinus), cause substantial endocrine dysregulation, and require multidisciplinary management to minimize morbidity [1, 4].

7.5 Role of Radiation Therapy (RT) in Pituitary Adenoma

The main indications for RT include:

- Residual tumor after incomplete resection, especially with cavernous sinus or parasellar invasion
- Recurrent tumor after initial surgery
- Persistent hormone hypersecretion in functioning adenoma (acromegaly, Cushing's disease, macroprolactinomas) refractory to surgery and/or medical therapy
- Patients unfit for surgery due to comorbidities or advanced age
- Select primary therapy in rare cases where surgery is contraindicated or declined [1, 6, 7, 9, 15]

7.6 Radiation Techniques

Modern RT for pituitary adenoma includes:

- *Conventional fractionated radiotherapy (CRT):* 45–54 Gy in 1.8–2.0 Gy fractions, using 3D conformal or IMRT for dose shaping. Image 7.1 shows Black Blood (BB) sequence diagnostic MRI sagittal section of a patient done in March 2022 showing signal diffusion restriction, size~4.7 x 4.1 x 3.8 (AP x TR x CC). The patient was initially diagnosed and operated in 2018, the patient developed recurrence in 2022, and operated in June 2022. Image 7.2 shows the planning CT with contouring volumes of the pituitary mass in the same patient. The patient was treated with conventional fractionation to a dose of 50.4Gy in 28 fractions. Image 7.3 shows the dose color wash of the same patient.
- *Fractionated stereotactic radiotherapy (FSRT):* Delivers highly conformal doses with sub-millimeter accuracy, suitable for larger or chiasm-adjacent tumors.

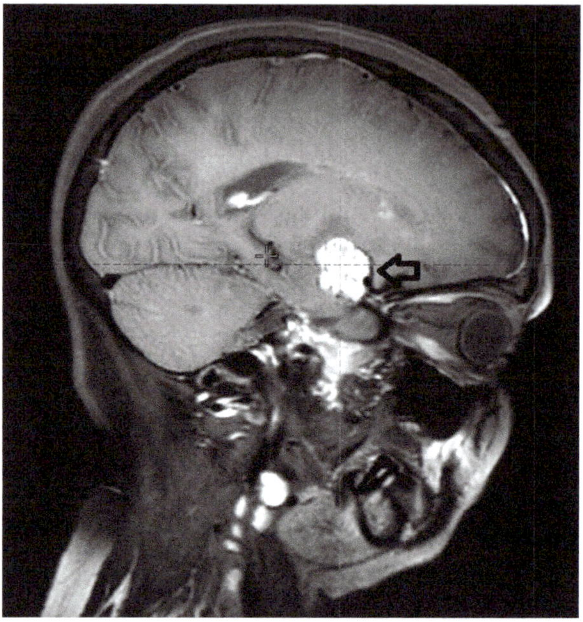

Image 7.1 Sagittal section of Black Blood (BB) sequence of MRI. This MRI image illustrates the typical appearance and dimensions of a pituitary mass, crucial for initial diagnosis, and treatment planning (This is an original image of diagnostic MRI of a patient, all copyrights reserved)

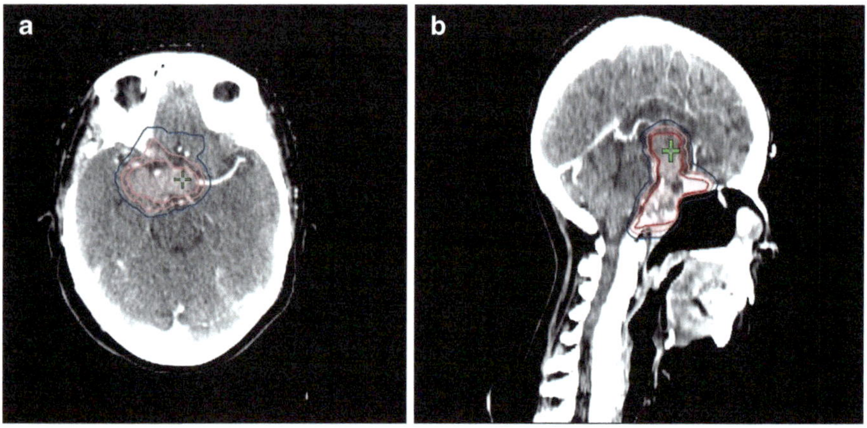

Image 7.2 (**a**) Axial view, (**b**) sagittal view. Planning CT showing contouring volumes of pituitary mass; innermost volume demonstrates GTV, middle volume demonstrates CTV, and outermost volume demonstrates PTV. (This is an original image of planning CT of the same patient, all copyrights reserved)

- *Stereotactic radiosurgery (SRS):* Single or few fractions (Gamma Knife, LINAC, CyberKnife, or proton SRS), best for small, well-defined tumors >2–3 mm from the optic apparatus. Image 7.4 shows the dose color wash of a patient treated with SRS.
- Proton therapy: Offers superior dose fall-off, sparing normal tissue, and is increasingly used in select centers [1, 9, 16–18].

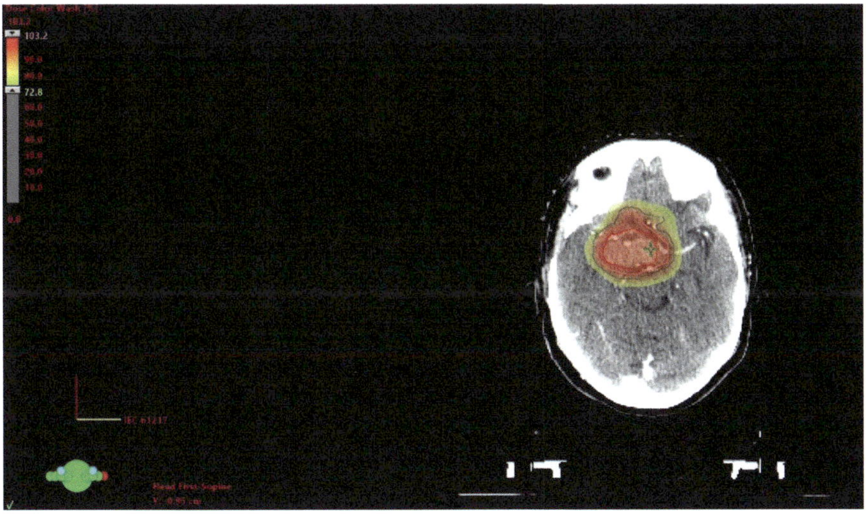

Image 7.3 Dose color wash axial section of the target volumes. (This is an original image of the plan created on planning CT of the same patient, all copyrights reserved)

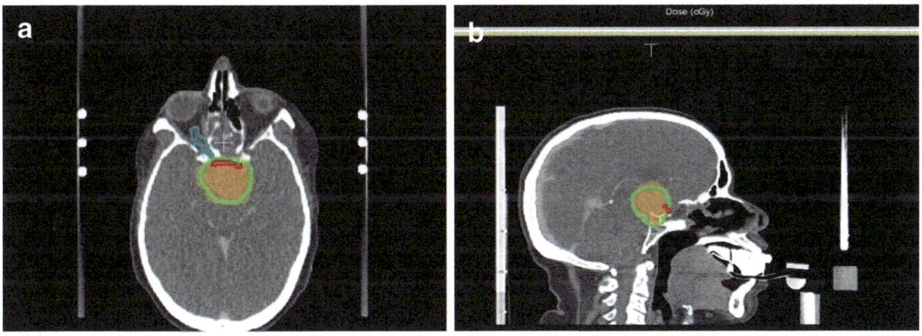

Image 7.4 Dose color wash: (**a**) axial section and (**b**) sagittal section of the target volumes for SRS. (This is an original image of the plan created on planning CT of a patient treated with SRS, all copyrights reserved)

RT provides durable tumor control in both non-functioning and functioning adenomas.

- Tumor control rates: 80–98% for non-functioning adenomas, 67–89% for functioning adenomas at 5–10 years [4, 6, 9, 19].
- Hormonal remission: 40–60% in acromegaly and Cushing's disease, 44–70% in macroprolactinomas, though normalization may take months to years [4, 6, 9, 20] .
- SRS/FSRT may achieve faster hormonal response and lower risk of late toxicity compared to CRT [5, 7, 21].

Compared to surgery, RT is noninvasive and avoids surgical risks, but has a slower onset of hormonal control and is less effective as primary therapy for microadenomas or when rapid decompression is needed (e.g., visual compromise). While medical therapy remains first-line, RT is employed when drugs fail or cannot be tolerated, or in macroprolactinomas producing mass effect. Medical therapy remains the first line of treatment for micro prolactinomas and as adjunct in functioning tumors [1, 4, 6].

RT is best suited for:

- Patients with residual or recurrent tumor after surgery, especially with cavernous sinus invasion or inoperable location
- Functioning adenomas (GH, ACTH, PRL) not controlled by surgery/medicine.

Table 7.1 shows the comparison of various radiation therapy techniques used for pituitary adenoma.

- Macroprolactinomas refractory to dopamine agonists and surgery
- Patients unfit for surgery due to comorbidities or advanced age
- Small, well-defined tumors (for SRS), with >2–3 mm from optic chiasm; FSRT/CRT for larger or chiasm-adjacent tumors [1, 5–7, 9]

Contraindications

- SRS is not suitable for large (>3 cm), irregular, or optic-adjacent tumors.
- CRT/FSRT may be preferred for extensive, invasive, or optic-involved tumors.

Limitations and Challenges

- Hormonal normalization may take years, especially in acromegaly and prolactinomas; bridging medical therapy is often needed [4, 6, 9].
- Acute side effects of radiation therapy for pituitary adenomas are generally mild and self-limited. Patients may experience transient fatigue, mild headache, scalp erythema, or nausea during or shortly after treatment, particularly with conventional fractionated RT or FSRT. Acute visual or neurological symptoms are rare with modern planning and dose constraints. Severe acute toxicities are uncommon, and most patients tolerate treatment well [4, 6, 7, 9].
- Hypopituitarism is the most common late effect (13–56% CRT, 10–30% SRS, 6–40% FSRT), requiring lifelong hormone replacement [4, 6, 7, 9].
- Visual loss is rare (<2%) with modern planning and dose constraints.
- Secondary malignancy is very rare (<1–2% at 10–20 years), especially with modern techniques [4, 7, 9].
- Cerebrovascular risk is increased, particularly with higher doses and older techniques; modern conformal RT reduces this risk [4, 9].

Table 7.1 Comparison of radiation therapy techniques for pituitary adenoma

Technique (references)	Typical dose and fractionation	Key dose constraints	Indications	Main outcomes	Common side effects	Notable late effects
Conventional fractionated RT (CRT/EBRT) [4, 6, 9]	45–54 Gy in 25–30 fractions (1.8–2.0 Gy/fraction)	Optic chiasm/nerve: <50–54 Gy; Brainstem: <54 Gy	Large, irregular, or chiasm-adjacent tumors; post-op residual/recurrent; not suitable for SRS	Tumor control: 80–98%; hormonal remission: 40–70% (functioning)	Hypopituitarism (13–56%); Rare visual loss (<2%)	Secondary malignancy (<1–2%); cerebrovascular disease (dose-dependent)
Fractionated stereotactic RT (FSRT) [4, 7, 18]	45–54 Gy in 25–30 fractions or hypofractionated (e.g., 25–30 Gy in 5 fractions)	Optic chiasm/nerve: <50–54 Gy; brainstem: <54 Gy	Tumors near optic apparatus or large/irregular; recurrent/residual; when SRS not feasible	Tumor control: 85–98%; hormonal remission: 40–70%	Hypopituitarism (6–40%); rare visual loss (<2%)	Very rare secondary malignancy; rare neurocognitive effects
Stereotactic radiosurgery (SRS) [5, 15, 21]	12–20 Gy (non-functioning); 15–30 Gy (functioning); single session or up to 5 fractions	Optic chiasm/nerve: <8–10 Gy (single fraction); minimum 2–3 mm from chiasm	Small, well-defined tumors >2–3 mm from optic chiasm; residual/recurrent; select functioning adenomas	Tumor control: 90–100%; hormonal remission: 40–60% (functioning)	Hypopituitarism (10–30%); rare visual loss (<2%)	Very rare secondary malignancy; rare cranial neuropathy
Proton therapy [16] (SRS or FSRT) [17]	SRS: 15–25 Gy (single fraction); FSRT: 45–54 Gy in fractions	Optic chiasm/nerve: <8–10 Gy; brainstem: <12 Gy	Tumors near critical structures; pediatric/young adults; re-irradiation	Tumor control: 90–98%; hormonal remission: 40–60%	Hypopituitarism (variable, similar to photon RT); rare visual loss	Theoretical lower risk of late effects due to reduced exit dose

Follow-Up

- Not all patients benefit equally; careful selection and multidisciplinary discussion are essential.
- Lifelong endocrine and imaging follow-up is required to monitor for recurrence and late effects [4, 6, 7, 9].
- Most data are from retrospective series; no RCTs directly compare RT modalities or RT vs. surgery/medicine [4, 6].

Conclusion

Radiation therapy remains a highly effective, safe, and essential component of the multidisciplinary management of pituitary adenomas, particularly for residual, recurrent, or refractory disease. Advances in RT techniques (FSRT, SRS, proton therapy) have improved precision and reduced toxicity. Careful patient selection, modern planning, and lifelong follow-up are critical to optimize outcomes and minimize risks.

7.7 RT-Associated Toxicity

Radiotherapy continues to be a cornerstone in the treatment of pituitary adenomas, particularly for incompletely resected, recurrent, or medically refractory tumors. However, its use is not without long-term risks. The most commonly reported complication is hypopituitarism, which affects up to 80% of patients within 5–10 years post-treatment, especially with older radiotherapy techniques and when RT follows surgery [4, 6, 9]. Growth hormone deficiency typically occurs first, followed by gonadotropin, ACTH, and TSH deficiency [9]. Injury may involve both the hypothalamus and remaining pituitary tissue, particularly when larger radiation fields are employed [9].

Another major toxicity is the risk of cerebrovascular syndrome. Multiple studies have reported a two- to fourfold increased risk of stroke and cerebrovascular mortality following cranial irradiation for pituitary adenomas [4, 17, 19]. The pathogenesis involves radiation-induced endothelial damage, microvascular inflammation, and accelerated atherosclerosis [4]. Notably, this risk appears to be dose- and technique dependent—older methods such as lateral opposing field CRT delivered excess dose to the temporal lobes, optic tracts, and vasculature [4, 6].

A rare but serious concern is the development of secondary intracranial tumors. A systematic review by Yamanaka et al. reported a latency of 13–21 years for radiation-induced gliomas, meningiomas, and sarcomas following pituitary RT, most arising in patients treated with CRT and multi-field techniques [20]. The cumulative incidence remains low (<2%), but long-term surveillance is warranted.

Recent advances in radiotherapy techniques have significantly reduced toxicity. Stereotactic radiosurgery (SRS) and fractionated stereotactic radiotherapy (FSRT) enable highly conformal dosing with steep dose fall-off, sparing surrounding normal tissue [5, 6, 17]. These modalities have demonstrated lower rates of hypopituitarism and vascular events, with some reports indicating no significant cerebrovascular complications even at long-term follow-up [5].

To minimize long-term risks, it is essential to:

- Adhere to optic pathway constraints (<10 Gy in SRS or <54 Gy in FSRT)
- Limit total dose and field size using modern imaging and planning
- Follow patients with lifelong endocrine and vascular monitoring
- Involve a multidisciplinary endocrine-neuro-oncologic care team

While radiotherapy is highly effective for tumor control, careful therapeutic planning using contemporary RT modalities is critical to mitigate late effects and preserve quality of life.

7.8 Future Directions

- The landscape of radiation therapy for pituitary adenomas is rapidly evolving, driven by advances in technology, improved understanding of radiobiology, and the emergence of precision medicine.
- Modern techniques such as fractionated stereotactic radiotherapy (FSRT), stereotactic radiosurgery (SRS), and proton therapy have demonstrated high rates of tumor control with reduced toxicity compared to conventional external beam radiotherapy [6, 7, 17, 18, 21].
- FSRT, in particular, offers excellent local control (up to 92%) and is suitable for both functioning and non-functioning adenomas, regardless of tumor size or proximity to the optic apparatus, with low rates of new hypopituitarism and visual toxicity [6]. SRS, especially with Gamma Knife, achieves rapid hormonal and radiological control, with tumor control rates exceeding 95% and hormonal remission in 40–50% of secreting adenomas [5, 15, 21].
- Proton therapy, leveraging the Bragg peak, allows for highly conformal dose delivery and further reduction in exit dose to normal tissues, with promising results in functional adenomas and a favorable safety profile [16].
- Ongoing research and future clinical trials are needed to refine dose constraints for critical neuroanatomical structures, such as the pituitary stalk and gland, to minimize the risk of hypopituitarism [15]. The relationship between target volume, margin dose, and late toxicity—especially in the context of SRS and proton therapy—remains an area of active investigation [15, 16].
- Prospective, multi-institutional registries and randomized trials comparing FSRT, SRS, and proton therapy will be essential to establish optimal treatment paradigms and long-term safety, particularly for rare but serious late effects such as secondary malignancies and cerebrovascular events.

Table 7.2 shows various studies done for use of radiomics, personalized medicine, and AI in the management of pituitary adenoma.

Table 7.2 Future directions with key focus areas and relevance to personalized medicine/AI

References	Focus area	Key findings	Relevance to personalized medicine/AI
Zheng et al. (2024) [22]	MRI radiomics in pituitary adenoma	Radiomics offers quantitative analysis by extracting high-throughput imaging data to establish biomarkers, demonstrating extensive applications in differential diagnosis, subtype identification, and treatment assessment of pituitary adenomas, with deep learning models showing high diagnostic accuracy and potential to reduce human error	Radiomics, through its quantitative analysis and integration with AI (e.g., CNNs), enables precision identification and individualized management strategies for pituitary adenomas by establishing imaging biomarkers and combining with clinical/genomic data, despite challenges in reproducibility and tailoring to individual variances
Dai et al. (2021) [23]	AI and deep learning in pituitary adenomas	AI and machine learning are widely applied in pituitary adenomas for diagnosis, prognosis, and treatment, demonstrating promise in image analysis and multi-omics data integration despite current challenges in data quality and model generalizability	AI and machine learning are crucial for advancing precision medicine in pituitary adenomas by improving personalized diagnosis, predicting outcomes, and guiding treatment through comprehensive data analysis
Bibault JE, et al. (2017) [24]	AI in radiation oncology	AI used for auto-segmentation, treatment planning, and outcome prediction in CNS tumors; optimizes dose distribution and reduces toxicity	AI-driven planning tailors RT to patient-specific anatomy and biology, improving outcomes
Toader C, et al. (2023) [25]	Precision medicine	Reviews molecular characteristics of pituitary adenomas, translating this into novel diagnostic, prognostic, and therapeutic strategies within precision medicine	Supports personalized medicine in pituitary adenomas by integrating genetic and molecular insights for tailored diagnostics, prognostics, and therapies, inherently relying on advanced computational methods like AI for complex data analysis

- Emerging indications for advanced radiation techniques include their use as primary therapy in select patients with small, well-defined, non-functioning adenomas, or in those with contraindications to surgery [5, 6]. The role of SRS and FSRT is also expanding in recurrent or residual functioning adenomas, especially when medical therapy is ineffective or not tolerated.
- Looking ahead, personalized medicine and artificial intelligence (AI) are poised to transform the field. AI-driven treatment planning, radiomics, and integration of clinical, imaging, and molecular data may enable individualized risk stratification and adaptive radiotherapy, optimizing outcomes while minimizing toxicity [23, 24]. The future of pituitary adenoma management will likely be

characterized by multidisciplinary, patient-centered care, leveraging technological innovation and data-driven decision-making to achieve durable tumor and hormonal control with the lowest possible risk.

7.9 Review of Literature

Radiation therapy (RT) has been a mainstay in the management of pituitary adenomas for decades, with a robust body of literature supporting its efficacy and safety. Both conventional fractionated radiotherapy (CRT) and modern techniques such as stereotactic radiosurgery (SRS), fractionated stereotactic radiotherapy (FSRT), and proton therapy have been extensively studied in retrospective and prospective cohorts.

- Brada et al. (1993) found 10-year progression-free survival rates of 97% for non-secreting adenomas [26]. However, CRT is associated with a significant risk of hypopituitarism (13–56%), and rare but serious late effects such as secondary malignancy (<1–2%) and cerebrovascular disease (up to 4% at 5 years) [1, 4, 19]. Large retrospective series have established the effectiveness of CRT in achieving durable tumor control. Becker et al. (2002) reviewed outcomes in over 1300 patients, reporting local control rates of 80–98% for non-functioning adenomas and 67–89% for functioning tumors, with 5-, 10-, and 15-year progression-free survival rates of 92%, 89%, and 79%, respectively [4].
- The advent of SRS and FSRT has allowed for more precise targeting, reducing exposure to surrounding brain structures. Ding et al. (2014) summarized multiple series, showing SRS tumor control rates of 90–100% for non-functioning adenomas and 40–60% hormonal remission for functioning tumors, with hypopituitarism rates of 10–30% [7]. Kopp et al. (2013) reported a 91.9% tumor control rate at a median follow-up of 57 months with FSRT and low rates of new hypopituitarism or visual toxicity [6].
- Losa et al. (2008) found that both CRT and SRS provided >90% 5-year progression-free survival in non-functioning adenomas, with SRS offering a lower risk of visual complications and a more favorable side effect profile in selected patients [1].
- Wattson et al. (2014) presented the largest series of functional pituitary adenomas treated with proton therapy, reporting a 98% local control rate and 3-year and 5-year hypopituitarism rates of 45% and 62%, respectively [16]. No cases of radiation-induced tumors or cerebrovascular accidents were observed, though longer follow-up is needed to confirm these findings.
- While randomized controlled trials are lacking, meta-analyses and large cohort studies provide high-level evidence. A meta-analysis by Minniti et al. (2007) found that SRS and FSRT achieved similar tumor control rates to CRT but with lower rates of late toxicity [27]. The absence of prospective randomized trials is a limitation, but the consistency of results across large retrospective series supports the efficacy of RT.

- Case reports and institutional series highlight the effectiveness of RT in challenging scenarios. For example, Castro et al. (2010) described a patient with a recurrent ACTH-secreting adenoma who achieved hormonal control and tumor stability after Gamma Knife radiosurgery, despite prior failed surgery and medical therapy [18]. Conversely, rare cases of late visual loss or secondary malignancy underscore the need for careful planning and long-term surveillance.

7.10 Long-Term Safety and Limitations

The most common late effect of RT is hypopituitarism, which may develop years after treatment and requires lifelong hormone replacement. Modern techniques have reduced the risk of visual loss (<2%) and secondary malignancy (<1–2%), but the risk of cerebrovascular events remains a concern, particularly with higher doses and older techniques [1, 4, 19, 28]. Lifelong follow-up with endocrine and imaging assessment is essential.

7.11 Conclusion

The literature consistently demonstrates that RT—especially with modern techniques—offers high rates of tumor control and acceptable safety for pituitary adenomas. Patient selection, individualized planning, and multidisciplinary care are critical to optimizing outcomes and minimizing risks.

References

1. Losa M, Picozzi P, Motta M, Valle M, Franzin A, Mortini P. The role of radiation therapy in the management of non-functioning pituitary adenomas. J Endocrinol Invest [Internet]. 2011 [cited 2025 Jul 21];34(8). Available from: https://doi.org/10.3275/7618.
2. Molitch ME. Diagnosis and treatment of pituitary adenomas: a review. JAMA. 2017;317(5):516.
3. Gheorghiu ML, Negreanu F, Fleseriu M. Updates in the medical treatment of pituitary adenomas. Horm Metab Res. 2020;52(01):8–24.
4. Becker G, Kocher M, Kortmann RD, Paulsen F, Jeremic B, Müller RP, et al. Radiation therapy in the multimodal treatment approach of pituitary adenoma. Strahlenther Onkol. 2002;178(4):173–86.
5. Rim CH, Yang DS, Park YJ, Yoon WS, Lee JA, Kim CY. Radiotherapy for pituitary adenomas: long-term outcome and complications. Radiat Oncol J. 2011;29(3):156.
6. Kopp C, Theodorou M, Poullos N, Astner ST, Geinitz H, Stalla GK, et al. Fractionated stereotactic radiotherapy in the treatment of pituitary adenomas. Strahlenther Onkol. 2013;189(11):932–7.
7. Ding D, Starke RM, Sheehan JP. Treatment paradigms for pituitary adenomas: defining the roles of radiosurgery and radiation therapy. J Neuro-Oncol. 2014;117(3):445–57.
8. Vandeva S, Daly AF, Petrossians P, Zacharieva S, Beckers A. Somatic and germline mutations in the pathogenesis of pituitary adenomas. Eur J Endocrinol. 2019;181(6):R235–54.
9. González-Virla B, Vargas-Ortega G, Romero-Gameros CA. Radiotherapy and mortality in pituitary adenomas. Arch Med Res. 2023;54(8):102900.

10. Vandeva S, Jaffrain-Rea ML, Daly AF, Tichomirowa M, Zacharieva S, Beckers A. The genetics of pituitary adenomas. Best Pract Res Clin Endocrinol Metab. 2010;24(3):461–76.
11. Beckers A, Aaltonen LA, Daly AF, Karhu A. Familial isolated pituitary adenomas (FIPA) and the pituitary adenoma predisposition due to mutations in the aryl hydrocarbon receptor interacting protein (AIP) gene. Endocr Rev. 2013;34(2):239–77.
12. WHO. WHO classification of tumours: endocrine and neuroendocrine tumours. 5th ed. Lyon: International Agency for Research on Cancer, WHO; 2025. 595 p
13. Asa SL, Mete O, Perry A, Osamura RY. Overview of the 2022 WHO classification of pituitary tumors. Endocr Pathol. 2022;33(1):6–26.
14. Villa C, Baussart B, Assié G, Raverot G, Roncaroli F. The World Health Organization classifications of pituitary neuroendocrine tumours: a clinico-pathological appraisal. Endocr Relat Cancer. 2023;30(8):e230021.
15. Castinetti F, Régis J, Dufour H, Brue T. Role of stereotactic radiosurgery in the management of pituitary adenomas. Nat Rev Endocrinol. 2010;6(4):214–23.
16. Wattson DA, Tanguturi SK, Spiegel DY, Niemierko A, Biller BMK, Nachtigall LB, et al. Outcomes of proton therapy for patients with functional pituitary adenomas. Int J Radiat Oncol Biol Phys. 2014;90(3):532–9.
17. Pomeraniec IJ, Taylor DG, Cohen-Inbar O, Xu Z, Lee Vance M, Sheehan JP. Radiation dose to neuroanatomical structures of pituitary adenomas and the effect of Gamma Knife radiosurgery on pituitary function. J Neurosurg. 2020;132(5):1499–506.
18. Castro DG, Cecílio SA, Canteras MM. Radiosurgery for pituitary adenomas: evaluation of its efficacy and safety. Radiat Oncol [Internet]. 2010 [cited 2025 Jul 21];5(1). Available from: https://ro-journal.biomedcentral.com/articles/10.1186/1748-717X-5-109
19. Brada M, Ashley S, Ford D, Traish D, Burchell L, Rajan B. Cerebrovascular mortality in patients with pituitary adenoma. Clin Endocrinol. 2002;57(6):713–7.
20. Yamanaka R, Abe E, Sato T, Hayano A, Takashima Y. Secondary intracranial tumors following radiotherapy for pituitary adenomas: a systematic review. Cancer. 2017;9(8):103.
21. Castinetti F, Nagai M, Morange I, Dufour H, Caron P, Chanson P, et al. Long-term results of stereotactic radiosurgery in secretory pituitary adenomas. J Clin Endocrinol Metab. 2009;94(9):3400–7.
22. Zheng B, Zhao Z, Zheng P, Liu Q, Li S, Jiang X, et al. The current state of MRI-based radiomics in pituitary adenoma: promising but challenging. Front Endocrinol [Internet]. 2024 [cited 2025 Jul 22];15. Available from: https://www.frontiersin.org/articles/10.3389/fendo.2024.1426781/full
23. Dai C, Sun B, Wang R, Kang J. The application of artificial intelligence and machine learning in pituitary adenomas. Front Oncol [Internet]. 2021 [cited 2025 Jul 22];11. Available from: https://www.frontiersin.org/articles/10.3389/fonc.2021.784819/full
24. Bibault JE, Burgun A, Giraud P. Intelligence artificielle appliquée à la radiothérapie. Cancer/Radiothérapie. 2017;21(3):239–43.
25. Toader C, Dobrin N, Tataru CI, Covache-Busuioc RA, Bratu BG, Glavan LA, et al. From genes to therapy: pituitary adenomas in the era of precision medicine. Biomedicine. 2023;12(1):23.
26. Brada M, Rajan B, Traish D, Ashley S, Holmes-Sellors PJ, Nussey S, et al. The long-term efficacy of conservative surgery and radiotherapy in the control of pituitary adenomas. Clin Endocrinol. 1993;38(6):571–8.
27. Minniti G, Jaffrain-Rea ML, Osti M, Cantore G, Enrici RM. Radiotherapy for nonfunctioning pituitary adenomas: from conventional to modern stereotactic radiation techniques. Neurosurg Rev. 2007;30(3):167–76.
28. Olsson DS, Nilsson AG, Bryngelsson IL, Trimpou P, Johannsson G, Andersson E. Excess mortality in women and young adults with nonfunctioning pituitary adenoma: a Swedish Nationwide study. J Clin Endocrinol Metabol. 2015;100(7):2651–8.

Schwannoma

8

Vikash Kumar and Sushma Sharma

8.1 Background

A schwannoma is a common, benign, slow-growing tumor composed entirely of well-differentiated Schwann cells, with an incidence of 3–5 per 100,000 population [1]. These tumors are usually encapsulated and derived from the myelin sheaths that cover peripheral nerves. Schwannomas account for 85% of cerebellopontine angle tumors, 29% of spinal nerve root tumors, and 8% of all intracranial tumors [2]. Although slow-growing, the growth rate is variable, averaging around 2.8 ± 1.3 mm per year. Malignant transformation is rare, occurring in less than 1% of cases, usually to neurofibrosarcoma. Due to their encapsulated nature, schwannomas often allow for a surgical cleavage plane, making surgical removal feasible and effective.

Approximately 90% of schwannomas are solitary and sporadic. Of the 5% that occur as multiple lesions but are not associated with NF2, are linked to schwannomatosis. Schwannomas can affect patients of any age, but most commonly present between the ages of 40 and 60 years [3]. Although most studies report no significant sex predilection, some have noted a slight female predilection. Among intracranial cases, 80–90% arise from the vestibular nerve. Bilateral vestibular schwannomas (VSs) are present in 5–10% of cases and are diagnostic of neurofibromatosis type 2 (NF2). Furthermore, about 60% of unilateral VSs and 90% of bilateral VSs exhibit NF2 gene mutations causing malfunction of its protein product, merlin (moesin–ezrin–radixin-like protein) [4].

Most schwannomas are located outside the central nervous system, classically within peripheral nerves of the skin and subcutaneous tissues. Intracranial schwannomas most often involve the eighth cranial nerve (vestibulocochlear nerve),

V. Kumar (✉)
Department of Radiation Oncology, Metro Cancer Institute, Faridabad, India

S. Sharma
Department of Neurology, Marengo Asia Hospital, Faridabad, India

K. Sood Sharma (ed.), *Radiation Therapy for Benign Disorders*,
https://doi.org/10.1007/978-981-95-6635-8_8

especially in the cerebellopontine angle. These tumors develop at the transition zone between central and peripheral myelination, primarily affecting the vestibular division; the cochlear division is rarely the site of origin. Schwannomas can also originate from the brachial and sciatic plexuses, although brachial plexus involvement accounts for less than 5% of upper extremity cases. Intraspinal schwannomas typically affect sensory nerve roots, with rare involvement of motor and autonomic nerves. Occasionally, schwannomas within the central nervous system lack a clear association with a specific nerve.

This section focuses on vestibular schwannomas—the most common type. Symptoms are usually related to mass effect on adjacent cranial nerves. These include sensorineural hearing loss and tinnitus (acoustic nerve involvement), vertigo and gait instability (vestibular nerve), facial paraesthesia (trigeminal nerve), facial paresis and taste changes (facial nerve), and ataxia (cerebellar peduncles). In cases of large tumors, compression of the fourth ventricle may lead to hydrocephalus [5].

The first major breakthrough in VS treatment occurred in the early twentieth century when Harvey Cushing introduced bilateral suboccipital craniotomy with subtotal resection, substituting digital enucleation and reducing mortality from 80% to less than 20% [6]. Later, Walter Dandy innovated a unilateral approach for complete or near complete tumor removal and pioneered pneumoencephalography to facilitate in diagnosis and localization [7]. In 1951, Leksell introduced stereotactic radiosurgery (SRS), and the first VS was treated in Stockholm in 1969, prompted by the high morbidity associated with surgery and Cushing's advocacy for noninvasive options [8]. In the beginning, radiation therapy (RT) was used as an adjuvant after incomplete resection, but in due course of time, SRS emerged as a primary alternative. Early SRS treatments delivered doses around 20 Gy, which led to notable toxicities such as facial nerve dysfunction (15%) and trigeminal neuropathy (15%). Dose de-escalation studies in the 2000s showed that reducing the dose to around 12 Gy preserved local control while significantly lowering toxicity rates [9].

Current management approaches include observation, microsurgery, radiosurgery, and fractionated stereotactic radiotherapy. SRS is widely accepted for small VSs, while larger tumors often require combined approaches. Over the past few years, a shift has been observed, with decreasing use of microsurgery, increasing preference for observation, and consistent use of radiation therapy.

8.2 Pathogenesis

Recent research into the pathobiology of NF2 and schwannomas has provided a more nuanced understanding of the complex interactions between various cell types within these tumors. Unlike other Schwann cell–derived tumors such as neurofibromas, which involve multiple fascicles of a nerve, schwannomas grow without entrapping axons beyond those directly associated with the originating Schwann cells.

Histologically, schwannomas comprise not only tumorigenic Schwann cells and axonal processes but also a heterogeneous population of non-neoplastic cells, including macrophages, T cells, endothelial cells, and occasionally perivascular B cells. These cell types engage in intricate paracrine and juxtracrine signaling mechanisms, contributing to tumor behavior and progression [10].

Unlike neurofibromas, peripheral nerve schwannomas are typically attached to nerve trunks and rarely invade the dura. They most commonly occur in the head and neck region or on the flexor surfaces of the extremities. Visceral and osseous schwannomas are particularly rare.

8.3 Role of Radiation Therapy (RT)

The baseline workup of vestibular schwannoma (VS) begins with a thorough clinical evaluation, including a detailed history, physical examination, baseline pure tone audiometry, and diagnostic imaging. Gadolinium magnetic resonance imaging (MRI) remains the gold standard for diagnosis. Typically, lesions enhance on T1-weighted images and are located near the internal auditory canal, which may appear expanded. Some tumors are purely intracanalicular. Differential diagnosis includes other cerebellopontine (CP) angle tumors: meningiomas, which typically do not involve the internal auditory canal, and epidermoid cysts, which have distinct imaging characteristics. In general, MRI findings are sufficient to diagnose VS, negating the need for histopathological confirmation. The Koos staging system (Stages I–IV) is used to classify tumors based on size and proximity to the brainstem [11] (Fig. 8.1 and Table 8.1).

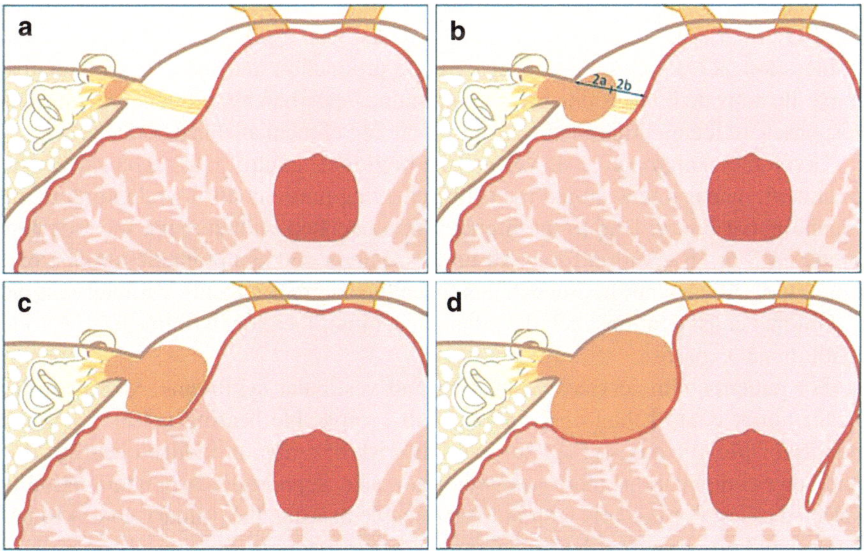

Fig. 8.1 Koos classification right-sided VS. (**a**) Koos 1; (**b**) Koos 2a and 2b; (**c**) Koos 3; (**d**) Koos 4. (*Source*: Pruijn et al. [12], Licensed under CC-BY 4.0)

Table 8.1 Koos classification system for vestibular schwannoma

Koos 1	Intracanalicular tumor
Koos 2a	Extending into cerebellopontine angle, < half of the shortest distance from porus to pons
Koos 2b	Extending into cerebellopontine angle, ≥ half of the shortest distance from porus to pons
Koos 3	Occupying cerebellopontine angle, touching pons or cerebellar peduncle, not compressing/displacing it
Koos 4	Compressing pons or cerebellar peduncle and/or shifting fourth ventricle

Management of schwannomas is individualized and depends on factors such as lesion size, symptomatology, patient comorbidities, and personal preferences. Treatment decisions are typically made in a multidisciplinary setting, with three main options: observation (wait and watch), microsurgical excision, and radiation therapy. Due to lack of randomized controlled trials, treatment selection is based on institutional experiences. Modern studies shows that local control exceeds 90% with surgical resection, fractionated stereotactic radiotherapy (FSRT), or SRS, with no significant differences among these modalities. For asymptomatic patients with Koos stage I or II tumors, a "wait-and-watch" strategy with annual MRI and audiometry is often advised. Tumor growth rate, rather than absolute size, is a better predictor of future hearing decline [13].

Radiation therapy (RT) is believed to exert its effects by inhibiting tumor cell proliferation, suppressing cellular differentiation, and promoting fibroblast activity. Additionally, RT impacts the vascular endothelial cells of capillaries. At low dose per fraction, it elicits anti-inflammatory effects, while at higher single doses (>12 Gy/fraction), it causes endothelial damage leading to vascular sclerosis and obliteration. RT also modulates nitric oxide production and induces an oxidative burst in activated macrophages and granulocytes, thereby influencing immune responses, reducing inflammation, and producing clinical analgesic effects.

Given the benign nature of VS and the high local control rates achievable with treatment, management should focus on achieving tumor control while minimizing cranial nerve injury. Due to the higher risk associated with surgery, most centers prefer SRS or observation for small tumors. Larger and symptomatic tumors, particularly those causing hydrocephalus, usually require microsurgical intervention. Additional considerations include patient age, tumor location, baseline hearing, and institutional expertise.

For patients with serviceable hearing and vestibular symptoms, SRS provides better tumor control than observation, with comparable hearing preservation and quality-of-life outcomes [14]. However, the risk of radiation-induced hearing loss and other complications increases with tumor size, supporting early intervention in selected cases. For patients with non-serviceable hearing, the primary goal is tumor control and preservation of adjacent cranial nerve function.

For large (Koos III/IV) VS, local control after radiosurgery depends upon marginal dose, tumor volume, and prior microsurgery; higher marginal doses favor tumor control, whereas large tumor and prior surgery negatively impact outcomes. Koos III tumors are usually symptomatic and warrant immediate intervention. The choice between RT and surgery depends on the size of the cisternal component of the tumor. For Koos IV lesions, decompression of the brainstem and cranial nerves becomes the priority, making surgery the preferred option [15]. RT may serve as a second-line treatment for patients who are not surgical candidates or may be integrated into combination strategies when residual tumor remains.

Despite excellent tumor control and low complication rates with SRS and FSRT, long-term hearing decline remains a major concern. Studies have shown that SRS offers superior hearing preservation compared to surgery, though hearing function may still decline to approximately 25% over 10 years [16].

8.4 Stereotactic Radiosurgery (SRS)

Radiosurgery has proven to be an excellent alternative to microsurgery for the management of vestibular schwannomas (VS) and is widely considered as a standard-of-care option in current practice. Given the steep learning curve associated with microsurgical techniques, the operative risks involved, and the benign nature of the disease, SRS offers a better favorable risk-to-benefit ratio for many patients.

This modality is especially suitable for patients who are high-risk surgical candidates, those with small tumors (<30 mm in diameter), Koos stage I or II tumors, individuals with serviceable hearing, and those who prefer a non-surgical approach. Although no randomized clinical trials have directly compared SRS with microsurgery, numerous studies suggest that SRS achieves comparable local control, with potentially more favorable rates of hearing preservation [17].

Most series demonstrate local control rates between 90% and 95%, while facial nerve deficits and trigeminal neuropathy occur in approximately 0–6% and 1–12% of cases, respectively [18] (Table 8.2).

The main concern with SRS remains long-term hearing preservation. Data from large series and meta-analyses report serviceable hearing preservation rates between 55% and 65% following treatment [25]. Favorable prognostic factors for hearing preservation include younger age, good hearing status at the time of SRS, early intervention post-diagnosis, smaller tumor volume, lower marginal radiation dose (<13 Gy), and reduced cochlear dose.

Tumor volume has consistently emerged as a significant prognostic factor for local control. For example, Rueb et al. [19] reported a 100% radiological tumor control rate and 78% serviceable hearing preservation in 45 patients with a median

Table 8.2 Patient outcome data for stereotactic radiosurgery

		Number of patients						Toxicity			
Author	Year	Total	Prior surgery	Median follow-up (months)	Median dose (Gy)	Median volume (cc)	Local control	Hearing preservation	Trigeminal nerve dysfunction	Facial nerve dysfunction	Hydrocephalus
Rueb et al. [19]	2017	49	4	65	12.6	0.24	100%	78%	0%	2%	NA
Windisch [20]	2019	996	175	42	13	0.61	96.6% at 3 years	21.50%	3%	0.90%	0.50%
							92.3% at 5 years				
							90.8% at 10 years				
Johnson [18]	2019	871	NA	62	13	0.9	97% at 3 years	76.9% at 3 years	5.80%	1.60%	1.70%
							95% at 5 years	68.4% at 5 years			
							94% at 10 years	51.4% at 10 years			
Rueb [19]	2018	335	70	30	13	1.1	98% at 3 years	56% at 5 years	3.80%	3.60%	0.80%
							89% at 5 years				
							88% at 10 years				
Klijn [21]	2016	420	NA	60	11	1.4	91.3% at 5 years	65% at 3 years	3.10%	1%	1.20%
							84.8% at 10 years	42% at 5 years			
Yeole [22]	2021	34	8	34.7	12	10.9	85.30%	0%	12.50%	4%	NA

Mezey [23]	2020	103	22	74	12.5	13.6	78.60%	25.20%	8.70%	2.90%	14.60%
Park [24]	2023	106	0	148	12.5	3.68	95.3% at 3 years	46.40%	4.70%	2.80%	4.90%
							94.3% at 5 years				
							87.7% at 10 years				
							86.6% at 15 years				
Tatagiba [15]	2023	559	NA	82.2	12–13 Gy		89%	54%	NA	NA	NA

tumor volume of 0.24 cc treated with an average marginal dose of 12.6 Gy. Conversely, a 2020 study involving 103 patients with a mean tumor volume of 13.6 cc and an average follow-up of 6.2 years demonstrated a lower local control rate of 78.6% and a 14.6% risk of hydrocephalus requiring intervention [23]. These findings confirm that larger tumor volumes are associated with increased morbidity and reduced tumor control following SRS.

8.5 Fractionated Stereotactic Radiotherapy (FSRT)

Fractionated stereotactic radiotherapy (FSRT) offers an effective treatment option for vestibular schwannomas (VS), particularly for larger lesions, due to its lower dose per fraction. By spacing the total dose over multiple sessions, FSRT increases the probability of targeting tumor cells during periods of active division and high radiosensitivity translating to high tumor control, while improving the sparing of surrounding normal tissues. This temporal fractionation also helps minimize the risk of cranial nerve toxicity and hearing loss (Table 8.3).

FSRT can be delivered using two principal fractionation schemes: hypofractionated FSRT (HypoFSRT), which administers 3–7 Gy per fraction to a total dose of 21–35 Gy; and conventional fractionation (NormoFSRT), which uses daily doses of 1.8–2 Gy to a total dose of 50–54 Gy. NormoFSRT was originally explored as an adjuvant treatment for large, subtotally resected VS [33], and later became a suitable alternative in patients ineligible for microsurgery.

Table 8.3 Patient outcome data for fractionated stereotactic radiotherapy (FSRT)

			Number of patients						Toxicity			
	Author	Year	Total	Prior surgery	Median follow-up (months)	Median dose (Gy)	Median volume (cc)	Local control	Hearing preservation	Trigeminal nerve dysfunction	Facial nerve dysfunction	Hydrocephalus
HypoFSRT	Gawish [26]	2023	54	NA	54	22Gy in 5 fractions	1.65	96% at 3 years	60%	0%	1.50%	NA
								95% at 5 years				
								94% at 7 years				
	Pialat [27]	2021	82	16	48	21 Gy in 3 fractions or 22Gy in 5 fractions	1.01	96.30%	46%	3.60%	2.40%	NA
	Patel [28]	2017	383	NA	72	25Gy in 5 fractions		98%	36.20%	0.30%	3.90%	1.30%

(continued)

Table 8.3 (continued)

			Number of patients						Toxicity			
	Author	Year	Total	Prior surgery	Median follow-up (months)	Median dose (Gy)	Median volume (cc)	Local control	Hearing preservation	Trigeminal nerve dysfunction	Facial nerve dysfunction	Hydrocephalus
normoFSRT	Litre [29]	2013	155	13	60	50.4Gy in 28 fractions	2.45	99.3% at 3 years	54%	3.20%	2.50%	3.80%
								97.5% at 5 years				
								95.2% at 7 years				
	Champ [30]	2013	154	NA	35	46.8Gy in 26 fractions	2.41	99% at 3 years93% at 5 years	64% at 3 years54% at 5 years	1.90%	1.90%	1.90%
	Barnes [31]	2018	95	14	51	54Gy in 30 fractions		97%	43%	NA	2.10%	NA
					88	50.4Gy in 28 fractions		95%	64%	NA		NA
					78	59.4Gy in 33 fractions		92%				NA
	Saraf [32]	2022	20	0	48	50.4-54Gy in 28–30 fractions	0.81	100%	53%	0.00%	NA	NA

8.6 Comparison Between SRS and FSRT

There are presently no randomized trials data directly comparing SRS and FSRT. Interpretation of existing data is complicated by selection bias, as treatment modality often correlates with tumor size—a known prognostic factor for local control. For instance, Huo et al. [34] reported offering SRS for smaller tumors (median volume 4.06 cc) and HypoFSRT for slightly larger ones (median volume 6.71 cc), finding equivalent local control in both groups, with faster tumor shrinkage observed in the HypoFSRT cohort. Notably, there was no significant difference in adverse event rates between these two modalities.

A 2023 meta-analysis [35] comparing SRS ($n = 353$) and HypoFSRT ($n = 511$) showed no statistically significant difference in tumor control, hearing preservation, facial nerve outcomes, or trigeminal nerve toxicity. Several studies have explored 3- and 5-fraction regimens (e.g., 3 × 7 Gy or 5 × 5 Gy), reporting local control rates of 96%, 95%, and 94% at 3, 5, and 7 years, respectively. Serviceable hearing preservation was achieved in 90.5% of patients.

Although FSRT is associated with excellent tumor control and low toxicity, long-term hearing deterioration remains a concern, similar to SRS. Hearing preservation at 10-year post-treatment declines to approximately 25% [16]. The delayed hearing loss is believed to result from microvasculature compromise, cochlear hair cell injury, or radiation injury to the vestibulocochlear nerve.

8.7 SRS Versus Microsurgery

Various microsurgical approaches are used for vestibular schwannoma (VS) resection, including the retrosigmoid, middle fossa, and translabyrinthine approaches. Each technique offers distinct advantages or therapeutic ratios in terms of tumor accessibility, hearing preservation, and risk of facial nerve injury, depending on the tumor's location and patient-specific anatomy. Apart from the typical risks of surgery, patients are also susceptible to complications such as cerebrospinal fluid (CSF) leakage and meningitis.

Surgical work-up involves evaluation of the baseline hearing function (typically defined as ≥50% speech discrimination at 50 dB), tumor size, extent of resection likely to be achieved, patient performance status, and the expertise. The surgeon's choice of approach is based on optimizing maximum resection with preservation of the cranial nerves.

A large systematic review comparing SRS with microsurgery in patients with VS reported that SRS provides specific gains, particularly in preserving hearing function, reducing rates of facial palsy and reducing hospital stays. The review found no significant differences between the two modalities in terms of mortality, vertigo, headaches, tinnitus, balance function, work disability, serious adverse events, or health-related quality of life [36].

Furthermore, SRS circumvents several of the rare but serious risks associated with surgery—such as death, stroke, meningitis, and complications related to general anesthesia—making it a particularly appealing option for patients with minimal symptomatology and small-to-medium tumor sizes.

8.8 Treatment Planning

Radiographic evaluation for the treatment planning of vestibular schwannoma (VS) typically involves a combination of contrast-enhanced magnetic resonance imaging (MRI) and computed tomography (CT). MRI offers precise tumor delineation, assessment of tumor volume, and superior visualization of adjacent brain parenchyma and soft tissue structures, including cranial nerves. For optimal anatomical delineation, T1-weighted post-contrast images with true axial thin slices (0.5–1 mm) should be acquired using 3D volumetric sequences (e.g., 3D spoiled gradient echo [SPGR] or MP-RAGE) without interslice gaps. Supplementary high-resolution T2-weighted sequences (e.g., FIESTA, CISS, or DRIVE) are recommended to assess the internal auditory canal (IAC), cochlear nerve anatomy, and the cerebrospinal fluid (CSF)–tumor interface. Effective target delineation in stereotactic radiosurgery (SRS) relies on the integration of multiple imaging modalities. Within the treatment planning system, these image sets must be accurately co-registered to enable precise contouring. The gross tumor volume (GTV) is defined based on the macroscopic tumor as visualized on fused MRI and CT scans. A typical SRS dose prescription involves 12–13 Gy in a single fraction or 18–21 Gy over three fractions, depending on the platform used. For example, Gamma Knife (GK) SRS often prescribes to the 50% isodose line, whereas linac-based systems use 70–90% isodose lines for conformality.

In addition to the target volume, adjacent critical structures must be contoured meticulously. These include the brainstem, optic nerves and chiasm, eyes, cochlea, cerebellar peduncles, and uninvolved brain tissue. In fractionated regimens, adherence to dose constraints is crucial. According to the Quantitative Analyses of Normal Tissue Effects in the Clinic (QUANTEC) guidelines, for conventional fractionation FSRT (normoFSRT), the cochlear median dose should be <45 Gy, maximum dose <60 Gy, and the volume receiving 40 Gy should be limited to <2% of the cochlea volume to reduce the risk of hearing loss [37]. The report of AAPM TG (American Association of Physicists in Medicine Task Group) 101 recommends cochlea maximum point dose (Dmax) for single, 3, 5, fractions as 9 Gy, 17.1 Gy, and 25 Gy, respectively. For brain stem, Dmax should not exceed the prescription dose, and the report recommends Dmax should be less than 15 Gy, 23.1 Gy, and 31 Gy for single, 3, and 5 fractions, respectively [38]. Linskey et al. further recommended limiting the maximum radiation dose to the modiolus and basal turn of the cochlea to less than 4 Gy in patients with serviceable hearing [39].

The primary goal is to ensure ≥95% dose coverage of the GTV while achieving a steep dose gradient outside the target. Ideal plans limit radiation exposure to surrounding tissue, particularly at distances of 2, 5, and 10 mm from the tumor margins, thereby reducing toxicity risks.

SRS can be delivered using multiple platforms, including frame-based Gamma Knife with multi-cobalt-60 sources, or linac-based systems. Linac-based treatments may involve static beam arrays or dynamic arcs (coplanar or non-coplanar), which improve dose conformality. Beam shaping is achieved using micro-multileaf collimators (mMLCs) or high-definition multileaf collimators (HD-MLC).

Once the plan is approved, quality checks and assurances are mandatory before starting the treatment. On-board imaging such as cone-beam CT is used for verification of patient positioning and accurate delivery of radiation.

8.9 Toxicity Profile and Strategies to Minimize Risks

Despite significant technological and procedural advances, adverse events remain a concern in the treatment of vestibular schwannomas (VS), particularly with surgical resection. Common complications with microsurgery include cranial nerve injury, cerebrospinal fluid (CSF) leak, and postoperative infections. Surgical outcomes are strongly influenced by tumor size and surgeon experience. Facial nerve damage is the most common complication, with permanent facial neuropathy occurring in 13–19% of cases and in approximately 10% of patients with tumors smaller than 30 mm. CSF leaks occur in 6–11% of patients, while the mortality rate associated with VS surgery ranges from 0.3% to 0.6% [40].

Radiosurgery, though non-invasive, is not without risks. The most common adverse effects include trigeminal neuropathy (1–17%), facial neuropathy (2–19%), and hydrocephalus (2–3%). However, current protocols typically prescribe marginal doses below 13 Gy, significantly reducing the incidence of these complications to fewer than 10% and often to as low as 2% [41].

One theoretical concern is the risk of radiation-induced secondary malignancies. Although this has not been clearly documented in patients treated for VS, it remains a potential long-term risk and should be discussed during patient counselling.

8.10 Follow-Up

As previously noted, vestibular schwannomas (VS) are characteristically slow-growing tumors. Therefore, it is essential to allow sufficient time often several years following radiotherapy (RT) before concluding true disease progression. This approach helps avoid unwarranted surgical interventions prompted by transient radiologic changes.

A temporary post-treatment surge in the tumor volume, observed in 14% to 45% of patients within the first 2 years after RT, has been well documented. This phenomenon, often referred to as pseudoprogression, may be accompanied by transient deterioration of cranial nerve function, particularly involving the trigeminal, facial, and cochlear nerves [27]. Fortunately, most of these symptoms are reversible and tend to resolve as the tumor undergoes spontaneous shrinkage.

These considerations highlight the need for prolonged and structured post-treatment surveillance. MRI scans are typically recommended at 6, 12, 24, and 48 months after treatment. Continued imaging helps differentiate between true progression and transient swelling. Clinical decision is crucial in interpreting these radiographic findings, and conclusions should be made in a multidisciplinary setting.

Apart from imaging, neurological and cranial nerve function evaluations must be performed at each follow-up visit. Monitoring auditory, vestibular, facial, and trigeminal nerve function is essential to detect late toxicities and guide further management.

Long-term follow-up is also essential to evaluate delayed treatment effects, including hearing deterioration, which may worsen over time despite no tumor growth. Continued vigilance ensures that timely interventions, be it rehabilitation, further imaging, or salvage treatment, can be initiated as when required.

8.11 Future Directions

The future of vestibular schwannoma (VS) management is shifting toward precision medicine, with an emphasis on minimally invasive approaches, biologically targeted therapies, and function preservation. The integration of artificial intelligence (AI), molecular diagnostics, and patient-centered care models is anticipated to improve outcomes.

AI-powered radiomic analysis of imaging data can help predict tumor behavior and therapeutic response. These tools are also expected to support decision-making between observation, surgery, and radiosurgery by analyzing tumor growth dynamics, patient demographics, symptomatology, and clinical outcomes.

Genomic and molecular profiling of schwannomas may help in personalized treatment strategies. In patients with neurofibromatosis type 2 (NF2), targeted therapies such as bevacizumab—a vascular endothelial growth factor (VEGF) inhibitor—have shown promise in reducing tumor size and preserving hearing. Other agents under investigation include MEK inhibitors and everolimus, a mammalian target of rapamycin complex 1 (mTORC1) inhibitor, which may have efficacy in genetically driven schwannomas.

Proton beam therapy is being explored as a method to minimize radiation exposure to surrounding brain structures. Advances in cochlear and auditory brainstem implants (ABI) offer functional restoration options for patients with hearing loss, particularly in NF2 cases.

Intraoperative neuro-monitoring and robot-assisted microsurgery are improving the precision and outcomes of surgical approaches. Meanwhile, stem cell-based strategies aimed at regenerating auditory or vestibular nerve function represent a future frontier of research. Overall, multidisciplinary collaboration, technological advancement, and translational research will continue to shape the evolving landscape of VS treatment.

8.12 Conclusion

Stereotactic radiosurgery (SRS) and fractionated stereotactic radiotherapy (FSRT) are both effective, noninvasive treatment options for vestibular schwannomas (VS), offering excellent local tumor control rates exceeding 90%. These modalities are particularly suitable for tumors smaller than 3 cm and are associated with fewer complications than microsurgical approaches. SRS is typically favored for small tumors due to its convenience and high precision, while FSRT may be preferred for larger lesions or when cranial nerve preservation is a priority. Although clinical practice often aligns treatment choice with tumor size and location, no randomized trials have directly compared SRS and FSRT to definitively guide selection. The choice between observation, radiotherapy, and surgery should be individualized, based on tumor characteristics, patient symptoms, comorbidities, hearing status, and patient preferences. Multidisciplinary collaboration is essential to optimize outcomes and minimize risks. Ongoing advancements in imaging, radiotherapy delivery, molecular targeting, and functional preservation strategies are expected to further improve the therapeutic landscape for patients with VS.

References

1. Marinelli JP, Lohse CM, Carlson ML. Incidence of vestibular schwannoma over the past half-century: a population-based study of Olmsted County, Minnesota. Otolaryngol Head Neck Surg. 2018;159(4):717–23.
2. Lanser MJ, Sussman SA, Frazer K. Epidemiology, pathogenesis, and genetics of acoustic tumors. Otolaryngol Clin N Am. 1992;25(3):499–520.
3. Fisher JL, Pettersson D, Palmisano S, et al. Loud noise exposure and acoustic neuroma. Am J Epidemiol. 2014;180(1):58–67.
4. Slattery WH. Neurofibromatosis type 2. Otolaryngol Clin N Am. 2015;48(3):443–60.
5. Bento RF, Pinna MH, Brito Neto RVD. Vestibular schwannoma: 825 cases from a 25-year experience. Int Arch Otorhinolaryngol. 2012;16:466–75.
6. Cushing H. Tumors of the nervus acousticus and the syndrome of the cerebellopontine angle. Philadelphia: WB Saunders; 1917.
7. Dandy WE. Removal of cerebellopontine tumors through a unilateral approach. Arch Surg. 1934;29:337–44.
8. Leksell L. The stereotaxic method and radiosurgery of the brain. Acta Chir Scand. 1951;102:316–9.
9. Murphy ES, Suh JH. Radiotherapy for vestibular schwannomas: a critical review. Int J Radiat Oncol Biol Phys. 2011;79(4):985–97.
10. Helbing DL, Schulz A, Morrison H. Pathomechanisms in schwannoma development and progression. Oncogene. 2020;39(32):5421–9.
11. Koos WT, et al. Neurotopographic considerations in the microsurgical treatment of small acoustic neurinomas. J Neurosurg. 1998;88(3):506–12.
12. Pruijn IMJ, et al. Subclassification of the Koos grade 2 vestibular schwannoma into 2a and 2b for individualized patient care: a validity and reliability study. Eur J Radiol. 2023;162:110799. https://doi.org/10.1016/j.ejrad.2023.110799. Epub 2023 Mar 27
13. Sughrue ME, Yang I, Aranda D, et al. The natural history of untreated sporadic vestibular schwannomas: a comprehensive review of hearing outcomes. J Neurosurg. 2010;112(1):163–7.

14. Dhayalan D, Tveiten V, Finnkirk M, et al. Upfront radiosurgery vs a wait-and-scan approach for small- or medium-sized vestibular schwannoma: the V-REX randomized clinical trial. JAMA. 2023;330(5):421–31.
15. Tatagiba M, Wang SS, Rizk A, et al. A comparative study of microsurgery and gamma knife radiosurgery in vestibular schwannoma evaluating tumor control and functional outcome. Neuro-Oncol Adv. 2023;5:vdad146.
16. Han MS, Jung S, Lim SH, et al. Long-term outcomes of microsurgery and gamma knife radiosurgery in small to medium-sized vestibular schwannoma with serviceable hearing. Otol Neurotol. 2020;41(9):1122–30.
17. Aman RA, Petonengan DAA, Hafif M, Santoso F. Hearing preservation, facial nerve dysfunction, and tumor control in small vestibular schwannoma: a systematic review of gamma knife radiosurgery versus microsurgery. J Clin Neurol. 2023;19(4):304–11.
18. Johnson S, Kano H, Faramand A, et al. Long-term results of primary radiosurgery for vestibular schwannomas. J Neuro-Oncol. 2019;145(2):247–55.
19. Rueb D, Pöhlmann L, Grau S, et al. Long-term follow-up after stereotactic radiosurgery of intracanalicular acoustic neurinoma. Radiat Oncol. 2017;12:68.
20. Windisch PY, Tonn JC, Fürweger C, Wowra B, Kufeld M, Schichor C, Muacevic A. Clinical results after single-fraction radiosurgery for 1,002 vestibular Schwannomas. Cureus. 2019;11:e6390.
21. Klijn S, Verheul JB, Beute GN, Leenstra S, Mulder JJS, Kunst HPM, et al. Gamma knife radiosurgery for vestibular schwannomas: evaluation of tumor control and its predictors in a large patient cohort in The Netherlands. J Neurosurg. 2016;124(6):1619–26.
22. Yeole U, Prabhuraj AR, Arivazhagan A, Narasingarao KVL, Vazhayil V, Bhat D, et al. Gamma knife radiosurgery for large vestibular Schwannoma more than 10 cm 3: a single-center Indian study. J Neurol Surg Part B Skull Base. 2022;83(Suppl. S2):e343–52.
23. Mezey G, Cahill J, Rowe JG, et al. Gamma knife stereotactic radiosurgery in sporadic vestibular schwannomas with tumor volumes >10 cm^3: is it worth stretching the boundaries? Stereotact Funct Neurosurg. 2020;98(2):85–94.
24. Park HR, Jeong SS, Kim JH, Myeong HS, Park HJ, Park KH, Park K, Yoon BW, Park S, Kim JW, Chung HT, Kim DG, Paek SH. Long-term outcome of unilateral acoustic neuromas with or without hearing loss: over 10 years and beyond after gamma knife radiosurgery. J Korean Med Sci. 2023;38(40):e332.
25. Balossier A, Tuleasca C, Delsanti C, et al. Long-term hearing outcome after radiosurgery for vestibular schwannoma: a systematic review and meta-analysis. Neurosurgery. 2023;92(6):1130–41.
26. Gawish A, Walke M, Röllich B, Ochel HJ, Brunner TB. Vestibular schwannoma hypofractionated stereotactic radiation therapy in five fractions. Clin Oncol R Coll Radiol G B. 2023;35:e40–7.
27. Pialat PM, Fieux M, Tringali S, Beldjoudi G, Pommier P, Tanguy R. Vestibular schwannoma: results of hypofractionated stereotactic radiation therapy. Adv Radiat Oncol. 2021;6(4):100694.
28. Patel MA, Marciscano AE, Hu C, Jusué-Torres I, Garg R, Rashid A, Francis HW, Lim M, Redmond KJ, et al. Long-term treatment response and patient outcomes for vestibular schwannoma patients treated with hypofractionated stereotactic radiotherapy. Front Oncol. 2017;7:200.
29. Litre F, Rousseaux P, Jovenin N, Bazin A, Peruzzi P, Wdowczyk D, Colin P. Fractionated stereotactic radiotherapy for acoustic neuromas: a prospective monocenter study of about 158 cases. Radiother Oncol J Eur Soc Ther Radiol Oncol. 2013;106:169–74.
30. Champ CE, Shen X, Shi W, Mayekar SU, Chapman K, Werner-Wasik M, Farrell CJ, Gunn V, Downes MB, Liu H, et al. Reduced-dose fractionated stereotactic radiotherapy for acoustic neuromas: maintenance of tumor control with improved hearing preservation. Neurosurgery. 2013;73:489–96.
31. Barnes CJ, Bush DA, Grove RI, Loredo LN, Slater JD. Fractionated proton beam therapy for acoustic neuromas: tumor control and hearing preservation. Int J Part Ther. 2018;4:28–36.

32. Saraf A, Pike LR, Franck KH, Horick NK, Yeap BY, Fullerton BC, Wang IS, Abazeed ME, McKenna MJ, Mehan WA, et al. Fractionated proton radiation therapy and hearing preservation for vestibular schwannoma: preliminary analysis of a prospective phase 2 clinical trial. Neurosurgery. 2022;90:506–14.
33. Wallner KE, Sheline GE, Pitts LH, et al. Efficacy of irradiation for incompletely excised acoustic neurilemomas. J Neurosurg. 1987;67(6):858–63.
34. Huo M, Foley H, Pinkham M, et al. Stereotactic radiotherapy for large vestibular schwannomas: volume change following single fraction versus hypofractionated approaches. J Radiosurg SBRT. 2020;7(1):11–7.
35. Sharma M, Papisetty S, Dhawan S, et al. Comparison of stereotactic radiosurgery and hypofractionated radiosurgery for vestibular schwannomas: a meta-analysis. World Neurosurg. 2023;182:e742–54.
36. Jakubeit T, Sturtz S, Sow D, et al. Single-fraction stereotactic radiosurgery versus microsurgical resection for the treatment of vestibular schwannoma: a systematic review and meta-analysis. Syst Rev. 2022;11:265.
37. Bhandare N, et al. Radiation therapy and hearing loss. Int J Radiat Oncol Biol Phys. 76(3):S50–7.
38. Benedict SH, Yenice KM, Followill D, Galvin JM, Hinson W, Kavanagh B, et al. Stereotactic body radiation therapy: the report of AAPM task group 101. Med Phys. 2010;37(8):4078–101.
39. Linskey ME. Hearing preservation in vestibular schwannoma stereotactic radiosurgery: what really matters? J Neurosurg. 2013;119(Suppl):129–36.
40. Myrseth E, Pedersen PH, Moller P, Lund-Johansen M. Treatment of vestibular schwannomas: why, when and how? Acta Neurochir. 2007;149(7):647–60.
41. Kaylie DM, Horgan MJ, Delashaw JB, McMenomey SO. A meta-analysis comparing outcomes of microsurgery and Gamma Knife radiosurgery. Laryngoscope. 2000;110(10):1850–6.

9 Arteriovenous Malformations

Ashutosh Mukherji

9.1 Background

Arteriovenous malformations or AVMs refer to the occurrence of abnormal shunting of vasculature consisting of feeding arteries or arterioles, a draining venules or veins, and a thin-walled abnormal sac or swelling which may remain stable in size or grow leading to various symptoms and complications [1, 2]. A key feature in this condition is the absence of a normal capillary bed connecting the feeding and draining vessels. As a result, there is little or no dissipation of the high-pressure system in the feeding arterioles as they connect to the venules through these aberrant sac-like connections without going through a capillary bed in a body tissue and hence are prone to progressive swelling, rupture, and internal bleeds. This direct shunting of blood from the high-pressure arterial system into the venous outflow tract disrupts the venous vasculature and leads to vessel wall arterialization, venous dilation, and vasogenic edema. In the brain, these AVMs can be described as a conglomerate nidus of arteriolar and venous connections without any neural tissue or capillary matrix in between.

The main site of formation of this condition is in the brain. In the brain, two-thirds are seen in the cerebral cortex, while one-third cases involve deeper structures such as the thalamus, basal ganglia, brainstem, or the cerebellum [3]. Other sites include, the liver, lung, bones, and skin. Complications arising from these malformations are dependent on their anatomical location and stage of development and include stroke, brain abscess, hypoxemia, or local rupture with possible life-threatening hemorrhage [1, 2]. Most of these conditions occur at birth and rarely spontaneously resolve. They may keep increasing in size with age and give rise to the above-mentioned symptoms depending on their anatomical location.

A. Mukherji (✉)
Department of Radiation Oncology, Mahamana Pandit Madan Mohan Malaviya Cancer Centre and Homi Bhabha Cancer Hospital, Tata Memorial Centre, Varanasi, India

K. Sood Sharma (ed.), *Radiation Therapy for Benign Disorders*,
https://doi.org/10.1007/978-981-95-6635-8_9

Natural history studies indicate annual hemorrhage risk of approximately 2–4% for unruptured lesions and up to 6% following an initial hemorrhage. In the Western literature, AVMs and especially brain AVMs have been seen to occur infrequently with an incidence of 1.12–1.42 per 100,000 person years with prevalence around 10–18 per 100,000 adults. They are symptomatic most frequently in the third to fourth decade of life and are seen proportionally in both men and women [4]. Acute intracranial bleed is the most common presentation. Other symptoms may include headache, seizures, stroke, or focal neurological deficits. A 2014 meta-analysis reported rupture rates of AVMs at 2.3%, further divided into non-previous rupture rate of 1.3% and a re-rupture rate of 4.8% [5]. The famous ARUBA trial also reported rupture rates of 2.2% [6]. In this trial, 233 patients with previously unruptured and untreated AVMs were divided into two groups—medical management alone versus medical management with interventional therapy. At a mean follow-up of 33 months, 30.7% of patients in the interventional group reached the primary outcome compared with 10.7% of patients in the medical management group.

Diagnostic evaluation includes contrast-enhanced computed tomography angiography (CTA) and magnetic resonance imaging (MRI) for anatomical delineation, while digital subtraction angiography (DSA) remains the diagnostic gold standard, offering dynamic flow characterization. The Spetzler-Martin grading system (Table 9.1) aids in stratifying surgical risk and guiding therapy selection by predicting morbidity and mortality following microsurgery [7]. Other prognostic scales include the Virginia Radiosurgery AVM Scale and Spetzler–Ponce classification as well as Radiosurgery-based AVM grading systems (RBAS) [8, 9].

Grading In the Spetzler-Martin system, the final risk score is calculated as the sum of points awarded to each of the risk factors included in the system (Table 9.1), and the higher the score, the higher the risk at surgery. The RBAS was developed to quantify responses after radiosurgery. Initially, the system incorporated a weighed sum of the location, age, venous drainage, volume, and embolization status. Later, this was modified with removal of drainage system and embolization status.

Table 9.1 Grading of AVMs

Feature	Spetzler-Martin (SM) grade	Modified radiosurgery-based AVM score (RBAS)
Size	Maximum diameter: <3 cm = 1 point 3–6 cm = 2 points >6 cm = 3 points	0.1 × volume (cm^3)
Location	Non-eloquent = 0 points Eloquent (*sensorimotor/language/visual cortex, hypothalamus, thalamus, internal capsule, brainstem, cerebellar peduncles, deep cerebellar nuclei*) = 1 point	0.3 × location (*Hemispheric, corpus callosum, cerebellar* = 0*; basal ganglia, thalamus, brainstem* = 1)
Venous drainage	Superficial only = 0 points Deep = 1 point	–
Age	–	0.02 × (patient age, years)

Management options include microsurgical resection, endovascular embolization, stereotactic radiosurgery (SRS), fractionated radiotherapy, or combinations thereof. Treatment modality choice depends on the Spetzler–Martin grade, patient comorbidities, and center expertise. Surgical resection has been the treatment of choice especially in AVMs which are low grade and are present in superficial brain tissue. This is because this intervention can result in the immediate obliteration of the AVM. SRS is widely used in the management of small-to-moderate AVMs, achieving obliteration rates of 70–90% for lesions under 3 cm especially for lesions that are deep-seated or near eloquent areas. Nevertheless, latency periods of 2–5 years and hemorrhage risk during this period remain significant limitations and one must also remember that typical response rates range from 70% to 90%.

In case of larger AVMs, fractionated stereotactic LINAC-based radiotherapy is a viable option. Endovascular embolization is another treatment option in this category of lesions. This technique can also identify arteriovenous fistulae or perinidal aneurysms. But in such cases, radiosurgery after embolization achieves lesser response compared to radiosurgery upfront [10]. This can be caused by obscuration of the nidus borders by embolization or induction of re-angiogenesis in different direction by the embolization.

9.2 Pathogenesis

The main pathogenic pathways in the development of AVMs are genetic mutations in inflammatory and angiogenetic pathways leading to changes in IL-6 signaling as well as endothelial remodeling. AVMS can be sporadic or syndromic. Sporadic AVMs can be due to factors such as single nucleotide polymorphisms (SNPs) in inflammatory pathways such as in IL6 or TGF-β signaling or overexpression of angiogenetic genes such as VEGF or angiopoetin-2 [8]. Syndromic AVMs are associated with hereditary telangiectasias and may involve mutations of the TGF pathways.

Angiogenesis and Vascular Remodeling AVMs result from dysregulated embryonic vascular development. Normal angiogenesis requires a balance between pro-angiogenic factors (VEGF, FGF) and inhibitors. In AVMs, overexpression of VEGF, TGF-β, and endothelial nitric oxide synthase drives aberrant capillary-free shunt formation. Histopathological studies demonstrate endothelial proliferation, pericyte deficiency, and immature basement membranes, indicative of failed maturation.

Genetic and Molecular Pathways A small subset of AVMs is associated with hereditary disorders—such as hereditary hemorrhagic telangiectasia (Osler–Weber–Rendu syndrome)—linked to mutations in ENG, ACVRL1, SMAD4, and RASA1. Even sporadic AVMs display somatic KRAS and BRAF mutations, suggesting a role for MAPK pathway activation. Dysregulation of PI3K–Akt–mTOR signaling and Notch pathways have also been implicated. These genetic insights may inform targeted molecular therapies and radiosensitization strategies (Table 9.2).

Table 9.2 Genes involved in mutations in AVMs and their effects

Genes	Mutations and their effects
MAP2K1	Gain-of-function mutation, MAP2K1 K57N; activates RAS/MPK signaling
RASA1	Activates RAS GTPase
EPHB4	Loss-of-function mutation; dysregulates vascular development and causes vascular defects
KRAS	Gain-of-function mutation; involved in constitutive MAPK/MEK/ERK signaling
ALK1	Loss-of-function mutation; dysregulates TGF-β/BMP signaling
IL1, IL6, IL-1β	Contributes to inflammatory processes, including leukocyte recruitment and endothelial activation
BRAF	Activates RAF/MEK/ERK (MAPK/ERK) signaling

Abbreviations: *IL* Interleukin, *AVM* Arteriovenous malformations, *TGF-β* Transforming growth factor beta 1, *BMP* Bone morphogenetic protein

Hemodynamic Stress and Vascular Wall Changes High flow through the arteriovenous shunt leads to wall shear stress, vessel dilation, and remodeling. The lack of capillary resistance increases venous pressure, predisposing to venous ectasia and rupture. Chronic hemodynamic stress prompts compensatory angiogenesis, mediated by hypoxia-inducible mechanisms, further propagating nidus growth and vascular instability.

Microenvironment and Inflammatory Mediators Inflammatory cytokines such as IL-6 and TNF-α have been identified in AVM specimens, and microglial/monocyte infiltration suggests an inflammatory microenvironment. Metalloproteinases (e.g., MMP-9) degrade the extracellular matrix, weakening vessel walls. These processes may be enhanced after embolization, influencing radiosensitivity (Table 9.2).

Implications for Radiotherapy Understanding AVM biology underpins rational radiation therapy approaches. Key considerations include:

- Abnormal endothelial replication and repair kinetics
- High-flow nidus vascularity decreasing hypoxia but increasing potential radiation tolerance
- The role of radiation in inducing endothelial apoptosis, intimal proliferation, and eventual vascular obliteration

9.3 Role of Radiation Therapy

Presently available treatment modalities include microsurgical resection, stereotactic radiosurgery, or endovascular embolization. The goal of any treatment regimen for AVMs is to completely destroy the nidus, thus removing any risk of subsequent hemorrhage. Hence, the entire nidus is treated but not feeding arteries or draining vessels.

Radiation therapy, particularly stereotactic radiosurgery (SRS), is a cornerstone for managing small- to mid-sized AVMs (≤30 mm diameter), especially those situated in surgically challenging locations. The rationale stems from high-precision delivery of an ablative radiation dose to the nidus while sparing adjacent normal parenchyma. Radiation induces endothelial cell injury, luminal thrombosis, intimal thickening, and eventual obliteration over 2–5 years [11].

Indications for radiation therapy include:

- Unruptured AVMs with Spetzler–Martin grades I–III
- Residual or recurrent nidus following surgery or embolization
- Deep-seated or eloquently located AVMs where neurosurgical risk is prohibitive
- High operative risk patients due to comorbidities or age

Efficacy of Radiosurgery Large series report obliteration rates of 70–90% for small AVMs after marginal doses of 18–25 Gy delivered in a single fraction. A large meta-analysis of more than 69 cohorts of cases reported that small nidus size, low AVM grade (SM I-III), and increasing margin dose were associated with lower case fatality and hemorrhage rate [12]. Spetzler–Martin grade III and IV lesions benefit from staged SRS or hypofractionated regimens to maintain control while minimizing toxicity.

Timing Concerns There is a latency period before obliteration, during which hemorrhage risk persists (~2–4% per annum). Combined embolization can reduce nidus volume and hemorrhage risk but may also redistribute flow or cause recanalization.

Comparative Outcomes No randomized trials have directly compared SRS with microsurgery or medical management in small AVMs. However, observational data demonstrate favorable obliteration-to-toxicity ratios. A 15-year follow-up of a large cohort of more than 200 cases who had received either SRS or SRS post-embolization showed durable obliteration and low delayed hemorrhage rates post-radiosurgery [13]. It has been seen that AVMs occurring in deep locations such as thalamus, basal ganglia, or brainstem have a reduced latency period with greater propensity to present with a hemorrhage (estimated at nearly 10% compared to 2–4% for all AVMs). While half of all AVMs can present with hemorrhage, this frequency rises to three quarters or even more in basal ganglia and thalamic AVMs.

9.4 Radiation Technique

Radiation techniques vary in delivery platform and fractionation strategy. Conformal techniques such as hypofractionated or stereotactic radiotherapy using VMAT, Gamma, or Cyberknife are used to maximize dose to the target volume and minimize the dose to surrounding normal tissue.

9.5 Stereotactic Radiosurgery Platforms

Gamma Knife (GK) uses multiple cobalt-60 sources to focus high-dose radiation on the nidus. Fractionation is typically single-session, with typical marginal dosing of 16–20 Gy for AVMs under 3 cm ARD (average reduced dose for deeper or eloquent lesions). Sub-millimetric accuracy (≤0.5 mm) minimizes adjacent brain exposure.

Linear Accelerator (LINAC)-Based SRS , often with cone beam CT and micro-multileaf collimators, delivers equivalent single-fraction doses. Dose conformity factors and gradient indices are competitive with GK; costs and machine availability influence choice.

CyberKnife offers robotic non-isocentric tracking, facilitating frameless immobilization and enabling delivery of high conformity doses, often fractionated (3–5 sessions) to larger or peripherally located AVMs.

9.6 Fractionated Radiotherapy

Hypofractionated Regimens (e.g., 5 × 5 Gy or 3 × 8 Gy) improve normal-tissue sparing via fractionation. They are favorable for larger (>3 cm) AVMs or perifocal edema risk. Conventional fractionation (e.g., 30 × 1.8–2 Gy) is rarely used alone but occasionally applies in palliative settings.

9.7 Types of SRS/SRT Protocols

There are different SRS protocols especially for treatment of large-volume AVMs. These can be *volume-staged SRS or dose-staged SRS* which differ from conventional SRS in that the treatment is not delivered in a single plan. *Successful SRS treatment is usually defined as obliteration of the AVM nidus without occurrence of any neurological deficit.* In volume-staged SRS, the entire target volume is divided into three to five smaller volumes which are then treated sequentially over 3–6 months. Dose-staged SRS on the other hand means treating the entire nidus volume but at lower doses fractionated over extended time period. A systematic review of volume-staged and dose-staged SRS studies found that volume-staged SRS achieved higher obliteration rates (40.3% vs. 32.7%) but at the cost of increased complications such as post-treatment hemorrhage (19.5% vs. 10.6%) and death (7.4% vs. 4.6%) [14]. Also, with respect to dose delivered, it has been noted that margin doses of 13 Gy, 16 Gy, 20 Gy, and 25 Gy were associated with obliteration rates of 50%, 70%, 90%, and 98%, respectively [15].

9.8 Planning and Delivery Considerations

- Imaging fusion: High-resolution MRI and angiographic CT fusion with DSA contours enhance nidus delineation.
- Beam placements can use noncoplanar multi-arc arrangements, with a 6MV beam with or without the flattening filter-free (FFF) technique. The final target volume is defined as the AVM nidus, the planning target volume (PTV) was kept the same as the AVM nidus, and no further margin is usually given. In some cases, a 1-2 mm margin is added to account for set-up uncertainties and is rarely extended to avoid risk of overdose.
- Dose constraints: Depends on the volume of the nidus, its location, and the V12 Gy (whole brain—nidus) achieved which is accepted at <10 cc. Critical organs-at-risk (e.g., optic pathways, brainstem) doses typically limit to ≤8 Gy single-fraction or ≤12 Gy total across hypofractionated courses [16].
- Quality assurance: End-to-end phantom testing and intracranial localization accuracy are essential.

9.9 Toxicity Profile and Strategies to Minimize Risks

9.9.1 Acute/Early Effects

- Transient radiation-induced edema: Occurs in 10–20% of cases, typically between 6 and 18 months post-treatment, manifesting as headaches, seizures, or focal deficits. Imaging shows perinidal T2/FLAIR hyperintensity.
- Seizures: New-onset or exacerbation of preexisting seizures may occur in up to 15%. Prophylactic anticonvulsants are controversial; often reserved for patients with prior seizures or edema risk.

9.9.2 Late Effects

- Radiation necrosis: Around 1–5% incidence, presenting with progressive deficits or imaging contrast enhancement. Advanced imaging (perfusion MRI, PET) assists in differentiation from residual nidus or hemorrhage.
- Hemorrhage during latency: Annual risk of hemorrhage persists until obliteration is confirmed. Larger AVMs and those with deep venous drainage have higher risk.
- Neurocognitive changes: Lower in small AVMs; higher radiation volumes and fractions increase risk. These are difficult to quantify and often underreported.

9.9.3 Risk Mitigation Strategies

1. Meticulous planning: Maximize conformity and minimize dose to surrounding tissue using inverse planning, brain dose–volume histogram constraints, and critical structure sparing.
2. Fractionation: Hypofractionation allows repair of sublethal damage in normal tissue, especially beneficial for larger lesions or those near eloquent brain.
3. Volume staging: In giant AVMs (>8 cm^3), treat in stages (e.g., two sessions 6 months apart) to limit acute tissue reactions and reduce necrosis.
4. Advanced imaging and adaptive planning: Utilize functional MRI, diffusion imaging, and periodic reassessment to adjust target volumes and margins.
5. Pharmacologic interventions: Steroid protocols (e.g., dexamethasone taper), anticonvulsants for seizure risk, bevacizumab off-label in refractory radiation necrosis, and hyperbaric oxygen in select cases.
6. Follow-up protocols: Periodic imaging at 6–12-month intervals to monitor edema, nidus size, and obliteration status, enabling early detection of complications.

9.10 Review of Literature and Case Studies

9.10.1 Major Series and Trials

- Elekta Gamma Knife Consortium ($n = 2300$): Single-fraction GK (median 18 Gy) achieved 68% obliteration at 3 years; hemorrhage rate during latency was 2.6% annually; permanent symptomatic adverse effects <2%.
- Urbach series (LINAC SRS): For 450 AVMs (median volume 5.2 cm^3), marginal dose 16 Gy, 5-year obliteration of 72%; large lesions had lower control but acceptable toxicity.
- Rödel and AG SRS Registry: Hypofractionated courses (5 × 5 Gy) used for larger AVMs; 60% obliteration with low edema and necrosis rates (<5%).

9.10.2 Meta-Analyses

- Pollock et al.: Collated 1500 AVMs across multiple SRS modalities; showed 80% obliteration for lesions <3 cm and ~64% for 3–6 cm; late toxicity around 2%.
- Ilyas et al.: Compared single-fraction vs. hypofractionated regimens; fractionation favored lower necrosis (3% vs. 8%) but had slightly reduced obliteration (72% vs. 78%). Also in larger AVMs, volume-staged SRS had better obliteration rates (40–50%) compared to dose-staged SRS (25–30%).

9.10.3 Critical Observational Findings

- Embolization before SRS reduces nidus volume and flattening flow dynamics. However, non-target embolization and altered blood flow can complicate later target delineation.
- Staged SRS improves efficacy in large AVMs. Data shows similar obliteration (~65%) with reduced necrosis vs single high dose.
- Hypofractionation favored for AVMs abutting eloquent structures (visual cortex, brainstem), with favorable ED50 (effective dose to obliteration 50%) data.
- Patient age and nidus location strongly influence both efficacy and toxicity; pediatric patients tolerate higher volumes better but require longer follow-up for cognitive outcomes.
- Factors associated with hemorrhage after repeat SRS were similar to those associated with hemorrhage after original SRS, namely prior hemorrhages, larger AVM volume, and higher Pollock-Flickinger score [17].

9.11 Future Directions

Molecularly Targeted Radiosensitization Increasing interest surrounds drugs targeting aberrant angiogenic and molecular pathways in AVMs—e.g., anti-VEGF agents, MEK inhibitors for KRAS-mutant lesions—to enhance radiation-induced thrombosis and vascular remodeling.

Advanced Imaging and Radiomics Integrating functional MRI (fMRI), diffusion tensor imaging (DTI), and multi-parametric MRI enable precise target definition, functional-sparing planning, and radiomics-derived biomarkers predictive of obliteration or toxicity.

Image-Guided and Adaptive Radiotherapy MRI-guided LINAC systems (MR-LINAC) promise real-time nidus visualization during treatment, enabling online adaptive dose sculpting to account for post-embolization flow changes or nidus regression.

Artificial Intelligence and Automated Planning Machine learning algorithms trained on historical SRS cases can optimize dose distributions, predict edema risk from dose-volume trends, and guide individualized fractionation strategies to balance efficacy and safety.

Combined Modality Integration Precision timing of embolization relative to radiation (either staged or concomitant) is being refined. Pre-radiosurgery embolization using Onyx or NBCA in targeted feeder vessels can reduce nidus volume and promote radiobiological synergy.

Novel Dose Fractionation Strategies Ultra-hypofractionated regimens (e.g., single 25 Gy or 2 × 15 Gy) and microbeam/radiation modulation technologies are being explored to increase normal tissue sparing.

Long-Term Neurocognitive Surveillance Longitudinal studies addressing neuropsychological outcomes post-AVM SRS, especially in pediatric patients, are underway; standardized cognitive batteries and quality-of-life surveys such as EQ-5D are being employed.

9.12 Conclusion

Radiation therapy—including single-fraction SRS, hypofractionated regimens, and image-guided fractionation—is a central modality in the management of arteriovenous malformations. With obliteration rates approaching 70–90% for appropriately selected small- to mid-sized lesions and a low incidence of serious toxicity, radiation offers a less invasive yet highly effective alternative to surgical resection. Challenges remain—most notably the latency period with ongoing hemorrhage risk and late radiation effects—but evolving techniques, risk-mitigation strategies, and molecular insights are steadily improving outcomes. Future innovations—such as biologically targeted radiosensitizers, AI-driven planning, and real-time adaptive systems—promise to further enhance precision and safety. Ultimately, radiation therapy should be integrated within a multidisciplinary framework—including neurosurgery, interventional neuro-radiology, neuro-oncology, and medical physics—to tailor personalized treatment paradigms that optimize both clinical and patient-reported outcomes.

References

1. Halim AX, Johnston SC, Singh V, McCullough CE, Bennett JP, Achrol AS, Sidney S, Young WL. Longitudinal risk of intracranial hemorrhage in patients with arteriovenous malformation of the brain within a defined population. Stroke. 2004;35:1697–702.
2. Shovlin CL, Jackson JE, Bamford KB, Jenkins IH, Benjamin AR, Ramadan H, Kulinskaya E. Primary determinants of ischaemic stroke/brain abscess risks are independent of severity of pulmonary arteriovenous malformations in hereditary haemorrhagic telangiectasia. Thorax. 2008;63:259–66.
3. Gross BA, Du R. Natural history of cerebral arteriovenous malformations: a meta-analysis. J Neurosurg. 2013;118(2):437–43.
4. Ozpinar A, Mendez G, Abla AA. Epidemiology, genetics, pathophysiology, and prognostic classifications of cerebral arteriovenous malformations. Handb Clin Neurol. 2017;143:5–13.
5. Kim H, Al-Shahi Salman R, McCulloch CE, Stapf C, Young WL. Untreated brain arteriovenous malformation: patient-level meta-analysis of hemorrhage predictors. Neurology. 2014;83(7):590–7.
6. Mohr JP, Parides MK, Stapf C, Moquete E, Moy CS, Overbey JR, et al. Medical management with or without interventional therapy for unruptured brain arteriovenous malformations (Aruba): a multicenter, non-blinded, randomised trial. Lancet. 2014;383(9917):614–21.

7. Spetzler RF, Martin NA. A proposed grading system for arteriovenous malformations. J Neurosurg. 1986;65(4):476–83.
8. Pollock BE, Flickinger JC. Modification of the radiosurgery – based arteriovenous malformation grading system. Neurosurgery. 2008;63(2):239–43.
9. Pollock BE. Development and testing of a radiosurgery-based arteriovenous malformation grading system. Prog Neurol Surg. 2013;27:58–66.
10. Kano H, Kondziolka D, Flickinger JC, Park KJ, Iyer A, Yang HC, et al. Stereotactic radiosurgery for arteriovenous malformations after embolization: a case-control study. J Neurosurg. 2012;117(2):265–75.
11. Pollock BE, Flickinger JC, Lunsford LD, Maitz A, Kondziolka D. Factors associated with successful arteriovenous malformation radiosurgery. Neurosurgery. 1998;42(6):1239–47.
12. Van Beijnum J, van der Worp HB, Buis DR, Al-Shahi Salman R, Kappelle LJ, Rinkel GJ, et al. Treatment of brain arteriovenous malformations: a systematic review and meta-analysis. JAMA. 2011;306(18):2011–9.
13. Andrade-Souza YM, Ramani M, Scora D, Tsao MN, terBrugge K, Schwartz ML. Embolization before radiosurgery reduces the obliteration rate of arteriovenous malformations. Neurosurgery. 2007;60(3):443–52.
14. Ilyas A, Chen CJ, Ding D, Taylor DG, Moosa S, Lee CC, et al. Volume-staged versus dose-staged stereotactic radiosurgery outcomes for large brain arteriovenous malformations: a systematic review. J Neurosurg. 2018;128(1):154–64.
15. Flickinger JC, Pollock BE, Kondziolka D, Lunsford LD. A dose-response analysis of arteriovenous malformation obliteration after radiosurgery. Int J Radiat Oncol Biol Phys. 1996;36(4):873–9.
16. Flickinger JC, Kondziolka D, Maitz AH, et al. An analysis of the dose-response for arteriovenous malformation radiosurgery and other factors affecting obliteration. Radiother Oncol. 2002;63:347–54. https://doi.org/10.1016/S0167-8140(02)00103-2.
17. Kano H, Kondziolka D, Flickinger JC, Yang HC, Flannery TJ, Awan NR, et al. Stereotactic radiosurgery for arteriovenous malformations, part 3: outcome predictors and risks after repeat radiosurgery. J Neurosurg. 2012;116(1):21–32.

Trigeminal Neuralgia and the Role of Radiosurgery

10

Shyam Singh Bisht, Arkaja Tripathy, and Kushal Narang

10.1 Background

Trigeminal neuralgia (TN) or tic doulourex is a debilitating pain syndrome characterized by sudden, severe, electric shock-like facial pain, usually in one or more branches of the trigeminal nerve (Cranial Nerve V). Pain episodes are typically paroxysmal, lasting for seconds, often triggered by innocuous stimuli like smiling, brushing teeth, gentle touch, or blow of cold air over face. It's a rare condition with incidence of 4–5 per 100,000 people/year, with female preponderance (2:1). It is usually seen post 50 years of age [1].

Historically, treatment consisted of surgical interventions like partial nerve section/alcohol injections in the early twentieth century. Further understanding that vascular compression over root entry zone (REZ) of trigeminal nerve was the most common underlying mechanism led to new treatment pathways. The introduction of microvascular decompression (MVD) to relieve neurovascular compression revolutionized the surgical management of TN and is still widely used today. SRS as a treatment modality for TN was first introduced by Lars Leksell in 1971 with the development of Gamma Knife. It involves delivering high dose of radiation over a small part of trigeminal nerve. It offers a noninvasive treatment option, causing controlled nerve injury and disrupting pain transmission. Apart from Gamma Knife, CyberKnife has also been used extensively in last two decades for TN radiosurgery. Presently, the first line of therapy remains pharmacotherapeutic agents with the reservation of MVD, SRS, or other minimally invasive treatment choices like radiofrequency rhizotomy/glycerol injections for the refractory cases.

S. S. Bisht (✉) · A. Tripathy · K. Narang
Division of Radiation Oncology, Medanta—The Medicity, Gurugram, India

K. Sood Sharma (ed.), *Radiation Therapy for Benign Disorders*,
https://doi.org/10.1007/978-981-95-6635-8_10

10.2 Anatomy and Pathophysiology of Trigeminal Neuralgia

The trigeminal nerve (CN V) originates at the pons, where sensory and motor roots emerge separately: sensory fibers relay through three nuclei—mesencephalic (proprioception), principal sensory (touch), and spinal trigeminal (pain/temperature) nuclei—while the motor nucleus (solitary) innervates the muscles of mastication. From the pons, the nerve travels through the prepontine cistern (cisternal segment) into Meckle's cave. The nerve then enters Meckel's cave, a CSF-filled dural pouch containing the trigeminal (Gasserian) ganglion, which then divides into three branches: V1 (ophthalmic), V2 (maxillary), and V3 (mandibular). V1 and V2 pass through the cavernous sinus, where tumors, inflammation, or vascular lesions can cause cranial neuropathies responsible for around 2–5% of TN cases. V1 branch exit via the superior orbital fissure and V2 branch through foramen rotundum. V3 branch, carrying both sensory and motor fibers, exits through the foramen ovale to reach the infratemporal fossa. Peripherally, V1 branch supplies the forehead and cornea, V2 branch supplies the midface and upper teeth, and V3 the lower face, lower teeth, and mastication muscles.

Neurovascular compression (NVC) may occur at the REZ which lies approximately 2–6 mm from the pons as this area has a thin myelin sheath and is thus vulnerable to compression (most commonly caused by the superior cerebellar artery) accounting for approximately 75–90% of cases. Vascular compression may be seen in more than three-fourth of the cases of classical TN, but 36% of the cases with vascular loop in REZ may be asymptomatic. Thus, vascular loop in REZ has high sensitivity but poor specificity, and atrophy of nerve in that region increases the specificity. It is postulated that the chronic compression at REZ results in demyelination and remyelination of touch/temperature fibers of trigeminal nerve (type A fibers). This dysmyelination results in abnormal electrical current–like situation triggered by facial stimuli, which is spilled over to the poorly myelinated pain fibers, resulting in facial pain-like condition. Anatomical variations like smaller cisternal cross-sectional area can increase the likelihood of neurovascular conflict; lesser nerve dimensions in cisternal space, and smaller nerve-brainstem angle are also considered contributing factors in trigeminal neuralgia (TN) as they might increase the possibility of conflict.

Other pathologies along the course of trigeminal nerve includes multiple sclerosis plaques or strokes at the brainstem (1–3% of TN cases), tumors (schwannomas, meningiomas) in the cisternal or Meckel's cave segments; cavernous sinus syndromes affecting V1/V2 brsnches and rare causes such as dental injuries, perineural tumor spread (<1%), or trauma [2].

10.3 How to Diagnose TN

Classic TN is defined by neurovascular compression with morphologic changes in the nerve, secondary TN arises from identifiable structural lesions like MS or tumors (15%), and idiopathic TN is diagnosed when no clear cause is found on imaging (10%).

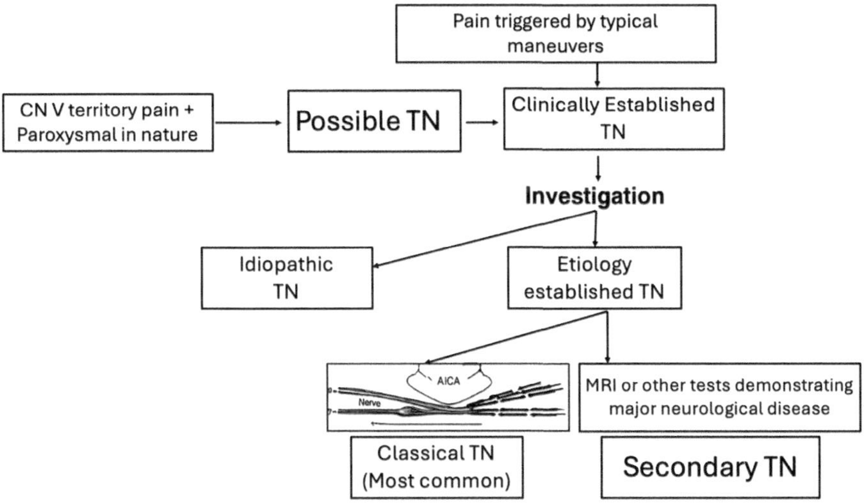

Fig. 10.1 Diagnostic algorithm for the diagnosis of Trigeminal neuralgia

TN can also be categorized as type 1 (purely paroxysmal, electric shock-like pain) or type 2 (includes constant pain), distinctions important for prognosis and treatment (Fig. 10.1). Optimal MRI evaluation to determine the involved segment and etiology should include high-resolution 3D T2-weighted sequences such as fast imaging employing steady-state acquisition (FIESTA) or constructive interference in steady state (CISS) to clearly visualize the trigeminal nerve within the cerebrospinal fluid and detect subtle nerve-vessel conflicts. Thin-slice post-contrast 3D T1-weighted imaging with fat suppression is essential for identifying enhancing lesions like schwannomas or meningiomas, while additional axial and coronal T2-weighted images through the pons help detect demyelinating plaques. Time-of-flight or contrast-enhanced MR angiography should also be performed to delineate vascular anatomy and identify aneurysms or arteriovenous malformations impacting the trigeminal pathway [3].

10.4 Treatment

Pharmacotherapy The treatment of TN begins with initiating preventive pharmacotherapeutics. First-line options include carbamazepine and oxcarbazepine. Additional rescue therapy may be necessary to provide short-term relief. If the clinical response to medications is inadequate or poorly tolerated, alternative oral agent may be used including gabapentin, lamotrigine, or baclofen. Next step involves interventions for refractory pain including microvascular decompression, rhizotomy, radiosurgery, or peripheral neurectomy. Conversely, if the initial or alternative preventive therapy leads to a favorable response, the effective treatment should be continued for at least 6–8 weeks before attempting a gradual taper over weeks; therapy should be resumed promptly if symptoms recur. Additionally, for acute or short-term rescue therapy, options include a short-term increase in preventive therapy (if not already at maximum dose), sumatriptan, phenytoin/fosphenytoin, IV lidocaine. These measures aim to manage acute exacerbations or provide relief during the titration of preventive treatments.

Microvascular Decompression (MVD) is considered the gold-standard surgical treatment for medically refractory trigeminal neuralgia (TN) because it directly addresses the underlying cause—neurovascular compression—by microsurgically repositioning or padding the offending vessel away from the trigeminal nerve at the root entry zone. Pooled data from recent meta-analyses show that MVD achieves immediate pain relief in about 83–96% of patients and sustained pain freedom in 72–80% at long-term follow-up (up to 10 years). However, complications include facial numbness (5–20%), hearing loss, CSF leak, or, rarely, serious events like brainstem infarction or death [4, 5].

Rhizotomy includes percutaneous procedures targeting the trigeminal nerve via the foramen ovale under imaging guidance, using radiofrequency thermocoagulation (heat lesion), balloon compression (mechanical injury), or glycerol rhizolysis (chemical injection). Initial pain relief is achieved in about 90% of patients, but pain-free rates decline over time: 68–85% at 1 year, 54–64% at 3 years, and ~50% at 5 years. Major complications are rare but include aseptic meningitis (0.2%), maxillary artery injury, dural tears, and risk of oculomotor nerve injury. Postoperative dysesthesia occurs in 12%, and long-term issues include trigeminal sensory loss in ~50%, corneal numbness with keratitis risk in ~4%. Facial numbness is more common after rhizotomy [6]. Table 10.1 shows the differences between SRS, MVD, and rhizotomy.

Peripheral neurectomy can be performed on the branches of the trigeminal nerve, which are the supraorbital, infraorbital, alveolar, and lingual nerves. Neurectomy is accomplished by incision, alcohol injection, radiofrequency lesioning, or cryotherapy.

Stereotactic Radiosurgery Stereotactic radiosurgery (SRS) is indicated for medically refractory trigeminal neuralgia, especially in patients unable or unwilling to undergo open surgery, and in those with recurrent pain after prior procedures. It is also an option for select cases of secondary TN without a mass lesion requiring resection. It demonstrates high initial efficacy, with large series and reviews reporting initial pain relief rates of 70–90%, depending on patient selection and criteria for success. Treatment outcome is measured using the Barrows Barrow Neurological Institute (BNI) Pain Intensity Score (Table 10.2). Clinically, outcomes classified as BNI I to IIIb are considered successful, whereas Grades IV to V suggest inadequate pain control or recurrence. Even though initial pain control rates are high, the pain control durability declines over time. Positive predictors of pain relief include neu-

Table 10.1 Comparison of MVD, SRS, and percutaneous rhizotomy for the treatment of TN

Feature	Microvascular decompression (MVD)	Stereotactic radiosurgery (SRS)	Percutaneous rhizotomy
Mechanism	Microsurgical separation of offending vessel from nerve root	Focused radiation induces nerve injury at REZ	Lesioning trigeminal root/ganglion via heat, compression, or glycerol
Pain relief (initial)	~90–95% pain relief	70–90% pain relief	~90% immediate pain relief
Pain relief (long term)	70–80% pain-free at 5 years	50–60% pain-free at 3–5 years	50% pain-free at 5 years
Recurrence rate	~20–30% at 5 years	30% at 5 years	~50% at 5 years
Complications	Major risks: Hearing loss, CSF leak, infarct (<2% serious); facial numbness uncommon	Facial numbness (10–30%), bothersome dysesthesia rare (<1%)	Facial numbness common (~50%), anesthesia dolorosa (4%)
Anesthesia requirement	General anesthesia, craniotomy required	None; outpatient or day-case	Sedation/local anesthesia; outpatient procedure
Hospital stay	3–7 days typical	OPD procedure	OPD procedure
Suitability	Best for healthy, low-risk patients	Suitable for elderly/high-risk patients	Suitable for patients needing immediate pain control or with limited options
Repeatability	Technically feasible but more difficult after first MVD	Repeatable with caution; risk of increased numbness	Repeatable but with increased risk of sensory complications

Table 10.2 Barrow's Neurological Institute Pain Intensity Scale used for response assessment after treatment in Trigeminal Neuralgia

Grade	Description
I	Complete pain relief, no medication required
II	Occasional pain, no medication required
IIIa	No pain, continue medication
IIIb	Persistent pain, controlled with medication
IV	Some pain, not controlled with medication
V	Severe pain or no relief

rovascular conflict, higher dose to REZ, shorter duration of pain (<3 years), type I TN, dose >75Gy. Previous failed MVD, multiple sclerosis, secondary TN are negative predictor for long-term pain control [7, 8].

SRS may also be used in recurrent TN after initial radiosurgery. Other treatment options include MVD or percutaneous rhizotomy. Repeat SRS can provide renewed pain relief in ~61% of patients, but with an increased risk of facial numbness compared to initial treatment. Microvascular decompression offers durable control but requires open surgery, while rhizotomy provides alternative percutaneous lesioning options [9].

10.5 Effect of SRS

SRS for TN precisely targets the trigeminal nerve's root entry zone (REZ) with 80–90 Gy of focused radiation. This results in selective injury to hyperexcitable, demyelinated nerve fibers by damaging sodium channels, blocking abnormal pain signal conduction. The demyelinated areas of the nerve are more sensitive to radiation-induced conduction block than intact fibers; hence, radiosurgery is especially effective in classical TN where neurovascular compression has already damaged myelin. The effect of radiation is seen over few days to weeks. It induces focal axonal degeneration and demyelination, reducing ectopic discharges and cross-talk transmission that cause paroxysmal pain. Ultimately, this partial denervation interrupts the pathological pain circuits in the trigeminal pathway, leading to significant, long-lasting pain relief [10].

10.6 Planning of SRS

The most established target is the retrogasserian portion or the cisternal segment of the trigeminal nerve, typically 4–6 mm in length, 3–4 mm anterior to the pons. Some target slightly longer nerve segments (up to 8 mm) to improve coverage in recurrent or atypical cases, but this increases the risk of facial numbness. Studies suggest Retrogasserian target as the ideal choice in SRS as it balances the efficacy with safety by maximizing dose to the pain-generating fibers while sparing the brainstem. Root entry zone target was historically used for classic TN but is associated with higher risk of dysesthesia if target is extended too close to the pons, similarly targeting Gasserian ganglion is not recommended now. Primary SRS (first-time radiosurgery) typically prescribes 70–90 Gy to the maximum dose point, with many series advocating 80–85 Gy for best pain control. Secondary/repeat SRS often reduces the prescription to 60–70 Gy to limit cumulative radiation toxicity to the brainstem and minimize sensory complications; doses above 75 Gy in repeat SRS have been linked to higher hypesthesia. Similar pain control but a higher incidence of sensory deficits is seen with higher cumulative doses. If we look at the dose constraints, while plan evaluation, the brainstem should receive a Dmax of less than 16 Gy, as doses exceeding 25 Gy correlate with increased risk of facial numbness; additionally, the volume of brainstem receiving ≥12 Gy should be limited to less than 28 mm^3 [11]. The temporal lobes should have a Dmax below 40 Gy, and the hippocampus should receive less than 6-10 Gy to minimize neurocognitive risks. Within the trigeminal pathway, the Gasserian ganglion can tolerate up to 45 Gy, but the motor root should receive less than 60 Gy to avoid motor dysfunction. The internal carotid artery (ICA) should be kept under 30 Gy to reduce the risk of radiation-induced vasculopathy. VII and VIII cranial nerve complex should also be delineated.

Gamma Knife planning utilizes a rigid stereotactic frame for immobilization and submillimeter accuracy. Planning involves a single 4-mm isocenter shot placed on the nerve segment and the 50% isodose line typically covers the target, with sector blocking to protect the brainstem. GK's mechanical precision yields very steep dose gradients—ideal for sparing nearby structures.

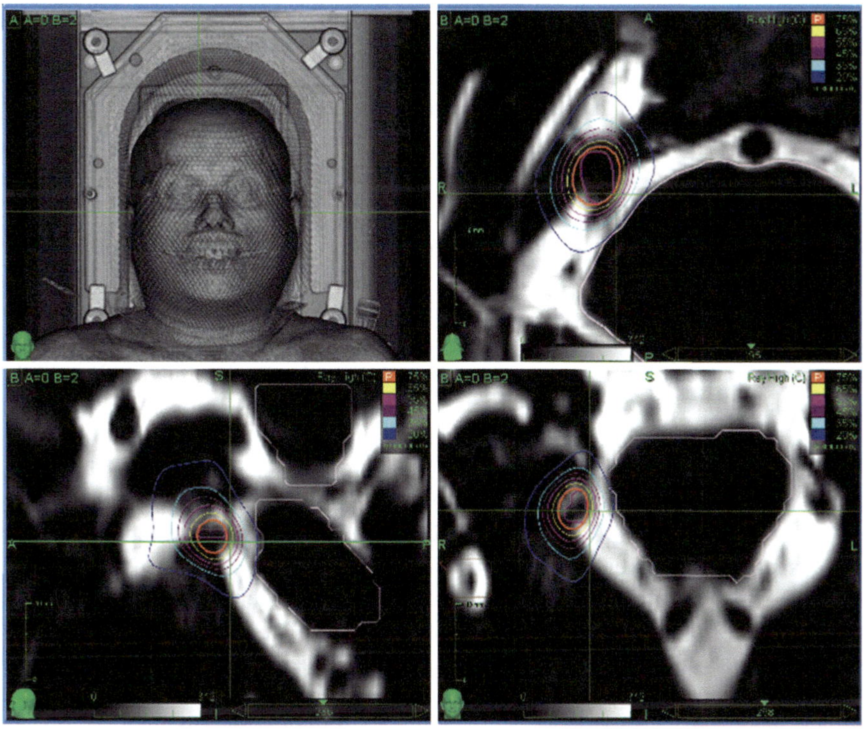

Fig. 10.2 CyberKnife Radiosurgery plan of trigeminal neuralgia case. (Courtesy-Radiation Oncology, Medanta The Medicity)

CyberKnife (CK) planning uses frameless, mask-based immobilization with real-time X-ray skull tracking for submillimeter accuracy. Planning in CK systems leverages non-isocentric delivery with 100+ beam directions to sculpt dose around the trigeminal nerve target, allowing longer target segments if needed (Fig. 10.2). CK plans often prescribe dose at the 70% isodose line, with maximum dose around 85Gy at the centre of target.

LINAC-based SRS uses either conical collimators (5 mm) or micro-multileaf collimators (MLCs) to deliver a single isocenter plan. Planning integrates CT-MRI fusion with high-resolution T2 MRI (FIESTA/CISS) for nerve visualization. Immobilization can be achieved with a stereotactic frame or mask-based system. Treatment delivery is arc based. LINAC-based treatment requires rigorous QA [12].

10.7 Complications of Treatment

MVD complications include hearing loss in 1–3% of patients due to cochlear nerve manipulation, facial weakness or numbness from nerve injury, and cerebrospinal fluid (CSF) leaks or pseudomeningocele formation from dural defects. Less

Table 10.3 Barrow's Neurological Institute Facial Numbness Scale

Grade	Description
I	No facial numbness
II	Mild facial numbness, not bothersome
III	Facial numbness that is bothersome but not disabling
IV	Facial numbness that is very bothersome or disabling

common but serious risks include infection, meningitis, stroke, or brainstem injury, with mortality rates below 0.2%. Complication rates can be reduced through meticulous microsurgical technique, use of intraoperative neuromonitoring, avoiding excessive cerebellar retraction by employing CSF drainage for brain relaxation, and ensuring a watertight dural closure to prevent CSF leaks. Performing MVD in high-volume skull base centers with experienced surgeons also significantly lowers the risk of complications and improves outcomes.

Stereotactic radiosurgery (SRS) for trigeminal neuralgia most commonly causes facial sensory loss, with hypesthesia occurring in about 10–30% of patients and, rarely, bothersome dysesthesia or anesthesia dolorosa. Flickinger et al. found that there is increase in toxicity (numbness) with the use of two isocenters/longer length of target which is called as Flickinger effect. Corneal numbness leading to keratitis can occur if V1 fibers are affected, while very rare but serious complications include radiation injury to the brainstem or adjacent cranial nerves (III, IV, VI) can occur. Radiation-induced secondary tumors are theoretically possible but extremely rare. Strategies to reduce SRS complications include limiting the maximum brainstem dose to under 16 Gy, minimizing high-dose volumes (e.g., keeping brainstem volume receiving ≥12 Gy below 28 mm^3), targeting a precise 4–6 mm retrogasserian nerve segment, and ensuring steep dose gradients for rapid falloff. In repeat SRS, lowering the prescription dose to 60–70 Gy further reduces the risk of sensory complications.Facial sensory disturbance is the most common adverse effect, with 10–30% developing new or bothersome facial numbness (Table 10.3), usually mild. In some patients, numbness progresses to troublesome dysesthesias. The risk of bothersome numbness correlates with longer nerve segments treated and higher doses (>85 Gy).

Potential causes of radiosurgical failure in trigeminal neuralgia in some cases may be misdiagnosis, inaccurate targeting due to MR distortion or neural motion, vascular misidentification, prolonged treatment duration, and anatomical variants in CN V.

10.8 Key Studies

Regis et al. in 2015 published the long-term safety and clinical efficacy of GKRS in classical TN in 497 patients and found that 91.34% achieved initial pain relief, with a median time of 10 days (range 1–459 days). About 37.2% became pain-free within

48 h, 42.8% within 30 days, and 20% after 30 days. However, 34.4% experienced pain recurrence with a median delay of 24 months. The study also highlighted that while most patients achieved pain relief, a significant portion experienced some degree of hypesthesia (numbness) following radiosurgery [13].

A systemic review by Zachary Mendelson et al. compared microvascular decompression (MVD) and Gamma Knife surgery (GKS) for treating trigeminal neuralgia (TN), evaluating their effectiveness in pain relief. Based on 18 studies (2650 patients) for MVD and 25 studies (2846 patients) for GKS, it was found that MVD showed significantly higher rates of pain-free outcomes compared to GKS. However, the pain-free recurrence rates were similar between the two. Similar were the findings in the meta-analysis published by Sharma et al. The findings suggest that MVD may provide more durable and effective pain relief than GKS; however, the dilemma remains in elderly patients and in those without an obvious vascular compression [4, 5].

The systematic review by Tulesca et al., endorsed by the International Society of Stereotactic Radiosurgery (ISRS), analyzed 65 studies encompassing 6461 patients treated for classical trigeminal neuralgia (TN) with stereotactic radiosurgery (SRS), including 45 Gamma Knife (GKS), 11 LINAC, and 9 CyberKnife (CK) studies. Most studies were retrospective, with only one prospective trial. The mean prescribed doses ranged from 71.1 to 90.1 Gy for GKS, 83.3 Gy for LINAC, and 64.3–80.5 Gy for CK, with slight differences in isodose prescription levels (100% for GKS, 80–90% for others). Initial pain freedom without medication varied: GKS (28.6–100%, mean 53.1%), LINAC (17.3–76%, mean 49.3%), and CK (40–72%, mean 56.3%). Sensory complications like hypesthesia occurred in 21.7% (GKS), 27.6% (LINAC), and 29.1% (CK), with higher rates when targeting the root entry zone. Recurrence rates were lowest in CK (mean 25.8%) and highest in LINAC (32.2%). The review supports that SRS is a safe, effective treatment for drug-resistant TN, although more high-quality comparative data is needed [7].

Tuleasca et al. conducted a study at Timone University Hospital, Marseille, analyzing the safety and efficacy of repeat Gamma Knife surgery (GKS) for recurrent trigeminal neuralgia (TN). Out of 737 TN patients treated between 1992 and 2010, 497 had initial pain cessation. Among them, 157 patients (34.4%) experienced recurrence, and 13 patients (1.8%) underwent a second GKS, with data from 9 patients (≥1-year follow-up) included in final analysis. A median dose of 90 Gy was delivered to the retrogasserian cisternal segment. Initial pain relief was achieved in 88.9%, with a median latency of 6.5 days. However, hypesthesia occurred in 33.3% at 6 months and 50% at 1 year, persisting long term. A systematic review of 20 studies (626 patients) showed pain relief in 60–100%, with new hypesthesia in 11–80%. The study concluded that repeat GKS offers comparable pain relief to initial treatment but at the cost of higher sensory complications and highlighted the need for clearer selection criteria, optimal targeting, and dose recommendations [14].

10.9 Future Directions

Future directions in the radiation treatment of trigeminal neuralgia (TN) emphasize precision targeting, technological innovation, and individualized planning to improve outcomes and reduce toxicity. High-resolution imaging techniques such as 3D FIESTA MRI, diffusion tensor imaging (DTI), and tractography allow for precise localization of the affected trigeminal nerve segment, particularly the retrogasserian zone, minimizing radiation to adjacent structures like the brainstem and cranial nerves. Dose modulation strategies, including lower doses for repeat radiosurgery (60–70 Gy) and hypofractionated stereotactic radiotherapy (HSRT) in secondary TN may be explored in near future. Technological advances like MRI-guided radiotherapy and robotic radiosurgery platforms (e.g., CyberKnife) offer enhanced dose conformity and real-time visualization, allowing safer treatment near critical neurovascular structures.

Other areas under research include novel sodium channel blockers such as vixotrigine and eslicarbazepine being studied for their selective action and improved side effect profiles. Early-phase trials show these drugs may reduce paroxysmal attacks without the cognitive or systemic toxicities associated with older antiepileptics. Additionally, interest is growing in botulinum toxin type A (BoNT-A) for refractory TN, with studies reporting meaningful pain relief and minimal invasiveness, although further large-scale trials are needed to standardize administration. Other emerging targets include TRP channels, P2X3 receptors, and inflammatory mediators, which could lead to more targeted and potentially disease-modifying therapies. Neuromodulation also offers a promising non-destructive alternative for patients with refractory TN or contraindications to invasive procedures. Techniques such as motor cortex stimulation (MCS) and deep brain stimulation (DBS) are under investigation, particularly in cases of secondary TN or post-surgical failures [15, 16].

10.10 Summary

Trigeminal neuralgia (TN) is a debilitating facial pain syndrome often managed initially with pharmacologic agents. For refractory cases, interventions such as microvascular decompression (MVD), stereotactic radiosurgery (SRS), or rhizotomy are recommended. Among these, SRS has emerged as a key noninvasive modality, particularly suited for elderly or surgically unfit patients. Targeting the retrogasserian segment with 80–90 Gy, SRS offers excellent initial and sustained pain relief with minimal toxicity. Outcomes are best in classical TN (with neurovascular compression), early-onset disease, and with the use of high-precision platforms like Gamma Knife or CyberKnife, which ensure targeting accuracy, steep dose gradients and reduced toxicity. Repeat SRS remains an option for recurrences, showing renewed pain control in ~60%, though with increased side effects.

Future directions focus on enhancing targeting accuracy through advanced imaging (3D FIESTA, DTI) and optimizing dosing, especially in repeat or secondary TN. MRI-guided SRS and robotic systems improve conformity and reduce off-target exposure. Emerging pharmacologic options (e.g., vixotrigine, BoNT-A) and neuromodulation techniques like DBS/MCS are also being explored. With these innovations, SRS continues to hold a pivotal role, balancing efficacy, safety, and patient quality of life, particularly in medically or surgically challenging TN cases.

References

1. MacDonald BK, Cockerell OC, Sander JW, Shorvon SD. The incidence and lifetime prevalence of neurological disorders in a prospective community-based study in the UK. Brain. 2000;123(Pt 4):665–76. https://doi.org/10.1093/brain/123.4.665. PMID: 10733998.
2. Graff-Radford S, Gordon R, Ganal J, Tetradis S. Trigeminal neuralgia and facial pain imaging. Curr Pain Headache Rep. 2015;19(6):19. https://doi.org/10.1007/s11916-015-0495-y. PMID: 26017711.
3. Docampo J, Gonzalez N, Muñoz A, Bravo F, Sarroca D, Morales C. Neurovascular study of the trigeminal nerve at 3t MRI. Neuroradiol J. 2015;28(1):28–35. https://doi.org/10.15274/NRJ-2014-10116. PMID: 25924169; PMCID: PMC4757119.
4. Sharma R, Phalak M, Katiyar V, Borkar S, Kale SS, Mahapatra AK. Microvascular decompression versus stereotactic radiosurgery as primary treatment modality for trigeminal neuralgia: a systematic review and meta-analysis of prospective comparative trials. Neurol India. 2018;66(3):688–94. https://doi.org/10.4103/0028-3886.232342. PMID: 29766927.
5. Mendelson ZS, Velagala JR, Kohli G, Heir GM, Mammis A, Liu JK. Pain-free outcomes and durability of surgical intervention for trigeminal neuralgia: a comparison of gamma knife and microvascular decompression. World Neurosurg. 2018;112:e732–46. https://doi.org/10.1016/j.wneu.2018.01.141. Epub 2018 Jan 31. PMID: 29382615.
6. Lopez BC, Hamlyn PJ, Zakrzewska JM. Systematic review of ablative neurosurgical techniques for the treatment of trigeminal neuralgia. Neurosurgery. 2004;54(4):973–82; discussion 982-3. https://doi.org/10.1227/01.neu.0000114867.98896.f0. PMID: 15046666.
7. Tuleasca C, Régis J, Sahgal A, De Salles A, Hayashi M, Ma L, Martínez-Álvarez R, Paddick I, Ryu S, Slotman BJ, Levivier M. Stereotactic radiosurgery for trigeminal neuralgia: a systematic review. J Neurosurg. 2019;130(3):733–57. https://doi.org/10.3171/2017.9.JNS17545. Epub 2018 Apr 27. PMID: 29701555.
8. Singh R, Davis J, Sharma S. Stereotactic radiosurgery for trigeminal neuralgia: a retrospective multi-institutional examination of treatment outcomes. Cureus. 2016;8(4):e554. https://doi.org/10.7759/cureus.554. PMID: 27182468; PMCID: PMC4858443.
9. Berti A, Ibars G, Wu X, Sabo A, Granville M, Suarez G, Schwade JG, Jacobson RE. Evaluation of CyberKnife radiosurgery for recurrent trigeminal neuralgia. Cureus. 2018;10(5):e2598. https://doi.org/10.7759/cureus.2598. PMID: 30013862; PMCID: PMC6039152.
10. Gorgulho A. Radiation mechanisms of pain control in classical trigeminal neuralgia. Surg Neurol Int. 2012;3(Suppl 1):S17–25. https://doi.org/10.4103/2152-7806.91606. Epub 2012 Jan 14. PMID: 22826806; PMCID: PMC3400477.
11. Zhang M, Lamsam LA, Schoen MK, Mehta SS, Appelboom G, Adler JK, Soltys SG, Chang SD. Brainstem dose constraints in nonisometric radiosurgical treatment planning of trigeminal neuralgia: a single-institution experience. World Neurosurg. 2018;113:e399–407. https://doi.org/10.1016/j.wneu.2018.02.042. Epub 2018 Feb 14. PMID: 29454124.
12. Ma L, Kwok Y, Chin LS, Yu C, Regine WF. Comparative analyses of linac and gamma knife radiosurgery for trigeminal neuralgia treatments. Phys Med Biol. 2005;50(22):5217.

13. Régis J, Tuleasca C, Resseguier N, Carron R, Donnet A, Gaudart J, Levivier M. Long-term safety and efficacy of gamma knife surgery in classical trigeminal neuralgia: a 497-patient historical cohort study. J Neurosurg. 2016;124(4):1079–87. https://doi.org/10.3171/2015.2.JNS142144. Epub 2015 Sep 4. PMID: 26339857.
14. Tuleasca C, Carron R, Resseguier N, Donnet A, Roussel P, Gaudart J, Levivier M, Régis J. Repeat gamma knife surgery for recurrent trigeminal neuralgia: long-term outcomes and systematic review. J Neurosurg. 2014;121(Suppl):210–21. https://doi.org/10.3171/2014.8.GKS141487. PMID: 25434955.
15. Islam J, Elina KC, Park YS. Recent update on trigeminal neuralgia. J Korean Soc Stereotact Funct Neurosurg. 2022;18(1):9–19.
16. Branco R, Silva BG, Pereira A, Amorim I, Jacinto J. What is new and effective in treating refractory trigeminal neuralgia? Cureus. 2024;16(11):e73110. https://doi.org/10.7759/cureus.73110. PMID: 39650988; PMCID: PMC11622163.

Paragangliomas

11

Ashutosh Mukherji

11.1 Background

Paragangliomas are neuroendocrine neoplasms arising from extra-adrenal paraganglia and are classified based on anatomical origin: sympathetic (typically along the abdominal sympathetic chain) or parasympathetic (especially at head and neck sites, which account for the majority of all paragangliomas) [1, 2]. More than three-fourths of paragangliomas located outside of the head and neck are sympathetic, secreting norepinephrine, unlike the more differentiated intraabdominal adrenal medulla tumors neuroblastoma and pheochromocytoma which primarily secrete epinephrine [3]. Paragangliomas are rare. According to an old study by Beard et al [4] they had an annual incidence of about 0.2-0.6 per 100,000 before year 2000 which later increased after 2010 to 0.6 per 100,000 due ti improved imaging. The combined incidence of paragangliomas and pheochromocytomas is estimated at 500-1600 annually in the US [4, 5].

Paragangliomas commonly present in the fourth to fifth decades (mean ~47 years), but hereditary cases typically manifest about a decade earlier. As mentioned in previous paragraph, these tumors can arise from both sympathetic and parasympathetic neural crests. Sympathetic origin tumours can be distributed from the base of skull down to the bladder or prostate. Parasympathetic tumours (eg. glomus jugulare or carotid body tumours) are more commonly seen in head and neck areas, and are mostly hormonally silent but can cause symptoms due to mass effect. More than 70% of the parasympathetic paragangliomas are in the head and neck region; of these, 5% of the temporal ones and 15% of the carotid body tumors could turn malignant [6]. Pain is the most common symptom of malignant

A. Mukherji (✉)
Department of Radiation Oncology, Mahamana Pandit Madan Mohan Malaviya Cancer Centre and Homi Bhabha Cancer Hospital, Tata Memorial Centre, Varanasi, India

K. Sood Sharma (ed.), *Radiation Therapy for Benign Disorders*,
https://doi.org/10.1007/978-981-95-6635-8_11

transformation. Regional spread in head and neck paragangliomas is seen to the neck nodes, and distant metastases while rare is seen to the lung and bones [6].

Clinical presentation of these tumors can depend on their site of origin. Sympathetic paragangliomas near the adrenal can give rise to symptoms such as episodic hypertension, tachycardia, sweating, and headache [3]. Those in the head and neck areas can be further divided based on location. Temporal or tympanic canal tumors can present with hearing loss, tinnitus, and disequilibrium and on examination are seen as a bluish swelling or mass behind the eardrum. Carotid body tumors usually occur at the carotid bifurcation presenting as a slow growing mass lesion with associated carotid bruit and may be pulsatile in nature. Their further growth into the parapharyngeal space can involve cranial nerves (especially Cr. N X and XII) and may even involve the sympathetic plexus on progression [7]. Glomus jugulare tumors are paragangliomas growing at the skull base and can involve Cr. N. IX to XII as well as Horner's syndrome on further progression. They are usually associated with bone destruction and can invade superiorly into middle cranial fossa and inferiorly into the jugular fossa. They usually present as an intraoral parapharyngeal mass displacing the tonsil anteriorly [7]. Other locations in the head and neck where paragangliomas (PGL) are known to occur are the glossopharyngeal paraganglia, jugular tympanic area, larynx, nasal cavity, trachea, thyroid gland and the orbit [8].

Various factors can affect the chosen treatment modality for paragangliomas. These include the location and extent of the tumor, patient age and health, the anticipated morbidity of the treatment alternatives, and preferences of the patient and physician. In case of very small (<1 cm diameter) non-secretary, asymptomatic head and neck paragangliomas, observation can be a management option. These are followed up with serial MR or CT scans every 6 months, and in case there is an increase in the lesion size, surgery is contemplated.

Historically, surgical extirpation has been the treatment modality of choice. This offers a complete chance of cure by complete removal of the tumor. However, the intricate neurovascular anatomy and proximity to cranial nerves often result in significant morbidity, including cranial nerve deficits or vascular injury. Over recent decades, radiation therapy (RT) has been incorporated into management—particularly for unresectable, residual, recurrent, or surgically high-risk tumors. With advancements such as stereotactic radiosurgery (SRS) and intensity-modulated RT (IMRT), tumor control has improved significantly while minimizing adverse effects. The benign nature and indolent behavior of many paragangliomas provide a unique rationale for applying RT in benign disease contexts, balancing tumor control against potential long-term toxicity. Cure after radiation therapy is often defined as sustained non-progression of the residual mass if any.

11.2 Pathogenesis

Paragangliomas originate from paraganglionic cells derived from the neural crest associated with autonomic ganglia. Sympathetic variants can secrete catecholamines, whereas head and neck parasympathetic types are largely non-functional. Many paragangliomas are sporadic, but between 30% and 50% of cases harbor germline mutations in susceptibility genes such as SDHB (have the highest potential for malignant transformation), SDHD, or associated with syndromes such as Carney-Stratakis dyad, neurofibromatosis type 1 (NF1), von Hippel-Lindau (VHL), and multiple endocrine neoplasia types 2A and 2B (MEN2) [9] which drive tumorigenesis via mechanisms including abnormal cellular metabolism, angiogenesis, and pseudohypoxic pathways.

Molecular alterations—particularly succinate dehydrogenase (SDHx) dysfunction—stabilize hypoxia-inducible factors, promoting angiogenic signaling and cellular proliferation. Aberrant catecholamine secretion potentiates cardiovascular sequelae and may impact microenvironment interactions.

The rationale for radiation therapy lies in its capacity to inflict DNA double-strand breaks leading to apoptosis, mitotic catastrophe, and cessation of tumor cell proliferation. SRS delivers high-dose focal irradiation with submillimeter accuracy, maximizing tumor cell death while preserving adjacent structures. RT-induced endothelial damage and vascular disruption further impair tumor blood supply, which is pivotal given the rich vascularity of these tumors. Moreover, RT modulates tumor microenvironment and may deter vasculogenesis—key processes in paraganglioma maintenance and growth.

Given the typically indolent nature, effective local control via RT—achieving tumor stabilization or regression—can arrest progression, palliate symptoms, and prevent mass-related neurovascular compromise.

11.3 Histopathology

Paragangliomas usually present with three typical histological patterns:

1. Zellballen pattern: the "*chief cells*" are arranged in a nest-like pattern with surrounding fibrovascular stroma. The chief cells are usually epithelioid or rarely spindle shaped with round hyperchromatic and chromatin clustered nuclei. These cells stain for synaptophysin, neuron specific enolase, CD56, CD57, and PGP9.5.
2. Angiomatous pattern: consisting of large spindle cells or crescent-shaped cells and capillaries.
3. Polyhedral cells with columnar architecture and abundant cytoplasm that form the adenomatous pattern.

Imaging The basic requirements for imaging in case of paragangliomas are a CT and MRI scan. In a jugular-tympanic or jugular glomus paraganglioma, a CT provides a better assessment of the contact of the tumor with the temporal bone, while an MRI provides a better contrast and orientation of extent of soft tissue involvement by the tumor [10, 11]. Ultrasound of the neck nodal mass reveals a hypervascular, solid, well-defined, hypoechoic tumor. Classic CT scan findings include a homogenous mass lesion with intense contrast uptake and delayed wash-out, with presence of cystic changes, necrosis, and internal calcifications.

In MRI, on T1-weighted images, these tumors display intermediate signal intensity with dispersed areas of signal void indicating high flow vascularity. In T2-weighted scans, there is a "*salt and pepper*" appearance with a pronounced hypervascular pattern. Paragangliomas showed the highest uptake when assessing the SSTR expression, so the Ga-DOTATE PET/CT proved to be of use in differentiating them from other tumors such as schwannoma, meningioma, esthesioneuroblastoma, which proved to have a lower uptake [11].

A biopsy taken from the lesion is however the gold standard for establishing the diagnosis. However, care must be taken during biopsy to avoid hemorrhage because of the highly vascular nature of the mass lesion. Also, intra-operative release of catecholamines and resultant hypertension is another risk that needs to be accounted for.

Surgical Treatment In case of head and neck small paragangliomas showing growth or in case of the following situations, surgical excision remains the treatment of choice:

- Tympanic paragangliomas
- Jugular paragangliomas with troublesome conductive hearing loss, pulsatile tinnitus, or impending or actual facial nerve weakness
- Significant brainstem compression
- Secretory tumors
- Cranial nerve dysfunction related to tumor burden
- Clinical evidence of rapid growth
- Malignant disease
- Patient choice

In secretory tumors, preoperative management is important. This includes control of hypertension starting 7 days before surgery using either alpha-adrenergic blockers such as prazosin plus phenoxybenzamine or selective blockers like doxazosin [12]. In addition, a high sodium diet with high fluid intake can negate the vascular contraction caused by catecholamine release and resultant severe hypotension after tumor removal. This preoperative blockade is a vital recommendation in all catecholamine-secreting tumors [13]. In some cases, metyrosine (a catecholamine synthesis inhibitor) may be required where other drugs are ineffective or there is a large tumor burden which may require manipulation during surgery.

Other preoperative interventions include embolization and preoperative radiotherapy. Embolization is used in secretory head and neck paragangliomas with tumors larger than 3 cm being typical scenarios for use of embolization [13]. The advantages of this approach are lower blood loss, faster recovery, easier resection, and shorter intraoperative time. Preoperative radiotherapy is typically used in small, non-secretory, benign tumors in the skull base and neck in proximity to or abutting critical nerve or vascular structures.

Surgical techniques used for paragangliomas include minimally invasive laparoscopic or retroperitoneoscopic approach for abdominal tumors, radical or partial cystectomies, composite head and neck or skull base resections, or transcervical resection for carotid body tumors. The most significant complications or intraoperative risks during surgery are bleeding, stroke, and cranial nerve dysfunction. Various tumor classification systems, such as the Fisch or Glasscock-Jackson classification, can help assess resectability and guide surgical planning [14]. Local recurrence rate after surgery is 6.5% at 5 years, 16.1% at 10 years, and 17.1% at 15 years [15].

Staging of Paragangliomas Most tumors are staged for assessing operability. Commonly used systems are the Glasscock-Jackson classification Scheme [14] (Table 11.1) or the Fisch system [6] (Table 11.2) for assessing operability of glomus tumors or jugulo-tympanic tumors or Shamblin classification for carotid body tumors (Table 11.3) [16].

Table 11.1 Glasscock-Jackson classification scheme

Tumor class	Description
Type 1	Small tumor involving the jugular bulb, middle ear, or mastoid process
Type 2	Extending under internal auditory canal; may have intracranial extension
Type 3	Extending into petrous apex; may have intracranial extension
Type 4	Extending beyond petrous apex into clivus or infratemporal fossa; may have intracranial extension

Table 11.2 Fisch classification scheme

Tumor class	Description
Class A	Limited to mesotympanum; arise along the tympanic plexus on the cochlear promontory
Class B	Limited to mesotympanum, hypotympanum, and mastoid; bone over jugular bulb not eroded
Class C	Labyrinthine and apical compartments with:
Class C1	No invasion of the carotid artery, destruction of jugular bulb/foramen
Class C2	Invasion of the vertical carotid canal between foramen and the bend
Class C3	Invasion of the horizontal carotid canal short of foramen lacerum
Class C4	Extension to foramen lacerum and cavernous sinus
Class D	Represents intracranial extension with intra- or extradural extension
Class$De_{1/2}$	Tumors with *intracranial but only extradural extension*; De according to displacement of dura (De_1 = less than 2 cm, De_2 = more than 2 cm)
Class$Di_{1/2/3}$	Tumors with *intracranial and intradural extension*; $Di_{1/2/3}$ according to depth of invasion into posterior cranial fossa (Di_1 = less than 2 cm, Di_2 = between 2 and 4 cm, Di_3 = more than 4 cm)

Table 11.3 Shamblin classification for carotid body tumors [16]

Shamblin grade	Description
I	Tumors are small or localized and easily resected without vessel injury
II	Tumors adherent or partially surrounding the carotid vessels but with dissection still possible
III	Tumors intimately surround or encase the carotid vessels with impossible dissection

11.4 Role of Radiation Therapy

11.4.1 Indications

Radiation therapy (RT) is indicated in cases of:

- Inoperable or surgically unresectable tumors (due to proximity to cranial nerves or deep location)
- Residual or recurrent disease post-surgery
- Symptomatic mass effect causing cranial neuropathies
- Patients unfit for surgery

Head and neck lesions often benefit from RT when surgical morbidity is high, such as vagal or jugulotympanic tumors.

Definitive Radiation This is the most commonly used application of radiation in paragangliomas.

Doses range from 45 to 54 Gy in conventional fractionated radiotherapy or 25–30 Gy in 5–6 fractions or even 21 Gy in 3 fractions of stereotactic body radiotherapy. Most of the literature with respect to definitive irradiation comes from head and neck paragangliomas. Usually post-irradiation tumor response is slow [17] with a study reporting regression in 32% cases, progression in 9%, and a radiologically visible stable disease in nearly 60% cases.

Postoperative Radiation Can improve local control rates especially after sub-total resections. In a study, sub-total resections with post-op RT resulted in 69% local control compared to 86% for complete resections [18].

Radiation in Recurrent Disease Various studies have shown efficacy of conventionally fractionated radiotherapy in recurrent cases with local control rates as high as 83% [19]. There has been benefit of using newer treatment techniques such as IMRT. Doses range from 45 to 54 Gy with IMRT or 13–16 Gy with SRS/SRT (stereotactic radiation) [19].

11.4.2 Benefits vs Alternatives

RT offers local control rates of 90–100% at 5–10 years for carotid body and skull base paragangliomas, comparable to surgical outcomes but with much lower cranial nerve morbidity or mortality. Compared to surgery, RT avoids intraoperative risks, often allows preservation of nerve function, and is suitable for multifocal or bilateral disease. Conservative "wait-and-scan" approaches may be appropriate in asymptomatic, stable lesions, but RT offers definitive arrest of tumor progression when indicated.

11.4.3 Patient Selection

Ideal candidates include:

- Patients with progressive tumors on imaging
- Those with cranial nerve involvement or neurovascular compression
- Individuals with cystic or extensive tumors where surgery carries high morbidity
- Hereditary cases (e.g., SDHD mutations) characterized by multifocality or recurrence

Contraindications include pregnancy, untreated serious comorbidities, or prior maximal radiation exposure in the same location.

11.4.4 Limitations and Challenges

- Long latency for maximal tumor shrinkage
- Need for lifelong surveillance
- Potential late effects such as radiation-induced meningioma, carotid stenosis, or neurocognitive sequelae in skull base cases
- Uncertainty regarding radiation effects in genetic versus sporadic cases

11.5 Radiation Technique

11.5.1 Modalities

- *Stereotactic Radiosurgery (SRS)*: e.g., Gamma Knife or CyberKnife, delivering 1–5 fractions (SC < 3 cm)
- *Stereotactic Body RT (SBRT)*: Hypofractionated high-dose RT in multiple fractions.
- *Intensity-Modulated RT (IMRT)*: Conventional fractionation over weeks, precise shaping of dose to spare adjacent structures
- *Conventional EBRT*: 25–30 fractions, typically for larger macrosurgical fields.

Proton therapy is emerging, offering dosimetric advantages, particularly near critical structures

11.5.2 Immobilization and Imaging

- Thermoplastic mask for head/neck lesions, vacuum cradle for extracranial.
- Imaging for planning includes CT combined with MRI (for soft tissue delineation) and PET (e.g., 68-Ga-DOTATATE) for functional targeting.

11.5.3 Target Volume Delineation

- Accurate target volume delineation will require fusion of the simulation CT image with the diagnostic MRI scans, especially the contrast-enhanced T1-weighted MRI imaging, with a slice thickness no greater than 2 mm [20]
- During contouring, whether for SRT/SBRT or IMRT, the gross tumor volume (GTV) is marked out on the MR sequences, and then a clinical target volume (CTV) is added which is usually a 2–5 mm expansion radially keeping in mind anatomical barriers or the visible local extension to surrounding organs.
- A further 2–5 mm expansion gives the planning target volume (PTV) for IMRT. In case of SRT/SBRT, the PTV margin can be 0–1 mm.
- In LINAC-based stereotactic radiosurgery (SRS), the dose is prescribed to the 80% isodose line, while on Gamma Knife systems, dose is prescribed to the 50% isodose line.
- Since these tumors are non-malignant, elective nodal radiation is not required. In cases, where there is malignant transformation, first station nodes may be included.

11.5.4 Dose and Fractionation

- Head/neck paragangliomas: 45–54 Gy in 25–30 fractions; SRS: single 15–18 Gy.
- For malignant/metastatic cases: 65–70 Gy in 6.5 weeks in conventionally fractionated radiotherapy for malignant glomus tumors to the PTV, or 30–60 Gy delivered in hypofractionated schedules; BED $\geq$53 Gy_{10} associated with superior local control (81% vs 62%).
- IMRT regimens: median 74.4 Gy (BED) over ~13 fractions.

11.5.5 Organ Constraints

Constraints are based on standard QUANTEC data. Critical structures include the cochlea, cranial nerves, optic pathway, brainstem, and carotid arteries. Stringent dose constraints are essential—e.g., $\leq$8 Gy to cochlea in fractionated RT; $\leq$54 Gy to brainstem; carotid artery sparing to reduce stenosis risk. Special considerations apply to pediatric and hereditary cases—minimizing integral dose to avoid secondary malignancies over long survival periods.

11.6 Toxicity Profile and Strategies to Minimize Risks

Radiation therapy is generally well tolerated.

11.6.1 Acute Toxicities

- Transient mucositis or dermatitis in head/neck cases
- Fatigue
- Rare hypertensive crises—reported to occur acutely, but seldom in modern series
- Weight loss/nausea (reported in ~14% hospitalized patients during conventional RT)

11.6.2 Late Effects

1. Cranial nerve deficits (rare with SRS due to steep dose gradients), less than 10% patients report neuropathies [20]
2. Carotid artery stenosis and cerebrovascular events (~2 cases reported).
3. Secondary tumors (e.g., radiation-induced meningioma detected 15–18 years post-RT)
4. Hearing loss with petrous/parapharyngeal lesions especially with use of SRS

11.6.3 Mitigation Strategies

- Use of IMRT/SRS to conform dose and spare adjacent tissues
- Careful planning to limit dose to vulnerable structures (cochlea, vessels, brainstem)
- Consider FMISO-PET or proton RT in radiosensitive locations
- Long-term follow-up (>10 years) to monitor late sequelae
- Blood pressure monitoring during and after RT, particularly in functional tumors

11.7 Review of Literature and Case Studies

Head and Neck Paragangliomas In a retrospective cohort of 131 patients (156 tumors) treated with conventional EBRT (median 45 Gy in 25 fractions), the overall 5- and 10-year local control reached 99% and 96%, respectively. The cause-specific survival rates at 5 and 10 years were 98% and 97%, respectively; the distant metastases free rates at 5 and 10 years were 99% and 99%, respectively. Late complications included two vascular events and two radiation-induced meningiomas at 15–18 years post-RT. [7]

Meta-Analyses and Retrospectives Long-term data from 33 patients treated between 1967 and 1994 with EBRT or SRS showed a 10-year control rate of 92% and no radiation-induced malignancies [21].

Malignant/Metastatic Disease Less than 10% of paragangliomas have propensity for malignant transformation. *A Ki-67 value above 3%, tumor larger than 5 cm, SDH mutation presence, and necrosis in the histopathology indicate propensity for malignant transformation* [22]. *Metastatic disease is defined as occurrence of the paraganglioma in non-chromaffin organs*. Most common sites of disease metastases are bones, neck nodes, lungs, liver, and thyroid [23]. A series of 29 patients with 34 PGL/PCC lesions treated with CyberKnife radiosurgery (median dose 25 Gy associated with 97% lesion control) showed 8-year lesion control of 96% and symptom improvement in almost all symptomatic lesions [24].

Proton Therapy A small cohort ($n = 17$) treated with proton beam therapy for glomus jugulare tumors exhibited tumor control in all cases with limited acute toxicity. Prescribed dose was 50.4 RBE (RBE = 1.1); at median follow-up of 50 months, local control was 100% with stable size radiologically in 82% cases and reduction in size in 18%. One case developed grade 3 hearing impairment [25].

11.7.1 Specific Cases

- *Jugulotympanic Paraganglioma*: Treated with Gamma Knife SRS (single 15–18 Gy), reported 97% progression-free survival at 7 years and only 7.7% with grade 1–2 toxicity.
- *Hereditary SDHB-mutated REC*: Case reports have demonstrated effective RT outcomes with functional remission and stability over 5 years.

Overall, the accumulated literature demonstrates strong local control, symptom mitigation, and favorable safety profiles relative to surgical approaches, especially in complex or recurrent cases.

11.8 Future Directions

Advanced Delivery Techniques Proton beam therapy offers sharper dose fall-off with negligible exit dose—ideal for tumors adjacent to cranial nerves or brainstem. Carbon-ion therapy may also emerge as a potent treatment for radioresistant paragangliomas.

Stereotactic Developments Refinement of ultra-hypofractionated SBRT regimens, alongside robotics (CyberKnife®), may permit outpatient delivery and enhanced quality of life.

Molecular and Systemic Integration Integration of targeted agents like HIF2α inhibitors (belzutifan) and peptide receptor radionuclide therapy (PRRT) with RT could enhance tumor control in multi-focal or metastatic hereditary disease.

Personalized Radiotherapy Use of radiogenomics and AI can inform individualized RT—for example, predicting radiosensitive genomic signatures or planning to minimize late toxicity.

Future Trials Prospective multicenter trials evaluating SBRT vs IMRT, RT timing relative to surgery, and RT's role in hereditary vs sporadic cases are necessary. Focused endpoints should include functional preservation, QOL metrics, and long-term carcinogenesis.

11.9 Conclusion

Radiation therapy has become an essential modality in managing paragangliomas, particularly when surgery carries high morbidity or in cases of recurrent/postoperative disease. With local control rates consistently above 90% and a relatively low toxicity profile, RT—especially using SRS, SBRT, and IMRT—provides patients with effective tumor control while sparing critical structures. Emerging modalities like proton therapy and SBRT, along with targeted agents and AI-driven personalization, promise to improve both efficacy and safety. Future research, including prospective trials and genetic stratification, will refine indications and optimize long-term outcomes. Ultimately, RT represents a cornerstone of paraganglioma care and highlights the evolution of precision therapy in benign tumors.

References

1. Lenders JWM, Eisenhofer G. Update on modern management of pheochromocytoma and paraganglioma. Endocrinol Metab (Seoul). 2017;32(2):152–61.
2. Lam AK. Update on adrenal tumours. In 2017 World Health Organization (WHO) of endocrine tumours. Endocr Pathol. 2017;28(3):213–27.
3. Neumann HP, Pawlu C, Peczkowska M, Bausch B, McWhinney SR, Muresan M, Buchta M, Franke G, Klisch J, Bley TA, Hoegerle S, Boedeker CC, Opocher G, Schipper J, Januszewicz A, Eng C, European-American Paraganglioma Study Group. Distinct clinical features of paraganglioma syndromes associated with SDHB and SDHD gene mutations. JAMA. 2004;292(8):943–51.
4. Beard CM, Sheps SG, Kurland LT, Carney JA, Lie JT. Occurrence of pheochromocytoma in Rochester, Minnesota, 1950 through 1979. Mayo Clin Proc. 1983;58(12):802–4.
5. Al Subhi AR, Boyle V, Elston MS. Systematic review: incidence of PPGLs over 70 years. J Endo Soc. 2022;6:1–9.

6. Manolidis S, Shohet JA, Jackson CG, Glasscock ME 3rd. Malignant glomus tumors. Laryngoscope. 1999;109:30–4.
7. Gilbo P, Morris CG, Amdur RJ, Werning JW, Dziegielewski PT, Kirwan J, Mendenhal WM. Radiotherapy for benign head and neck paragangliomas: a 45-year experience. Cancer. 2014;120:3738–43.
8. Cleere EF, Martin-Grace J, Gendre A, Sherlock M, O'Neill JP. Contemporary management of paragangliomas of the head and neck. Laryngoscope Investig Otolaryngol. 2021;7:93–107.
9. Boedeker CC. Paragangliomas and paraganglioma syndromes. GMS Curr Top Otorhinolaryngol Head Neck Surg. 2011;10:Doc03.
10. Taïeb D, Varoquaux A, Chen CC, Pacak K. Current and future trends in the anatomic and functional imaging of head and neck paragangliomas. Semin Nucl Med. 2013;43:462–73.
11. Kuker R, Wang J, Nagornaya N, Bhatia RG, Quencer R, Serafini A. Ga-68 DOTATATE PET/CT in the evaluation of paragangliomas and other indeterminate lesions in the head and neck. Indian J Nucl Med. 2022;37:350–8.
12. Neumann HPH, Young WF, Eng C. Pheochromocytoma and Paraganglioma. N Engl J Med. 2019;381(6):552–65.
13. Lenders JW, Duh QY, Eisenhofer G, Gimenez-Roqueplo AP, Grebe SK, Murad MH, Naruse M, Pacak K, Young WF, Endocrine Society. Pheochromocytoma and paraganglioma: an endocrine society clinical practice guideline. J Clin Endocrinol Metab. 2014;99(6):1915–42.
14. Jackson CG, Glasscock ME, Harris PF. Glomus tumors. Diagnosis, classification, and management of large lesions. Arch Otolaryngol. 1982;108(7):401–10.
15. Parisien-La Salle S, Chbat J, Lacroix A, Perrotte P, Karakiewicz P, Saliba I, Le XK, Olney HJ, Bourdeau I. Postoperative recurrences in patients operated for pheochromocytomas and paragangliomas: new data supporting lifelong surveillance. Cancers (Basel). 2022;14(12)
16. Shamblin WR, ReMine WH, Sheps SG, Harrison EG. Carotid body tumor (chemodectoma): clinicopathologic analysis of ninety cases. Am J Surg. 1971;122:732–9.
17. Zabel A, Milker-Zabel S, Huber P, Schulz-Ertner D, Schlegel W, Wannenmacher M, Debus J. Fractionated stereotactic conformal radiotherapy in the management of large chemodectomas of the skull base. Int J Radiat Oncol Biol Phys. 2004;58(5):1445–50.
18. Ivan ME, Sughrue ME, Clark AJ, Kane AJ, Aranda D, Barani IJ, Parsa AT. A meta-analysis of tumor control rates and treatment-related morbidity for patients with glomus jugulare tumors. J Neurosurg. 2011;114(5):1299–305.
19. Elshaikh MA, Mahmoud-Ahmed AS, Kinney SE, Wood BG, Lee JH, Barnett GH, Suh JH. Recurrent head-and neck chemodectomas: a comparison of surgical and radiotherapeutic results. Int J Radiat Oncol Biol Phys. 2002;52(4):953–6.
20. Gigliotti MJ, Hasan S, Liang Y, Chen D, Fuhrer R, Wegner RE. A 10-year experience of linear accelerator-based stereotactic radiosurgery/radiotherapy (SRS/SRT) for paraganglioma: a single institution experience and review of the literature. J Radiosurg SBRT. 2018;5(3):183–90.
21. Krych AJ, Foote RL, Brown PD, Garces YI, Link MJ. Long-term results of irradiation for paraganglioma. Int J Radiat Oncol Biol Phys. 2006;65(4):1063–6.
22. Mete O, Wenig BM. Update from the 5th edition of the World Health Organization classification of head and neck tumors: overview of the 2022 WHO classification of head and neck neuroendocrine neoplasms. Head Neck Pathol. 2022;16:123–42.
23. Mediouni A, Ammari S, Wassef M, Gimenez-Roqueplo AP, Laredo JD, Duet M, Huy PT, Oker N. Malignant head/neck paragangliomas. Comparative study. Eur Ann Otorhinolaryngol Head Neck Dis. 2014;131:159–66.
24. Hong S, Kagawa K, Sato K, Ichi S. The long-term outcome of CyberKnife-based stereotactic radiotherapy for head and neck paragangliomas: a single-center experience. World Neurosurg. 2021;155:382–90.
25. Chartier J, Beddoka A, Cao KI, Feuvret L, Hermand P, Bolle S, Goudjil F, Sauvaget E, Choussy O, Dendale R, Calugaru V. Proton therapy to maintain local control of head and neck paragangliomas. Acta Oncol. 2023;62(4):400–3.

12 Juvenile NP-Fibroma

Poonam Goyal and Vaishali

12.1 Background

Juvenile naso pharyngeal angiofibroma (JNA): it is a benign neoplasm, arises in nasopharynx, makes up for 0.05% to 0.5% of all head tumors, shows male predominance, occurs majorly in 14–25 year groups, and is more common in India than in the Western countries.

JNA is a benign but locally aggressive neoplasm. It is also known as juvenile angiofibroma (JAF), fibromatous, or angiofibromatous hamartoma of nasal cavity [1].

It arises from fibrovascular stroma located in the posterolateral wall of roof of nose where sphenoid process of palatine bone meets horizontal ala of vomer and root of pterygoid process of sphenoid bone [2]. The growth starts in submucosa of nasopharynx and can extend up to nasal septum and posterior space of the nose leading to airway obstruction. If it keeps growing, it can invade sphenoid sinus, nasal fossa, middle turbinate, pterygomaxillary fossa, and maxillary sinus' posterior wall and eventually invades infratemporal fossa and middle cranial fossa [3].

JNA is a highly vascular neoplasm. Primary arterial supply is from internal maxillary artery, a branch of external carotid artery. Other supplying arteries include ascending pharyngeal artery, middle meningeal artery, accessory meningeal artery, and facial artery branches [1].

According to Fisch classification JNA is classified into four types: [3].

P. Goyal (✉)
Narayana Hospital Jaipur, Jaipur, Rajasthan, India

Vaishali
Mahatma Gandhi Medical College, Jaipur, Rajasthan, India

K. Sood Sharma (ed.), *Radiation Therapy for Benign Disorders*,
https://doi.org/10.1007/978-981-95-6635-8_12

Type 1: tumor is restricted to nasal cavity and nasopharynx without bone destruction.
Type 2: tumor invades pterygomaxillary fossa and maxillary, sphenoidal, and ethmoid sinus with bone destruction.
Type 3: tumor invades the infratemporal fossa, the orbit, and the parasellar region but remains lateral to cavernous sinus.
Type 4: tumor invades cavernous sinus, the optic chiasma, and pituitary fossa.

12.2 Pathogenesis

Origin of JNA is not clear. Theories considered are [1] hormonal influence and [2] vascular malformation.

Histologically JNA arises from vascular endothelial cells or fibroblasts. It contains protein basic fibroblast growth factor (bfgf) which shows strong positivity for β-catenin. Sporadic angiofibromas are associated with mutation of CTTNB gene. Expression of vascular growth receptors (VEGFR-2) indicate the vascular nature of JNA.

Adolescent [10-19 year of age] which indicates towards increased levels of androgen production as the root cause. This hormonal influence could lead to proliferation of tissue as well as incidence of recurrence.

Chromosome 17 deletions are seen in JNA. These deletions are associated with TP53 suppressor gene and HER2 oncogene. JNA is also seen in associations with familial adenomatous polyposis (FAP) and Gardner syndrome.

Association of JNA with HPV has also been studied, which showed HPV-specific proteins and DNA in JNA tissue [1].

12.3 Diagnosis

Clinical presentation: it is painless and progressive, and shows unilateral nasal obstruction. It could also present with epistaxis, rhinorrhea, and pain. On examination, firm, friable mass is found in the nasopharynx and nose. It could invade adjacent structures causing further symptoms like impaired Eustachian tube function, facial deformity, proptosis, visual acuity impairment, and even cranial nerve palsy if it invades the intracranial region [3].

JNA is diagnosed based on clinical findings and imaging. Biopsy is not beneficial as it bleeds severely on manipulation [2].

Clinical examination: Nasal endoscopy reveals solid, brittle, reddish-purple formation in nasal passage.

Radiological investigation: X-ray shows forward bowing of the rear wall of the maxillary sinus. Computed tomography shows enhancing soft tissue mass within posterior nasal cavity by sphenopalatine foramen along with extension in nasopharynx, pterygopalatine fossa, and sinuses. Secondary changes like expansion of nasal cavity, pterygopalatine fossa, and forward bowing of the rear wall of maxillary sinus can be seen. In aggressive tumors, bone destruction of the skull base with extension into the intracranial cavity is observed.

On CT angiography, vascularity of the mass can be determined. Cerebral angiography could show vascular score. This can help in preoperative planning for selection of different arteries and their branches for management.

MRI provides better contrast resolution than CT. JNA typically appears heterogeneous, showing intermediate signal intensity on T1-weighted images and intermediate to high intensity on T2-weighted images. Flow voids can be seen on both sequences.

Diffusion-weighted imaging and ADC values generally show evidence of facilitated diffusion, with higher-than-normal ADC readings. MRI shows intense enhancement with gadolinium contrast administration. It also aids in identifying spread into the cavernous sinus, sphenoid sinus, or along nerves through the skull base and into the orbit.

Pathological examination: On gross examination, a rounded, well-defined, unencapsulated mass covered by mucosa is observed. Its color ranges from pale white to pink or wine-red, depending on the lesion's vascularity [3].

Microscopic examination: The lesion consists of a complex mixture of blood vessels and fibrous stroma. The fibrous stroma varies from loose and edematous to dense, acellular, and highly collagenized. Vessel size ranges from capillaries and veins to larger vessels. Capillaries with plump endothelial cell linings are observed at the growing edge of the tumor, while larger vessels are located at the base of the lesion [2].

12.4 Management

The preferred treatment for this condition is surgical resection. Due to the tumor's highly vascular nature, many patients undergo preoperative embolization to reduce the risk of intraoperative bleeding and associated complications. This procedure also allows better identification of the vascular supply, particularly the external and internal carotid artery feeders, which aids in surgical planning.

12.5 Role of Radiation Therapy

In addition to surgical resection, radiation therapy may be used as an adjuvant treatment for residual or recurrent disease. It is primarily considered for advanced tumors involving critical regions or with intracranial extension that may not be fully resectable. The use of radiation therapy remains controversial due to potential long-term morbidity and the risk of secondary neoplasms from high-dose exposure. However, some studies have reported favorable outcomes with primary radiotherapy, making it a viable alternative when complete surgical excision is not feasible. This approach can lead to long-term disease control along with tumor size regression. However, in such cases, a persistent tumor burden can remain a long-term complication of radiation therapy. Several radiotherapy options are available, including stereotactic radiosurgery (e.g., Gamma Knife), intensity-modulated radiotherapy (IMRT) with conformal techniques, and conventional external beam radiotherapy. Reported success rates are generally similar, primarily in advanced-stage disease, though various long-term complications can occur. Postoperative morbidity is also a consideration following radiation therapy. Radiation-induced changes in the surgical bed, including increased tissue friability, can lead to higher morbidity and complications such as delayed cerebrospinal fluid (CSF) leaks with rhinorrhea following surgical resection or stereotactic radiosurgery. Repair of these leaks often necessitates multiple additional endoscopic procedures. Although radiation therapy may cause tumor regression, preoperative radiotherapy can contribute to increased surgical morbidity. Another adjuvant treatment option is hormonal therapy using androgen receptor blockers, such as flutamide. This approach can help reduce tumor size before surgical resection or in cases of recurrence, but it is not curative on its own. Evidence for the use of chemotherapy or other cytotoxic drugs in the management of JNA is limited. More studies are required for the use of cytotoxic drugs as a therapy regimen [1].

12.6 Radiation Technique

External beam radiation is delivered using intensity-modulated radiotherapy (IMRT) with a conformal technique to minimize radiation exposure to adjacent structures such as the optic nerves, optic chiasm, lens, retina, brain, brainstem, spinal cord, and salivary glands compared to conventional radiotherapy. Many studies report typical radiation doses ranging from 30 to 50 Gy, administered in daily fractions of 1.8 to 2 Gy.

Stereotactic radiotherapy or radiosurgery has also been employed, but it is better suited for well-defined residual or recurrent disease. It carries a potentially higher risk of late complications due to the delivery of a single high radiation dose over a concentrated treatment area [1].

Radiation therapy dose: 36 Gy delivered at 1.8 Gy per fraction, with consideration for boosting gross tumor to 45 Gy in selected cases. Patients should be older than 18 years, with no gross tumor involvement of the orbit or cavernous sinus.

Radiation therapy technique: The preferred photon RT approach utilizes multiple non-coplanar fixed beams or segmental arcs. In the fixed-beam method, five beam angles with intensity modulation are employed. For RT simulation, the patient is positioned supine with the head extended so that the orbital floor is perpendicular to the treatment table. Immobilization is achieved using a plastic mask, and an oral stent is employed to displace the tongue inferiorly.

CT simulation is done and images are fused with MRI image for contouring and furthur planning.

CT images are obtained in 3-mm contiguous slices from the skull vertex to mid-neck, and MRI in 1-mm contiguous slices using a T1-weighted sequence (TR 1720 ms, TE 3.4 ms).

Target Definition

- GTV (gross tumor volume): tumor visible on CT and MRI.
- CTV (clinical target volume): includes the entire ipsilateral pterygopalatine fossa and inferior orbital fissure, with a 1.0 cm expansion of the GTV in all directions where there are no anatomical barriers to tumor spread. Regional lymphatics are not included in the CTV.
- PTV (planning target volume): CTV plus 1 mm, accounting for positioning accuracy using cone-beam CT and a real-time surface image-guided stereotactic system.

Target Dose Constraints

- 95% of the PTV should receive 100% of the prescribed dose.
- 99% of the PTV should receive at least 93% of the prescribed dose.
- No more than 20% of the PTV should receive over 110% of the prescribed dose.

Normal Structures: Key structures to contour include the lens, retina, optic nerves, optic chiasm, pituitary, hypothalamus, cochlea, brainstem, and spinal cord.

Normal structure doses are evaluated for PRV where PRV = normal structure plus 1 mm.

Follow-up clinic examination and MR scan: 3 months after completing RT; then every 6 months for 5 years; and then every 5 years thereafter [4].

12.7 Toxicity Profile and Strategies to Minimize Risk

Radiation therapy can cause toxicity leading to various complications. Acute complications include rhinitis, watering of eyes, redness, irritation, and dryness of eye. It can also lead to cataract. Chronic complications include delayed growth due to hypopituitarism, delayed bone maturation, radiation-induced secondary malignancy like sarcomas, basal cell carcinoma, metastatic thyroid carcinoma.

How to minimize these risks:

1. Follow the principle of ALARA.
2. Hot spot and cold spot checks should be done thoroughly.
3. Dose distribution of PTV should be assessed—slice by slice in axial and coronal cuts.
4. Total dose should not be exceeded beyond 50–55 Gy.
5. Following measures should be taken before starting radiation:
   (a) Thorough ophthalmologic examination.
   (b) Eye/nose/ear infection if present should be treated.
   (c) Pituitary hormone (growth hormone) analysis.
6. Long-term follow-ups with imaging and blood analysis should be done.

12.8 Review of Literature

In a study done by Economou et al., patients showed resolution of symptoms after neoadjuvant radiotherapy (78.5%) as compared to patients with surgical resection (76.5%) [5].

Another study by Lee et al., showed that patients treated with primary RT (30–55 Gy) had a local control rate of 85% at 2 years, and external beam radiation therapy represents an effective mode of treatment for patients with advanced JNA [6].

Cummings et al. in their study showed that a single course of external beam megavoltage radiation to 3000 cGy in 3 weeks is an effective first treatment for patients with juvenile nasopharyngeal angiofibroma [7].

Wiatrak et al. studied three cases of large JNAs with extensive intracranial extension that were primarily managed with external beam RT treated with 36.6, 40, and 50.4 Gy with good long-term outcomes concluding that external beam radiation therapy is required in the management of extensive juvenile nasopharyngeal angiofibromas with intracranial extension [8].

In another study done by Reddy et al., 85% of total cases had a complete response on physical examination following radiation therapy concluding that radiotherapy is an effective treatment for advanced JNA [9].

12.9 Future Direction

There is a growing focus on improved and minimally invasive surgical techniques. Research is ongoing on the role of hormone therapy and growth factor receptor inhibitors which may lead to the development of targeted therapy.

12.10 Summary and Conclusion

Juvenile nasal angiofibroma (JNA) is a benign but locally aggressive tumor generally associated with good prognosis.

Origin of juvenile nasal angiofibroma remains unclear, though hormonal influence and vascular malformations are thought to play a significant role.

Diagnosis is primarily based on thorough clinical examination, imaging, and biopsy.

Preop embolization followed by surgical resection is the treatment of choice.

Role of radiation is generally considered in residual disease after R1–R2 resection, unresectable tumors, intracranial extension cases, and medically unfit patients.

References

1. Tork CA, Simpson DL. Nasopharyngeal angiofibroma. StatPearls – NCBI Bookshelf; 2023, June 26. https://www.ncbi.nlm.nih.gov/books/NBK545240.
2. Goldblum JR, Lamps LW, McKenny J, et al., editors. Rosai and Ackerman's surgical pathology. 11th ed. Philadelphia: Elsevier.
3. Makhasana JS, Kulkarni M, Vaze S, Shroff A. Juvenile nasopharyngeal angiofibroma. J Oral Maxillofac Pathol. 2016;20(2):330.
4. Amdur RJ, Yeung AR, Fitzgerald BM, Mancuso AA, Werning JW, Mendenhall WM. Radiotherapy for juvenile nasopharyngeal angiofibroma. Pract Radiat Oncol. 2011;1(4):271–8.
5. Economou TS, Abemayor E, Ward PH. Juvenile nasopharyngeal angiofibroma: an update of the UCLA experience, 1960–1985. Laryngoscope. 1988;98(2):170–5. https://doi.org/10.1288/00005537-198802000-00010.
6. Lee JT, Chen P, Safa A, Juillard G, Calcaterra TC. The role of radiation in the treatment of advanced juvenile angiofibroma. Laryngoscope. 2002;112(7 Pt 1):1213–20. https://doi.org/10.1097/00005537-200207000-00014.
7. Cummings BJ, Blend R, Fitzpatrick P, Clark R, Harwood A, Keane T, et al. Primary radiation therapy for juvenile nasopharyngeal angiofibroma. Laryngoscope. 1984;94:1599–605.
8. Wiatrak BJ, Koopmann CF, Turrisi AT. Radiation therapy as an alternative to surgery in the management of intracranial juvenile nasopharyngeal angiofibroma. Int J Pediatr Otorhinolaryngol. 1993;28(1):51–61. https://doi.org/10.1016/0165-5876(93)90146-t.
9. Reddy KA, Mendenhall WM, Amdur RJ, et al. Long-term results of radiation therapy for juvenile nasopharyngeal angiofibroma. Am J Otolaryngol. 2001;22:172–5.

Salivary Pleomorphic Adenoma

13

Jhanja Mohapatra and Shweta

13.1 Background

Pleomorphic adenoma is the most common salivary gland tumour. Nearly, 85% of salivary gland adenoma arise from parotid gland, 10% from minor salivary gland, and 10% from submandibular gland [1]. Seventy percent of all salivary gland tumours arise from parotid gland, out of which 40% are pleomorphic adenoma [2]. Pleomorphic adenoma was first termed by *Willis*. It is a slow-growing, benign, mixed tumour having dual nature of origin from epithelial and myoepithelial components.

It is more common in females and in younger age group with 46 years as the mean age of presentation [3]. Annual incidence has been reported as 0.02–0.035 cases per 1000 population [3].

Earlier pleomorphic adenoma was managed by local excision or enucleation which led to recurrence, ranging from 20% to 45%. Also, there was a high chance of temporary or permanent facial nerve paralysis in the postoperative period. Treatment then evolved to superficial or total parotidectomy and extracapsular dissection, which resulted in decreased recurrence rate and postoperative complications [4].

Although radiotherapy is not the primary modality of treatment in benign diseases but it is used as an adjuvant therapy dates back to the discovery of X-rays. Key benefits of including radiotherapy in benign diseases include controlling local disease progression, reducing pain and inflammation, preventing or reducing disfigurement, decreasing risk of recurrence, minimizing functional impairments, and improving quality of life.

J. Mohapatra (✉)
Department of Radiotherapy, Dharamshila Narayana Super Speciality Hospital, New Delhi, India

Shweta
Department of Radiotherapy, Max Super Speciality Hospital, Noida, India

K. Sood Sharma (ed.), *Radiation Therapy for Benign Disorders*,
https://doi.org/10.1007/978-981-95-6635-8_13

Radiotherapy acts on cellular level and protein expression leading to reduced cell proliferation, cell death, and inhibition of inflammation.

13.2 Pathogenesis

Parotid gland, located superficial to and partly behind ramus of mandible, is divided into superficial and deep lobes with facial nerve embedded in between and emerging to its five branches. Superficial lobe is the main site of origin of adenomas and sometimes invade the deeper tissues. Exact pathogenesis of pleomorphic adenoma is unknown. But multiple genetic and environmental factors may contribute to the disease. Chromosomal abnormalities of *8q12* and *12q15* leads to expression of genes like *PLAG1* and *HMGA2*, implicated in tumour development [5]. Radiation exposure particularly to head and neck region may trigger the development of tumour. Smoking, alcohol consumption, poor dietary habits, and exposure to carcinogens like asbestos are associated with tumour development. *Simian virus 40 (SV40)* tag sequences have been identified in pleomorphic adenomas [6]. Epithelial mesenchymal transition plays a key role in the progression and development of pleomorphic adenoma. It is the process where epithelial cells transform to mesenchymal cells and contribute to the mixed nature of tumour. Pleomorphic adenomas present as round, well-demarcated, painless, slow-growing mass. At time of presentation, it is usually less than 6 cm in greatest dimension and does not involve facial nerve. Grossly, it appears as an irregular ovoid mass with well-defined borders, sometimes covered by an incomplete fibrous capsule or maybe unencapsulated. On cut section, mass may be rubbery, fleshy, or mucoid interspersed with areas of haemorrhage and infarction [7]. Pleomorphic adenoma has three cellular components: epithelial, myoepithelial, and mesenchymal. Histologically, it shows variable pattern of epithelium and polygonal-shaped myoepithelial cells, with pale eosinophilic cytoplasm, in loose fibrous stroma of myxoid, chondroid, or mucoid type.

Pleomorphic adenoma usually presents as a slow-growing painless lump often in superficial lobe of parotid gland. Mostly, it is asymptomatic but as it grows over many years, it may cause facial nerve involvement leading to difficulty in chewing or swallowing and hearing loss. Rarely, it can also undergo malignant transformation known as *carcinoma ex pleomorphic adenoma*.

Radiation therapy works through a complex of multicellular interaction affecting different cell types. Radiotherapy is effective in inhibiting cell proliferation, suppressing cell differentiation, and modulating inflammatory cascade. Radiation can induce apoptosis by expressing cytokines in macrophages, leukocytes, and endothelial and other cells. Ionizing radiation suppresses T lymphocytes responsible for chronic inflammatory processes, thus reducing inflammation. Radiation leads to modification of immune response and inflammation as well as analgesic effects through modulation of nitric oxide production and oxidative burst in macrophages and granulocytes. Radiation also acts by direct DNA damage leading to tumour cell death.

13.3 Surgical Management of Pleomorphic Adenoma

Surgery is the mainstay of treatment of pleomorphic adenoma.

13.3.1 Types of Surgery [8]

1. *Enucleation of tumour*: It has high risk of recurrence due to microscopic invasion and satellite nodules extending beyond the capsule.
2. *Partial/Superficial Parotidectomy*: Removal of superficial lobe of parotid gland indicated in superficial lobe tumours. It has the advantage of low recurrence rate and facial nerve preservation.
3. *Total Parotidectomy*: Indicated in tumours involving both superficial and deep lobe of parotid. Entire parotid gland is removed with facial nerve preservation.
4. *Radical parotidectomy*: entire gland including facial nerve is removed with simultaneous nerve grafting. It is mostly used when facial nerve is circumferentially involved by malignant tumour or there is already established facial nerve paralysis.
5. *Extracapsular dissection (ECD)*: Indicated in small, mobile, well-encapsulated tumours of superficial lobe of parotid gland. Tumour is removed with a small margin of healthy tissue without dissecting the entire gland. It has a slightly higher risk of recurrence.

13.3.2 Complications of Surgery

The primary complication associated with parotid surgery is temporary or permanent facial nerve paralysis, which can significantly impact the quality of life. Multiple studies have demonstrated a positive correlation between parotidectomy and postoperative facial nerve dysfunction [9]. Another relatively common complication is Frey syndrome. Also, in cases involving recurrent tumours, surgical intervention carries the further risk of inducing malignant transformation into parotid cancer.

13.4 Role of Radiotherapy in Pleomorphic Adenoma

Radiation therapy is one of the important modalities in the treatment of pleomorphic adenoma. It has a major role in postoperative adjuvant setting.

13.4.1 Indications of Postoperative Adjuvant Radiotherapy [10]

1. Residual disease.
2. Close or positive margin.

3. Intraoperative tumour spillage.
4. High-grade tumour.
5. Tumour involving deep lobe of parotid gland.
6. Recurrent disease.

In case of parotid surgery, anatomical proximity to facial nerve branches makes it difficult to get sufficient margin. Pleomorphic adenomas develop a false capsule rather than a true one which can be incomplete or very thin in places, increasing the risk of tumour spillage and microscopic residual disease [11]. There are not much available data regarding definition of safe margin, so 1 mm margin is considered as full integrity of tumour capsule.

Adverse pathology includes ≥3/10 mitoses per high power field, squamous metaplasia, and hypercellularity which increases the risk of recurrence after surgery [12].

Deep lobe of the parotid gland is situated behind the facial nerve which makes it very difficult for surgical access and facial nerve preservation.

Recurrence in pleomorphic adenoma of parotid gland is significantly associated with younger patient age (below 30 years), suboptimal resection (residual disease, positive and uncertain surgical margins, and uncontrolled tumour spillage), and unfavourable histologic characteristics.

Radiotherapy can also be considered in special circumstances where surgery is contraindicated for medical reasons and unresectable tumour.

Radiotherapy being a noninvasive treatment modality can reduce risk of facial nerve damage and recurrence rate. Radiation therapy also has an advantage of minimal cosmetic and functional impairment. Radiation therapy is usually well tolerated, but it has some temporary side effects like xerostomia, altered taste sensation, mucositis, and rare complications such as altered facial sensation, pain in temporomandibular joint, and atrophy of masseter muscle.

13.5 Techniques of Radiation Therapy

Radiation therapy is used as an adjuvant treatment to surgery given after 4–6 weeks of surgery or as definitive therapy in special situations as described above. Radiation therapy can be given either by external beam or interstitial brachytherapy.

For external beam radiotherapy, planning CT scan of head and neck region is obtained, preferably contrast CT scan with 2–3 mm slice thickness and fiducial markers. Patient is positioned supine with proper immobilization method using thermoplastic mask for daily reproducibility of treatment position.

Three-field technique using ipsilateral lateral field and anterior-posterior wedge pair field with an oblique direction to avoid exit dose to orbit and oral cavity is used to treat the parotid compartment [13]. *Field boundaries* (Fig. 13.1) are zygomatic arch superiorly, masseter muscle anteriorly, pterygoid muscle and ramus of mandible laterally, and posterior belly of digastric muscle inferiorly. Disadvantage of angled wedge pair technique (Fig. 13.2) is irradiation of normal tissues in high

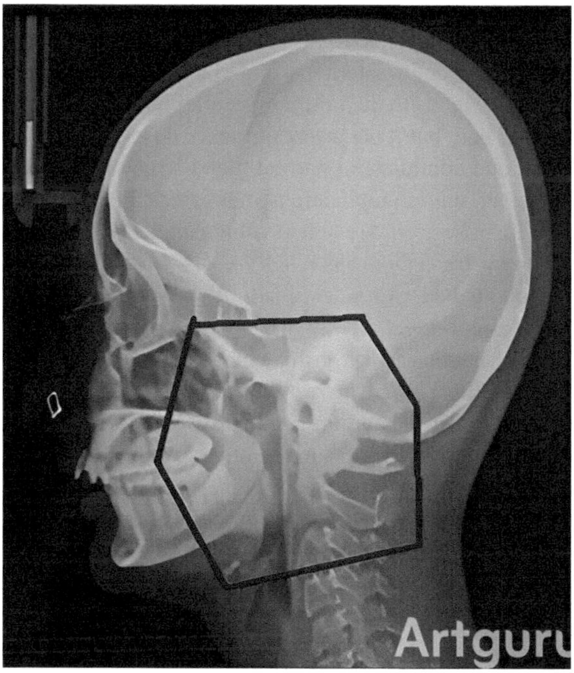

Fig. 13.1 Showing borders of 2D radiation field of parotid gland. (Original image, copyright reserved)

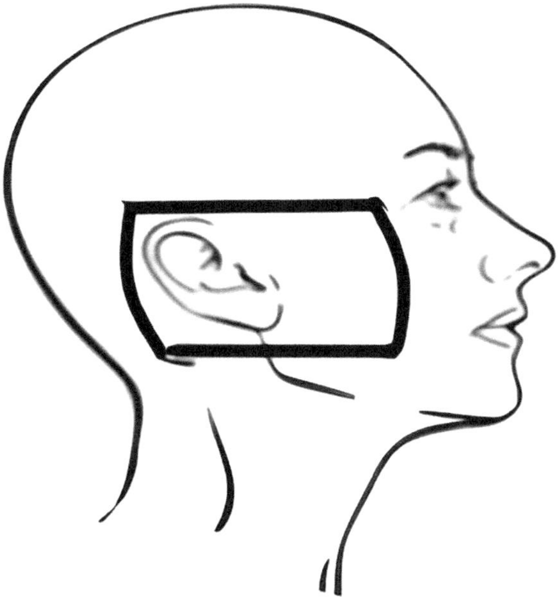

Fig. 13.2 Unilateral wedge pair field technique of photon beam

mastoid and retro-auricular area. To avoid this, combination of high-energy photon and high-energy electron is preferred which produces better dose homogeneity and less dose to contralateral parotid gland (Fig. 13.3). When the tumour involves deep lobe or extends to the midline, parallel photon fields are mandatory for coverage of tumour bed, but it has a risk of higher dose to normal organs like spinal cord, brain stem, and contralateral parotid gland which may lead to long-term complications. To avoid such complications, newer techniques like IMRT or arc therapy using IGRT can be used. Treatment volume includes *tumour bed, parotid compartment, or preoperative GTV + 5 mm margin*. CTV to PTV margin is 3–5 mm. Radiation dose to tumour bed is *50–54Gy with a dose rate of 1.6 to 1.8Gy/fraction* if no gross residual is present, and higher doses up to *60–66Gy in 2Gy per fractions* are used for residual disease or positive margin [10].

Interstitial brachytherapy can be used as monotherapy or as a boost to high-risk areas of positive margin, residual disease, local recurrent tumour, or unresectable disease after external beam radiotherapy. Single plane needle implant for superficial lobe tumour or a modified V plane with deep plane extending to retromandibular area for covering deep lobe of parotid is used. *Total dose of 60Gy is prescribed at 0.5 cm and delivered in 6–7 days* [14].

Dose constraints to be watched for in planning radiation therapy to parotid are:

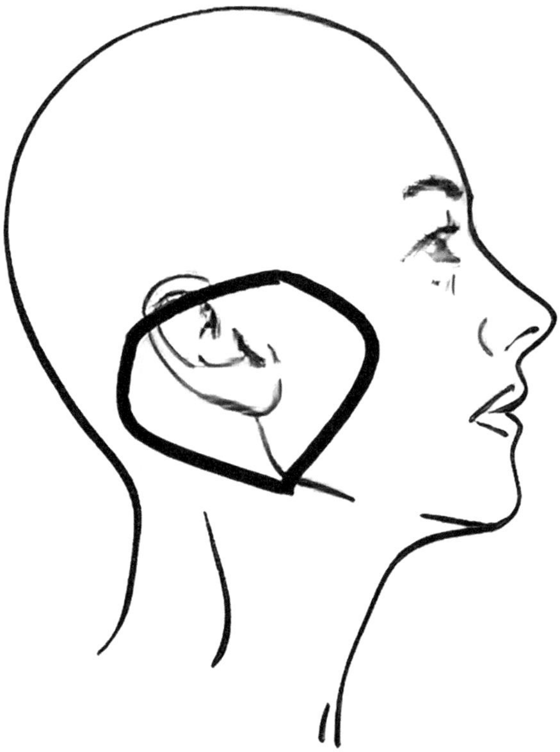

Fig. 13.3 Ipsilateral 16Mev electron plus 4–6MV photon beam field. (Original image, copyright reserved)

Contralateral parotid: Mean dose <20Gy.
Mandible: Max dose <70Gy.
Cochlea: Mean dose <45Gy.
Brain stem: Max dose <54Gy.
Spinal cord: Max dose <45Gy.

13.6 Radiation-Induced Toxicity

Toxicities for radiotherapy to parotid gland can be divided into acute and late.

Acute toxicities are mainly due to the effect of radiotherapy on skin and mucosa which includes dermatitis, mucositis, and xerostomia.

Radiation dermatitis also known as radiation-induced skin reaction is most common and can nearly be avoided. Risk of dermatitis is higher in head and neck cancer and seen in almost all the patients undergoing radiotherapy. Main pathophysiology is damage to the stem cells in the basal layer of skin, resulting in decreased repopulation. Risk increases with increase in volume of skin treated and radiation dose [15] Table 13.1 illustrates radiation induced skin toxicity.

Prevention of dermatitis can be done by avoiding tight clothing, shaving and smoking, reducing sun exposure, using better radiotherapy technique and planning.

Treatment of dermatitis includes using emollients and moisturizer, proper analgesic, early diagnosis and treatment of secondary infection, treatment break if required (mostly in grade III or higher).

Radiation-induced mucositis refers to erythema, oedema, and ulcerations of oral mucosa in patients undergoing radiotherapy. Reason behind this is rapid cellular turnover of basal epithelial layer of oral mucosa, making it susceptible for radiation injury. Oral mucositis leads to pain and decreased oral intake of patient resulting in nutritional deficiencies. This can sometimes be dose limiting [16] (Table 13.2).

Prevention is by pretreatment examination of oral cavity, maintaining oral hygiene, avoiding hot and spicy food, quit smoking and alcohol and using better radiation planning such as IMRT.

Treatment of oral mucositis includes benzydamine mouth gargles, local anaesthetic application, treatment of secondary infections, and pain control using a spectrum of analgesics like topical aspirin and lignocaine, morphine mouth gargles, or Doxepine oral rinses.

Table 13.1 CTCAE grading of radiation dermatitis

Grade 1	Grade 2	Grade 3	Grade 4	Grade 5
Faint erythema or dry desquamation	Moderated brisk erythema; patchy moist desquamation; mostly confined to skin folds and creases; moderate oedema	Moist desquamation in areas other than skin folds and creases; bleeding induced by minor trauma or abrasion	Life-threatening consequences; skin necrosis or ulceration of full thickness dermis; spontaneous bleeding from involved site; skin graft indicated	Death

Adapted from CTCAE version 6

Table 13.2 CTCAE grading of mucositis

Grade 1	Grade 2	Grade 3	Grade 4	Grade 5
Asymptomatic or mild symptoms; intervention not required	Moderate pain or ulcer that does not interfere with oral intake; modified diet indicated	Severe pain; interfering with oral intake	Life threatening consequences; urgent intervention indicated	Death

Adapted from CTCAE version 6

Table 13.3 CTCAE grading of dry mouth (xerostomia)

Grade 1	Grade 2	Grade 3	Grade 4	Grade 5
Symptomatic (e.g. dry or thick saliva) without significant dietary alteration; unstimulated saliva flow >0.2 ml/min	Moderate symptoms; oral intake alteration (e.g. copious water, other lubricants, diet limited to purees, and/or soft, moist food; unstimulated saliva flow 0.1 to 0.2 ml/min)	Impaired oral intake; tube feeding or TPN indicated; unstimulated saliva flow <0.1 ml/min	–	–

Adapted from CTCAE version 6

Xerostomia is the most prominent complication in head and neck radiotherapy due to radiation-induced damage to salivary glands. It alters the consistency, pH, and volume of saliva. 50–60% of decrease in salivary flow is seen in the first week, and after 7 weeks of radiotherapy, salivary flow reduces to approximately 20% [17] (Table 13.3).

Prevention of xerostomia can be done by salivary gland–sparing radiotherapy by focusing the beams better to target volume and reducing unnecessary irradiation to salivary gland. This is feasible by using better techniques such as 3D-CRT or IMRT. Amifostine which acts as a cytoprotectant has been useful in preventing xerostomia.

Treatment of xerostomia includes use of agents to maintain oral hygiene, such as fluoride agents and antimicrobials, saliva substitutes, and sialagogic agents for stimulating remaining gland.

Late toxicities include oedema, pain, altered taste sensation, trismus, hearing loss, osteoradionecrosis of mandible, or temporal bone necrosis [10].

13.7 Review of Literature

A retrospective study conducted by *Barton* et al [14] at Christie hospital, Manchester, included 187 cases of pleomorphic adenoma of parotid gland treated by radiotherapy during the period of 1951–1984. A total of 115 patients were given radiotherapy immediately after surgery and 72 recurrent patients received radiotherapy after resurgery. Radiotherapy was done in form of radium needle implant at the time of surgery and postoperative external beam radiotherapy with a head shell with three-field technique or wedge pair as standard. Median follow-up was 14 years. Of the

115 patients, 1 patient who received radiation immediately after surgery had recurrence. Among them, 41 patients who were given radiotherapy after incomplete clearance had no recurrence. One out of seventy-four patients who had local excision developed recurrence. Nine out of seventy-two recurrent patients who received radiation after surgery developed recurrence. This study concluded that radiotherapy should be given immediately after surgery to reduce recurrence, because in case of recurrent disease, there is risk of increased morbidity and further recurrence.

A study was conducted by *Malgorzata* et al [10] to define the recommendations for radiotherapy in patients with parotid gland pleomorphic adenoma after surgery. This study considered adjuvant radiotherapy in cases of suboptimal resection of primary tumour (residual tumour, intraoperative tumour spillage, closed or positive margin), high-grade tumour, younger age (<30 years), and recurrent disease. Newer techniques like IMRT, IGRT, and arc therapy were recommended with a dose of 50–54 Gy to tumour bed, parotid compartment or preoperative GTV +5 mm margin in case of complete resection of tumour, and 60–66 Gy in case of residual disease or positive margin. Specialized and personalized management of parotid adenoma should be evaluated by a multidisciplinary panel, considering the risk of recurrence and radiation-induced toxicity.

Audrey S. Wallace et al [18] conducted a retrospective study for radiotherapy in pleomorphic adenoma of head and neck at the University of Florida. This study included 25 patients, of whom 19 patients had pleomorphic adenoma of parotid treated by surgery followed by radiotherapy. Median follow-up period was 10.5 years. Radiotherapy was given by either interstitial brachytherapy or external beam. Local control was achieved in 72% of patients. The 5, 10, and 15 years overall local control rates were 76%, 76%, and 68% respectively. Adjuvant radiotherapy should be used in patients presented with positive margin or multinodular recurrence.

A. K. Dawson [19] conducted a study on radiotherapy in recurrent pleomorphic adenoma which included 29 patients treated by excision and postoperative radiotherapy following recurrence. A total of 20 patients were with first recurrence, of whom 18 became free of recurrence. Eight patients had second recurrence following surgery, of whom 50% had no further recurrence. One patient presented after third recurrence and had no further recurrence before death after treatment. This concludes that the use of radiotherapy as an adjuvant to surgery reduces further recurrence rates.

In a study by *Dawson* et al [20] in 1950–1971, 311 patients with primary pleomorphic salivary adenoma of parotid gland were managed with combination of surgery and radiation therapy and followed for up to 10 years. Recurrence rates at 0–5 years and 5–10 years were 1 and 1.5%, respectively. Ten recurrent patients developed benign disease and four patients developed malignant parotid tumours. One tumour was probably radiation induced and other was spontaneous malignant transformation of benign pleomorphic adenoma. This study recommended that pleomorphic adenoma should be primarily treated with surgery, and radiation therapy should be reserved for high-risk and recurrent cases.

Ravindra Yaparpalvi et al [13] compared nine different techniques of radiotherapy in parotid gland tumours:

S. no	Beam energy	No of fields	Beam arrangement
1.	6 MV photon	1	Lateral
2.	12 Mev electron	1	Lateral
3.	16 Mev electron	1	Lateral
4.	6 MV photon & 12 Mev electron	2	Ipsilateral wedge pair
5.	6 MV photon & 16 Mev electron	2	Ipsilateral wedge pair
6.	18 MV photon & 20 Mev electron	2	Ipsilateral
7.	18 MV photon & 20 Mev electron	2	Ipsilateral (different weightage)
8.	6 MV photon	2	Ipsilateral oblique
9.	6 MV photon	3	AP/PA/lateral

Doses were calculated using 3D radiotherapy planning system and, dose volume histograms (DVH) were calculated for target area coverage and determination of dose to organs at risk (OARs). This study concluded that the ipsilateral wedge-pair, the three-field, and the mixed electron-photon beam techniques are optimal unilateral treatment techniques for parotid gland tumours.

13.8 Future Directions

Radiation therapy plays a significant role in the adjuvant treatment and management of recurrent pleomorphic adenoma. However, its clinical benefits are often accompanied by notable toxicities, such as xerostomia and mucositis, due to scattered dose to the contralateral parotid gland and adjacent mucosal structures.

Proton beam therapy (PBT) has emerged as a promising alternative, primarily due to its Bragg peak property, which allows for sharp dose fall-off beyond the tumour target. This physical characteristic enables better sparing of surrounding organs at risk (OARs), including the oral cavity, sublingual glands, and the contralateral parotid gland [21].

Studies evaluating the use of proton therapy in major salivary gland malignancies have demonstrated favourable outcomes, including effective tumour control and reduced rates of acute toxicities. These findings support the potential application of proton therapy in pleomorphic adenoma.

Given its dosimetric advantages and early clinical evidence, proton beam therapy may be a valuable modality for selected cases of pleomorphic adenoma, especially where traditional photon therapy poses a high risk of toxicity to adjacent critical structures.

Radiotherapy for inoperable salivary gland tumours is often technically challenging due to the complex patterns of tumour spread and the proximity to critical structures such as the facial nerve, mandible, and brainstem. In cases of recurrent tumours, reirradiation with conventional photon therapy offers a limited therapeutic window, making it difficult to deliver a tumoricidal dose without exceeding the tolerance levels of surrounding healthy tissues. However, several studies have shown that high linear energy transfer (LET) radiation modalities, such as *neutron therapy and carbon ion therapy*, may help overcome these limitations by providing superior biological effectiveness and better dose conformity [22, 23].

Use of *artificial intelligence (AI)* is increasing in radiotherapy in head and neck cancer. It helps the clinician to reduce treatment planning time and improve plan quality. The ultimate goal is to improve patient outcomes by tailoring therapies to individual needs and enhance patient outcome.

13.9 Conclusion

Pleomorphic adenoma is the most common benign tumour of the salivary glands. It is a slow-growing lesion with a risk of recurrence following primary treatment and, in rare cases, may undergo malignant transformation. The primary treatment is surgical excision, typically performed via superficial or total parotidectomy. Adjuvant radiotherapy may be considered in high-risk cases, such as those involving high-grade histology, incomplete resection, intraoperative tumour spillage, or deep lobe involvement, to reduce the risk of recurrence. In cases of recurrent disease, surgical intervention becomes more challenging, making radiotherapy a more favourable option. Radiotherapy can be administered through either interstitial needle implantation or external beam radiotherapy (EBRT). With advancements in techniques such as intensity-modulated radiotherapy (IMRT) and arc therapy, radiation treatment has become more precise and better tolerated, with reduced side effects. Furthermore, high linear energy transfer (LET) radiation modalities such as proton beam therapy, carbon ion therapy, and neutron therapy offer superior dose distribution and the potential for decreased toxicity, especially in complex or radioresistant cases.

References

1. Almeslet AS. Pleomorphic adenoma: a systematic review. Int J Clin Pediatr Dent. 2020;13(3):284.
2. Spiro RH. Salivary neoplasms: overview of a 35-year experience with 2,807 patients. Head Neck Surg. 1986;8(3):177–84.
3. Bokhari MR, Greene J. Pleomorphic adenoma.
4. Guerra G, Testa D, Montagnani S, Tafuri D, Salzano FA, Rocca A, Amato B, Salzano G, Orabona GD, Piombino P, Motta G. Surgical management of pleomorphic adenoma of parotid gland in elderly patients: role of morphological features. Int J Surg. 2014;(12):S12–6.
5. Debnath SC, Adhyapok AK. Pleomorphic adenoma (benign mixed tumour) of the minor salivary glands of the upper lip. J Maxillofac Oral Surg. 2010;9:205–8.
6. Martinelli M, Martini F, Rinaldi E, Caramanico L, Magri E, Grandi E, Carinci F, Pastore A, Tognon M. Simian virus 40 sequences and expression of the viral large T antigen oncoprotein in human pleomorphic adenomas of parotid glands. Am J Pathol. 2002;161(4):1127–33.
7. Asha MN, Mutgi A, Sujith MS. The world's biggest benign Parotid Tumour 'pleomorphic adenoma': a rare case report. IOSR J Dent Med Sci. 2014;13(2):8–12.
8. Quer M, Guntinas-Lichius O, Marchal F, Vander Poorten V, Chevalier D, León X, Eisele D, Dulguerov P. Classification of parotidectomies: a proposal of the European Salivary Gland Society. Eur Arch Otorrinolaringol. 2016;273:3307–12.

9. Kadletz L, Grasl S, Grasl MC, Perisanidis C, Erovic BM. Extracapsular dissection versus superficial parotidectomy in benign parotid gland tumors: the Vienna Medical School experience. Head Neck. 2017;39(2):356–60.
10. Wierzbicka M, Fijuth J, Składowski K, Jurkiewicz D, Burduk P, Miłoński J, Niemczyk K, Pietruszewska W, Rogowski M, Stodulski D, Mikaszewski B. Adjuvant radiotherapy in parotid gland pleomorhic adenoma–recommendation. Otolaryngol Pol. 2022;76(5)
11. Wong WK, Shetty S. Classification of parotidectomy: a proposed modification to the European Salivary Gland Society classification system. Eur Arch Otorrinolaringol. 2017;274(8):3175–81.
12. Alzumaili B, Xu B, Saliba M, Abuhashem A, Ganly I, Ghossein R, Katabi N. Clinicopathologic characteristics and prognostic factors of primary and recurrent pleomorphic adenoma: a single institution retrospective study of 705 cases. Am J Surg Pathol. 2022;46(6):854–62.
13. Yaparpalvi R, Fontenla DP, Tyerech SK, Boselli LR, Beitler JJ. Parotid gland tumors: a comparison of postoperative radiotherapy techniques using three dimensional (3D) dose distributions and dose-volume histograms (DVHS). Int J Radiat Oncol Biol Phys. 1998;40(1):43–9.
14. Barton J, Slevin NJ, Gleave EN. Radiotherapy for pleomorphic adenoma of the parotid gland. Int J Radiat Oncol Biol Phys. 1992;22(5):925–8.
15. Pazdrowski J, Gornowicz-Porowska J, Kaźmierska J, Krajka-Kuźniak V, Polanska A, Masternak M, Szewczyk M, Golusiński W, Danczak-Pazdrowska A. Radiation-induced skin injury in the head and neck region: pathogenesis, clinics, prevention, treatment considerations and proposal for management algorithm. Rep Pract Oncol Radiother. 2024;29(3):373–90.
16. Bell A, Kasi A. Oral mucositis. In StatPearls [Internet]. StatPearls Publishing; 2023 May 29.
17. Dirix P, Nuyts S, Van den Bogaert W. Radiation-induced xerostomia in patients with head and neck cancer: a literature review. Cancer. 2006;107(11):2525–34.
18. Wallace AS, Morris CG, Kirwan JM, Werning JW, Mendenhall WM. Radiotherapy for pleomorphic adenoma. Am J Otolaryngol. 2013;34(1):36–40.
19. Dawson AK. Radiation therapy in recurrent pleomorphic adenoma of the parotid. Int J Radiat Oncol Biol Phys. 1989;16(3):819–21.
20. Dawson AK, Orr JA. Long-term results of local excision and radiotherapy in pleomorphic adenoma of the parotid. Int J Radiat Oncol Biol Phys. 1985;11(3):451–5.
21. Hanania AN, Zhang X, Gunn GB, Rosenthal DI, Garden AS, Fuller CD, Phan J, Reddy JP, Moreno A, Chronowski G, Shah S. Proton therapy for major salivary gland cancer: clinical outcomes. Int J Part Ther. 2021;8(1):261–72.
22. Douglas JG, Einck J, Austin-Seymour M, Koh WJ, Laramore GE. Neutron radiotherapy for recurrent pleomorphic adenomas of major salivary glands. Head Neck. 2001;23(12):1037–42.
23. Vischioni B, Dhanireddy B, Severo C, Bonora M, Ronchi S, Vitolo V, Fiore MR, D'Ippolito E, Petrucci R, Barcellini A, Ciurlia E. Reirradiation of salivary gland tumors with carbon ion radiotherapy at CNAO. Radiother Oncol. 2020;145:172–7.

14 Neurofibromas

Pooja Nandwani Patel and Rahul Misra

14.1 Background

Neurofibromas are benign tumors that are made up of multiple cells. These cells include Schwann cells, fibroblasts, mast cells, perineural cells, macrophages, and T cells [1, 2]. Neurofibromas can occur in the skin, soft tissue, and nerves and roughly present as solitary lesions in 90% of cases. Multiple neurofibromas may be part of syndromes like neurofibromatosis-1 or NF-1 [3], and they need to be managed accordingly.

Usually, the general treatment approach for neurofibromas has been observation until they are symptomatic or can potentially lead to severe damage or cosmetic disturbances. The most common treatment for neurofibromas has been surgery where feasible. However, there have been few case reports on the use of radiation in neurofibromas. The main reason behind limited use has been the side effects associated with conventional radiation techniques used historically. However, with newer techniques like three-dimensional conformal radiotherapy (3DCRT), intensity-modulated radiation therapy (IMRT), stereotactic radiosurgery (SRS), and proton therapy, side effects to normal tissue can be avoided, allowing radiation treatment to stand as a valid alternative option. Another new advance has been research into the molecular background of neurofibromas leading to the use of newer drugs like MEK inhibitors which seem to have a promising future.

One of the reasons for renewed interest in radiotherapy has been the advancements in technology which can help in controlling the disease in a noninvasive manner with lesser morbidity as compared to surgery in certain conditions.

P. Nandwani Patel (✉)
Department of Radiation Oncology, Sterling Hospitals, Ahmedabad, India

R. Misra
Department of Radiation Oncology, Wockhardt Hospitals, Rajkot, India

K. Sood Sharma (ed.), *Radiation Therapy for Benign Disorders*,
https://doi.org/10.1007/978-981-95-6635-8_14

14.2 Pathogenesis

Neurofibromas have a tendency to appear after puberty. Benign neurofibromas are usually seen with Von Recklinghausen disease (neurofibromatosis type 1 [NF1]) or sometimes seen sporadically also. Von Recklinghausen described this as an autosomal dominant disorder with defect on chromosome 17 [4]. Mostly, the age of presentation is in childhood and patients have numerous cutaneous or subcutaneous neurofibromas, melanotic lesions in the iris known as Lisch nodule, café au lait spots, and freckling of skin folds. In addition, children with NF1 can present with optic gliomas and astrocytoms in very early years of their life [5]. Certain osseous lesions such as sphenoid wing dysplasia and scoliosis also occur as part of the NF1 syndrome. Most adolescents and adults later on develop dermal and plexiform neurofibromas and rarely manifest to malignant peripheral nerve sheath tumor (MPNST). Leukemias and pheochromocytomas are more likely to occur in patients with NF1 [6]. There are no known predictive factors to determine the number or types of cutaneous neurofibromas in a patient with NF1. In fact there is a strong variability in cutaneous neurofibromas burden even between members of a family harboring the same NF1 mutation. There is some retrospective evidence to suggest that there is an increase in burden of cutaneous neurofibromas during pregnancy. This suggests that neurofibromas may have a hormone responsive element.

People with NF1 mutation have also been reported to have low serum vitamin D levels, but it is still not clear that these factors are causative or correlative. Schwann cells may be the primary causative cells behind neurofibromas, as in these cells there is loss of both NF1 alleles. There is no clear consensus regarding classification system for neurofibromas. These benign tumors also have different morphological characteristics, can occur as sporadically or multiple, and have different growth rates also. A commonly used classification system divides neurofibromas into five different types.

1. Localized cutaneous neurofibromas: These are the most common type of neurofibromas, seen commonly in patients with NF1, occur at multiple locations, and are mostly slow growing in nature [1, 3].
2. Localized intraneural neurofibroma: This is the second most common neurofibroma seen, and the most common site of location is cervical spine.
3. Diffuse cutaneous neurofibromas: These neurofibromas mostly involve the dermis and subcutaneous tissue. The most common site of presentation is head and neck region, and these are many of the times indolent in behavior [7].
4. Plexiform neurofibromas: These neurofibromas are the least common, are usually component of NF1, and rarely occur sporadically [1, 8]. These neurofibromas have the highest chance of malignant transformation. These tumors grow as focal growths or may extend longitudinally along the nerves and involve multiple nerve fascicles.
5. Soft tissue neurofibroma: These neurofibromas are unusual types of all neurofibromas and are rarely seen as component of NF1. These tumors cause cosmetic issues as they infiltrate soft tissues and muscles. They were previously also known as elephantiasis neurofibromatosis [1, 7].

14.3 Role of Radiation Therapy (RT) and Radiation Technique

Many neurofibromas do not require treatment. However, when they lead to cosmetic issues or may cause compression of nerve roots leading to symptoms or may have malignant transformation, surgery is usually the treatment of choice. In adulthood, neurofibromas may also gradually disappear on their own without treatment and their rate of growth also slows down. This has been demonstrated by a prospective study of 47 adults with NF1 [9]. Radiation therapy has mainly been used in case of recurrent disease or when surgery carries excessive morbidity. However, there have been some recent case reports of using SRS/ SBRT in the treatment of neurofibromas. One other factor preventing the use of radiotherapy is the recent evidence that MEK inhibitors may offer a good treatment alternative for certain types of neurofibromas.

Most studies have used conventional external beam radiotherapy (EBRT) [10–12]. Some studies have used brachytherapy and intraoperative radiotherapy [13]. Recent studies have used SRS [14, 15] in the treatment of neurofibromas with doses ranging from 10 to 24 Gy and median dose of 12 Gy. Conventional postop RT has been used post-surgery in doses ranging between 45 and 54 Gy. However, sometimes these doses have been boosted to 72 Gy using radium needle implants.

14.4 Toxicity Profile and Strategies to Minimize Risks

The role of radiation therapy has not been majorly tested in historic times with conventional radiation machines which were not very precise and carried a serious risk of side effects. With improved technology radiation, treatment was explored with the use of newer techniques like three-dimensional conformal radiotherapy (3DCRT) and stereotactic radiosurgery (SRS) limiting dose to normal tissue. Chopra et al [14] reported that the patients did not develop any major treatment-related complications. Robertson et al [10] reported that the patient tolerated treatment well and experienced only mild xerostomia, taste deficit, and dysarthria. His dysarthria improved with speech therapy while his xerostomia and taste deficits improved subjectively over the first year after treatment.

14.5 Review of Literature and Case Studies

Most of the studies discuss about the spontaneous regression of neurofibromas. The management of neurofibroma will depend on many factors including growth, location, symptoms if any, or any cosmetic disturbances. However, when treatment is required, surgery has most commonly been used. There have been some targeted medicines attempted but mostly still are many investigational. Radiotherapy mostly has been used in cases where the tumors are unresectable or are producing symptoms. Some studies have used SRS in radical setting and conventional RT in the adjuvant setting.

In 1975, Russell and Suit et al [13] treated one patient with neurofibroma with surgery followed by EBRT at a dose of 46 Gy followed by brachytherapy with radium implant at a dose of 26 Gy. The patient was tumor-free 2 years post-treatment. In 1981, Greenberg et al [11] treated three patients with neurofibroma with hyperfractionated RT at doses ranging from 48.4 Gy to 64 Gy. Two out of three patients had their disease controlled. Patients who received 48.4 Gy had limitations of pushing further dose because of close proximity of spinal cord. In 1984, Smalley et al [12] used a combination of EBRT and intraoperative RT to treat a case of neurofibroma. The patient had relief of discomfort and developed metastases 10 months postradiation treatment. 20 months post radiation treatment while still on chemotherapy the patient had local control.

In 2005, Chopra et al [14] treated four patients with neurofibroma with radiation therapy. The first patient, 41-year-old female, had plexiform neurofibroma at orbit and maxillary sinus. The tumor was excised four times and then radiation option was explored with dose of 50 Gy in 30 fractions, one fraction daily, five days a week. With follow-up even after 14.8 years, the disease was under control. The second patient was a 9-year-old female child with plexiform neurofibroma at parapharyngeal space and was diagnosed case of NF1. She was operated twice and then received radiation therapy with 50.4 Gy in 42 fractions; twice daily fractionation was given. At follow-up of 7.9 years, the patient died because of intercurrent disease. The third patient was a 24-year-old female with neurofibroma tumor with myxoid features located at long thoracic nerve. Surgery was attempted twice followed by radiation therapy with dose of 50 Gy in 30 fractions, one fraction daily, five days a week. Even at 13.3 years of follow–up, the disease was under control. The fourth patient was a 12-year-old male child with neurofibroma at spinal cord C3 region. Subtotal resection was done followed by stereotactic radiosurgery (SRS) radiation treatment of 12.5 Gy in one single session. At 1.7 years of follow-up, the tumor showed no relapse.

Suit et al [13] treated a case of neurofibroma located in the neck region with 75 Gy with disease controlled at follow-up. In 2009, Wentworth et al [15] treated six patients with SRS with doses ranging from 10 Gy to 24 Gy. Five year progression-free survival was 100 percent. Roberston et al [10] shared his experience of treating neurofibroma presenting at base of tongue region. The biopsy was suggestive of plexiform neurofibroma and he was a high risk case for surgery . Hence taking into consideration the post surgical morbidities, option of radiation treatment was explored. Patient was planned with three-dimensional conformal radiation therapy (3DCRT) with five fields targeting the base of tongue lesion with 60 Gy in 30 fractions. Patient has great relief from local pain at lesion site with minimal transient xerostomia. In subsequent follow-ups with radiographic examinations including magnetic resonance images, the disease remained in control at 3 years. This was the first case where unlike radiation treatment being explored in adjuvant setting, radiotherapy was given in upfront setting considering the risks and morbidities associated with surgery. Many new studies talk about the role of MEK inhibitors in treating neurofibromas [16].

14.6 Future Directions

With handful of case reports exploring the role of radiation with good local control rates and taking advantage of better targeted machines and techniques like three-dimensional conformal radiotherapy (3DCRT), intensity-modulated radiation treatment (IMRT), stereotactic radiosurgery (SRS), and proton therapy, better results can be expected as more dose can be pushed without much damage to nearby normal structures. Research into the molecular basis behind neurofibromas may also hold a promising future. Role of MEK inhibitors also holds a promising future.

14.7 Conclusion

The management of neurofibromas depends on various factors like symptoms, location, and growth pattern of these tumors. Treatment is usually advocated because of discomfort or cosmetic disturbances with surgery being the first preference of choice. With tumors relapsing after surgery or incomplete excision or difficult locations, radiation therapy with advanced conformal techniques can be explored. MEK inhibitors are gaining ground. However more work needs to be done in the field of treating neurofibromas with newer techniques like SRS and Proton.

References

1. Woodruff JM. Pathology of major peripheral nerve sheath neoplasms. In: Weiss SW, Brooks JSJ, editors. Soft tissue tumors. Baltimore: Lippincott Williams & Wilkins; 1996. p. 129–61.
2. Lott IT, Richardson EP. Neuropathological findings and the biology of neurofibromatosis. Adv Neurol. 1981;29:23–32.
3. Scheithauer BW, Woodruff JM, Erlandson RA. Tumors of the peripheral nervous system. In: Rosai JR, Sobin LH, editors. Atlas of tumor pathology. 3rd ed. Washington, DC: Armed Forces Institute of Pathology; 1999.
4. Cawthon RM, Weiss R, Xu GF, et al. A major segment of the neurofibromatosis type 1 gene: cDNA sequence, genomic structure and point mutations. Cell. 1990;62:193–201.
5. Listernick R, Charrow J, Greenwald MJ, et al. Natural history of optic pathway tumors in children with neurofibromatosis type 1: longitudinal study. J Pediatr. 1994;125:63–6.
6. Gutmann D. The neurofibromatoses: when less is more. Hum Mol Genet. 2001;10:747–55.
7. Freidman JM, Gutmann DH, MacCollin M, et al. Neurofibromatosis: phenotype, natural history and pathogenesis, 3rd ed. Baltimore: Johns Hopkins Press; 1999.
8. Korf BR. Plexiform neurofibromas. Am J Med Genet. 1999;89:31–7.
9. Merker VL, Cai W, Bredella MA, Muzikansky A, Thalheimer RD, Herr HP, Morris ME, Chang CY, Harris GJ, Plotkin SR, Jordan JT. Ten-year follow-up of internal neurofibroma growth behavior in adult patients with neurofibromatosis type 1 using whole-body MRI. Neurology. 2023;100(7):e661. Epub 2022 Nov 4.
10. Robertson TC, Buck DA, Schmidt-Ullrich R, et al. Isolated plexiform neurofibroma: treatment with three-dimensional conformal radiotherapy. Laryngoscope. 2004;114:1139–42.
11. Greenberg HM, Goebel R, Weichselbaum RR, et al. Radiation therapy in the treatment of aggressive fibromatosis. Int J Radiat Oncol Biol Phys. 1981;7:305–10.

12. Smalley SR, Rubin J, Leifermann KM. Neuro-fibrosarcoma and the sign of Leser-Trelat. CA Cancer J Clin. 1984;34:295–8.
13. Suit HD, Russell WO. Radiation therapy of soft tissue sarcoma. Cancer. 1975;36:759–64.
14. Chopra R, Morris CG, Friedman W, Mendenhall W. Radiotherapy and radiosurgery for benign neurofibromas. Am J Clin Oncol. 2005;28(3):317–20.
15. Wentworth S, et al. Clinical experience with radiation therapy in the management of neurofibromatosis-associated central nervous system tumors. Int J Radiat Oncol Biol Phys. 2009;73(1):208–13.
16. Dombi E, et al. Activity of selumetinib in neurofibromatosis type 1-related plexiform neurofibromas. N Engl J Med. 2016;375(26):2550–60.

Pterygium

15

Manisha Himthani and Nikhat Anjum

15.1 Background

Pterygium is a chronic, degenerative, and often recurrent ocular surface disease characterized by the invasion of fibrovascular tissue from the conjunctiva onto the cornea. It typically presents in individuals with high exposure to solar ultraviolet (UV) radiation [1], wind, and environmental irritants such as dust and smoke. This condition is more prevalent in equatorial and subtropical regions, earning it the colloquial designation "surfer's eye" [2]. Epidemiological studies estimate prevalence rates ranging from 2% to 30%, with a marked male predilection likely due to occupational and outdoor exposure patterns (Image 15.1).

Historically, the surgical excision of pterygium using the bare sclera technique was widely practiced. However, its efficacy was limited by high recurrence rates, reported as high as 30–89%. The recognition of these recurrence patterns led to the incorporation of adjunctive therapies, including conjunctival autografting (Image 15.2), limbal conjunctival transplantation, and the intraoperative or postoperative use of antimetabolites such as mitomycin C (MMC).

Despite their efficacy, each of these approaches carries risks, ranging from surgical complexity and extended operative times to significant ocular complications like scleral melting and cataract formation.

Radiation therapy, particularly in the form of localized beta-irradiation, emerged as a potential adjunctive or alternative treatment for pterygium. The first clinical applications of radiotherapy for pterygium date back to the 1950s [3]. Over the

M. Himthani (✉)
Department of Radiation Oncology, Dharamshila Narayana Super Speciality Hospital, New Delhi, India

N. Anjum
iCare eye Hospital, Noida, Uttar Pradesh, India

K. Sood Sharma (ed.), *Radiation Therapy for Benign Disorders*,
https://doi.org/10.1007/978-981-95-6635-8_15

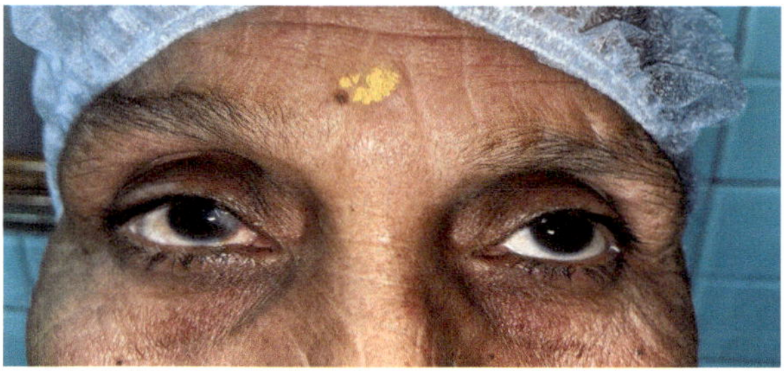

Image 15.1 A 74-year-old female with pterygium of right eye originating from nasal conjunctiva partially encroaching cornea. (Original image copyright protected ©)

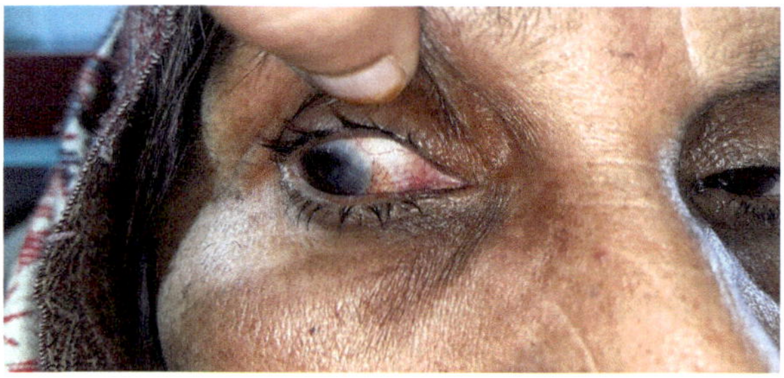

Image 15.2 Postsurgical excision with clear corneal and limbal conjunctival autograft in place (Surgeon: Dr. Nikhat Anjum). (Original image copyright protected ©)

decades, the technique has evolved, and its safety and efficacy have been reinforced through numerous studies and clinical experiences. The simplicity of application, minimal patient discomfort, and favorable long-term outcomes have made radiation therapy an asset in comprehensive pterygium management.

15.2 Pathogenesis

The pathogenesis of pterygium is multifactorial, with chronic exposure to ultraviolet (UV) radiation being the most consistent etiologic factor. UVB radiation is particularly damaging, initiating a cascade of events including oxidative stress, DNA damage, and induction of pro-inflammatory mediators. These factors synergistically disrupt the normal ocular surface architecture, primarily the limbal barrier, allowing for conjunctival tissue migration and subsequent corneal invasion.

Histologically, pterygium tissue reveals a complex interplay of epithelial hyperplasia, stromal fibrovascular proliferation, elastotic degeneration, and chronic inflammatory cell infiltration. The breakdown of the limbal stem cell niche is thought to be critical, leading to conjunctivalization of the cornea. Studies have demonstrated overexpression of key growth factors such as vascular endothelial growth factor (VEGF), basic fibroblast growth factor (bFGF), transforming growth factor-beta (TGF-β), and matrix metalloproteinases (MMPs), all of which contribute to angiogenesis, fibroblast activation, and extracellular matrix remodeling.

In recent years, the role of bone marrow-derived progenitor cells has also been implicated. Immunohistochemical analyses reveal the expression of stem cell markers including CD34 and c-Kit in pterygium tissue, suggesting a reparative yet pathologic cellular recruitment in response to chronic injury. Additionally, anti-apoptotic proteins such as surviving and cyclooxygenase-2 (COX-2) have been found to be upregulated in pterygium samples, indicating that resistance to programmed cell death may also play a role in lesion persistence and recurrence.

Radiation therapy exerts its therapeutic effect by interfering with these molecular and cellular processes. Beta-irradiation using Strontium-90 results in localized ionization, causing direct DNA damage and cell cycle arrest, particularly in rapidly dividing cells like fibroblasts and endothelial cells. This results in reduced cellular proliferation, suppression of angiogenesis, and modulation of the inflammatory milieu, thereby arresting disease progression and preventing recurrence.

15.3 Role of Radiation Therapy

Radiation therapy plays a crucial role in reducing the recurrence of pterygium post-surgery. It is particularly effective when administered as early postoperative adjuvant therapy, ideally within 24–48 h of surgical excision. The rationale is to target the proliferative phase of wound healing, thereby suppressing fibrovascular ingrowth and recurrence.

Indications for radiation therapy in pterygium include:

- Primary pterygium in high-risk individuals (younger age, extensive lesion, high UV exposure)
- Recurrent pterygium with previous failed surgical attempts
- Contraindications to antimetabolites like MMC (e.g., allergy, thin sclera, poor ocular surface)
- Limited access to skilled ophthalmic surgeons capable of performing conjunctival or limbal grafting

Beta-irradiation offers several advantages over other adjuvant modalities. Unlike MMC, which has a risk profile including secondary glaucoma, scleromalacia, and endophthalmitis, radiation is associated with minimal long-term toxicity when applied correctly. Compared to autografting, radiation is less resource-intensive, requires minimal surgical expertise, and is more reproducible across different settings.

Radiation therapy is not without limitations. It requires specialized equipment and trained personnel. Additionally, the long-term carcinogenic potential, although not substantiated in ophthalmologic applications, remains a theoretical concern, particularly in younger patients. Therefore, careful patient selection and adherence to standardized dosing protocols are essential.

In recent years, radiation therapy has also been explored as a primary treatment modality in select cases where surgery is contraindicated. In such scenarios, although complete lesion regression may not occur, significant symptomatic relief and lesion stabilization have been reported.

15.4 Radiation Technique

The preferred modality of radiation in pterygium treatment is beta-irradiation using Strontium-90 (90Sr), a pure beta-emitting radionuclide with a half-life of 28.8 years (Image 15.3). 90Sr decays to yttrium-90, which also emits beta particles, providing a dual source of localized radiation.

The treatment is delivered via a handheld applicator—typically a concave disc or plane source with diameters ranging from 10 to 23 mm (Image 15.4). The applicator is gently placed over the surgically exposed scleral bed, ensuring direct contact with the treatment area. Beta particles from 90Sr have a maximum tissue penetration of 2–3 mm and negligible depth beyond 5 mm, which makes them ideal for superficial ocular lesions while sparing intraocular structures.

Dose and fractionation schedules vary, with commonly adopted regimens including:

- 30 Gy in 3 fractions (10 Gy per fraction on alternate days) [4]
- 35 Gy in 5–7 fractions over 10–14 days [5]
- 60 Gy in 6 weekly fractions [6]

Most protocols emphasize the importance of initiating radiation within 24 h post-excision to achieve maximal therapeutic benefit. Immobilization is achieved using eyelid retractors, and anesthesia is generally not required. Treatments are quick, painless, and can be conducted in an outpatient setting.

Shielding of adjacent ocular structures such as the lens is paramount to avoid long-term complications like cataract formation. Dosimetry is typically

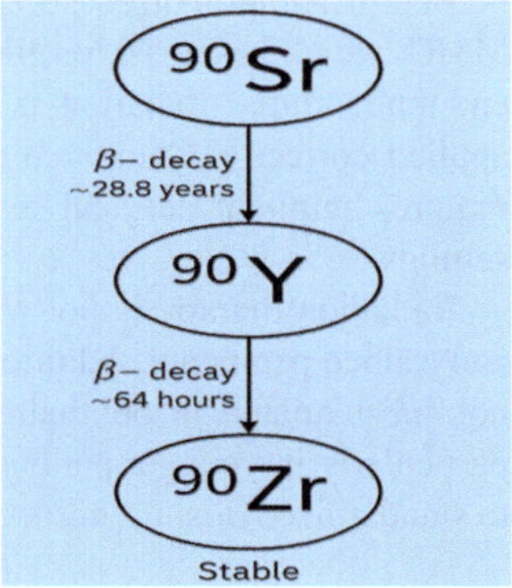

Image 15.3 Decay level scheme of Sr-90. (Original image copyright protected ©)

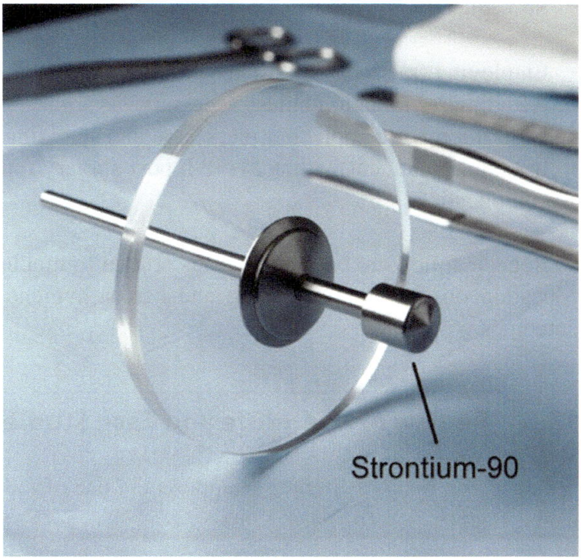

Image 15.4 Schematic representation of Strontium 90 eye applicator

surface-based, and modern applicators are pre-calibrated, reducing inter-operator variability. Accurate placement and consistency in duration and dose delivery are vital for achieving desired clinical outcomes.

15.5 Toxicity Profile and Strategies to Minimize Risks

When performed with adherence to recommended protocols, radiation therapy for pterygium is associated with a favorable safety profile. However, like any therapeutic intervention, it carries potential risks.

Common acute side effects include:

- Transient conjunctival hyperemia
- Mild ocular discomfort or foreign body sensation
- Watery eyes and photophobia

Late complications are rare but may include:

- Scleral thinning or dellen
- Conjunctival granuloma
- Cataract formation (especially with improper shielding or excessive dose)
- Scleromalacia in cases of reirradiation or high single-dose applications

Strategies to mitigate these risks include:

- Employing fractionated dosing schedules rather than single high doses
- Avoiding reirradiation unless necessary
- Ensuring precise applicator placement and shielding
- Initiating treatment within 24–48 h post-surgery for optimal efficacy and lower complications

Regular follow-up post-radiation is crucial to monitor for late sequelae. Patient education on symptom reporting and ocular hygiene further supports favorable outcomes.

15.6 Review of Literature and Case Studies

A substantial body of literature supports the use of radiation therapy in pterygium management:

- *Paryani et al.* (1994): Treated 825 lesions with 60 Gy in 6 weekly fractions. Recurrence was reported in only 1.7% of cases, with no major long-term complications.
- *Ali et al.* (2011): A systematic review of over 6000 cases across 17 studies revealed recurrence rates generally below 15% when radiation was initiated within 3 days postoperatively.
- *Viani et al.* (2012): Demonstrated 90% and 88% local control at 5 and 10 years, respectively, with a 35 Gy/7 fraction regimen, and minimal toxicity [5].
- *Isohashi et al.* (2007): Analyzed 1253 cases and concluded that initiating radiation within 48 h of surgery offered superior local control (above 90%) with minimal side effects [7].
- *Eng et al.* (2020): Reaffirmed the utility of beta-irradiation in benign ocular diseases, citing it as one of the most effective modalities in preventing recurrence of pterygium [8].

Randomized studies, such as those by Jürgenliemk-Schulz et al. [9] and Nakamatsu et al. [10], compared different fractionation regimens and validated the safety and efficacy of low to moderate dose radiation therapy. Notably, these trials also emphasized the importance of treatment timing, with earlier intervention correlating with better outcomes.

15.7 Future Directions

The landscape of radiation therapy in ophthalmology is poised for innovation. Several avenues are being explored:

- *Miniaturized and custom-contoured applicators*: These promise better conformity to irregular ocular surfaces, enhancing dose precision.
- *Integration with molecular therapies*: Combining radiation with anti-VEGF agents or COX-2 inhibitors could enhance therapeutic efficacy while reducing recurrence.
- *Artificial Intelligence (AI)*: AI-driven tools could assist in patient selection, recurrence risk stratification, and personalized dose planning.
- *Radio genomics*: Understanding genetic predisposition and molecular markers may guide individualized radiation protocols and predict response.

Proton therapy and stereotactic techniques, although promising, remain impractical for superficial lesions like pterygium due to high costs and logistical constraints. However, their precision offers potential applications in complex or recurrent ocular tumors, setting the stage for translational research in benign conditions.

15.8 Conclusion

Radiation therapy, especially using beta-irradiation with Strontium-90, remains an effective, safe, and accessible adjunct in the management of pterygium. It substantially reduces recurrence rates when appropriately timed and dosed. As a noninvasive outpatient procedure, it offers an excellent alternative in resource-limited settings and in patients unsuitable for other adjuvant therapies. With ongoing technological advancements and a deeper understanding of pterygium biology, radiation therapy is poised to play an even more refined role in ocular surface disorder management.

References

1. Zhou WP, Zhu YF, Zhang B, Qiu WY, Yao YF. The role of ultraviolet radiation in the pathogenesis of pterygia. Mol Med Rep. 2016;14(1):3–15.
2. Ding P, Wang R, He Y. Risk factors for pterygium: latest research progress on major pathogenesis. Exp Eye Res. 2024;243:109900.
3. Ali AM, Thariat J, Bensadoun RJ, Thyss A, Rostom Y, El-Haddad S, Gérard JP. The role of radiotherapy in the treatment of pterygium: a review of the literature including more than 6000 treated lesions. Cancer/Radiothérapie. 2011;15(2):140–7.
4. De Keizer RJ. Pterygium excision with free conjunctival autograft (FCG) versus postoperative strontium 90 (90Sr) beta-irradiation. A prospective study. Int Ophthalmol. 1997;21:335–41.
5. Viani GA, Stefano EJ, De Fendi LI, Fonseca EC. Long-term results and prognostic factors of fractionated strontium-90 eye applicator for pterygium. Int J Radiat Oncol Biol Phys. 2008;72(4):1174–9.
6. Paryani SB, Scott WP, Wells JJW, Johnson DW, Chobe RJ, Kuruvilla A, Schoeppel S, Deshmukh A, North Florida Pterygium Study Group. Management of pterygium with surgery and radiation therapy. Int J Radiat Oncol Biol Phys. 1994;28(1):101–3.

7. Isohashi F, Inoue T, Xing S, Eren CB, Ozeki S, Inoue T. Postoperative irradiation for pterygium. Strahlenther Onkol. 2006;182(8):437.
8. Eng TY, Abugideiri M, Chen TW, Madden N, Morgan T, Tanenbaum D, Wandrey N, Westergaard S, Xu K, Sudmeier LJ. Radiation therapy for benign disease: keloids, macular degeneration, orbital pseudotumor, pterygium, peyronie disease, trigeminal neuralgia. Hematology/Oncol Clin. 2020;34(1):229–51.
9. Jürgenliemk-Schulz IM, Hartman LJ, Roesink JM, Tersteeg RJ, van Der Tweel I, Kal HB, Mourits MP, Wyrdeman HK. Prevention of pterygium recurrence by postoperative single-dose β-irradiation: a prospective randomized clinical double-blind trial. Int J Radiat Oncol Biol Phys. 2004;59(4):1138–47.
10. Nakamatsu K, Nishimura Y, Kanamori S, Koike R, Tachibana I, Nishikawa T, Shibata T. Eine randomisierte klinische Studie zur postoperativen Strontium-90-Strahlentherapie für Pterygien: 30 Gy/3 Fraktionen versus 40 Gy/4 Fraktionen: treatment using 30 Gy/3 fractions vs. 40 Gy/4 fractions. Strahlenther Onkol. 2011;187:401–5.

Choroidal Haemangioma

16

Manisha Himthani and Nikhat Anjum

16.1 Background

Choroidal haemangiomas are benign vascular hamartomas arising from the choroidal vasculature. They are broadly classified into circumscribed and diffuse types, with the latter often associated with Sturge-Weber syndrome (Image 16.1) [1]. Although histologically benign, they may impair vision through subretinal fluid accumulation, exudative retinal detachment, or macular oedema (Image 16.2).

The true prevalence is unknown due to many asymptomatic cases, but symptomatic lesions are typically diagnosed in the second to fourth decades of life, with no gender predilection.

Historically, treatments ranged from observation to laser photocoagulation, transpupillary thermotherapy (TTT), and photodynamic therapy (PDT). However, each of these has limitations in treating deep lesions or those involving critical visual structures.

Radiation therapy entered the treatment landscape in the late twentieth century, initially via external beam radiotherapy and later through more targeted methods like plaque brachytherapy and proton beam therapy. The rationale lies in RT's ability to cause vascular sclerosis, reduce exudation, and stabilize or improve vision, while preserving the globe and ocular structures [2]. Its success in managing uveal melanomas also paved the way for use in benign ocular conditions, particularly when other modalities are insufficient or pose a higher risk.

M. Himthani (✉)
Department of Radiation Oncology, Dharamshila Narayana Super Speciality Hospital, New Delhi, India

N. Anjum
iCare eye hospital, Noida, Uttar Pradesh, India

K. Sood Sharma (ed.), *Radiation Therapy for Benign Disorders*, https://doi.org/10.1007/978-981-95-6635-8_16

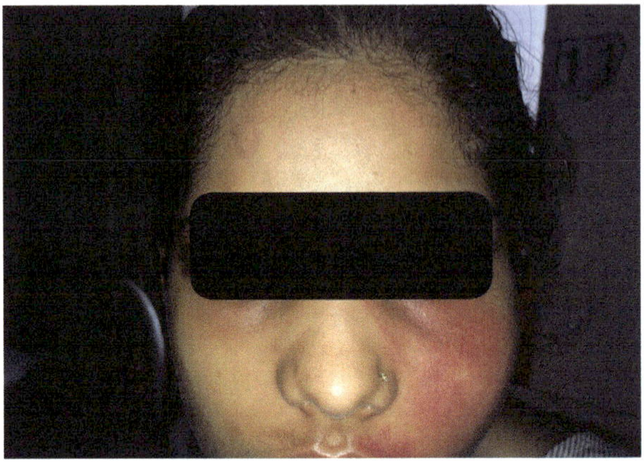

Image 16.1 Sturge-Weber syndrome triad: Port-wine stain (typically one side of the face); neurological symptoms: seizures, developmental delays; ocular involvement: glaucoma, choroidal haemangiomas. (Original photo: Copyright protected ©)

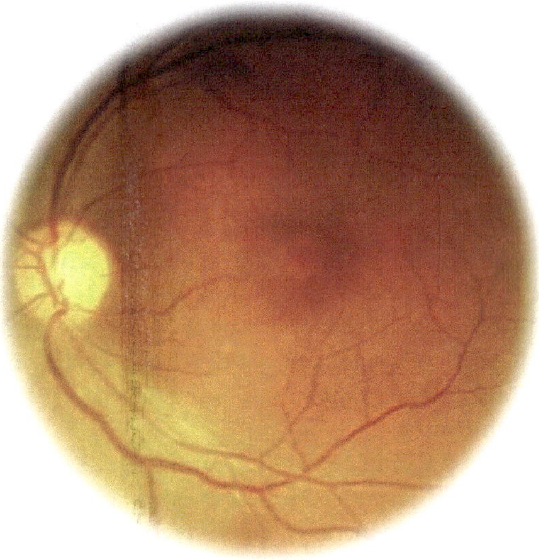

Image 16.2 Fundoscopy image of choroidal haemangioma

16.2 Pathogenesis

Choroidal haemangiomas consist of vascular channels lined by endothelium, lacking the atypia seen in malignancies [3]. The circumscribed variant typically involves the posterior pole, whereas diffuse haemangiomas are often present from birth and progress gradually.

At a molecular level, increased expression of angiogenic factors such as vascular endothelial growth factor (VEGF) contributes to vascular permeability and exudation. Secondary changes in the retinal pigment epithelium and outer retina result from chronic subretinal fluid, leading to irreversible vision loss if untreated.

Radiation therapy acts through vascular endothelial damage and subsequent occlusion of abnormal vessels. Ionizing radiation induces DNA damage in endothelial cells, leading to apoptosis and vessel wall fibrosis. This results in decreased exudation and stabilization of the retinal architecture. RT also reduces inflammatory cytokines and VEGF expression, contributing to the resolution of retinal detachment.

This mechanism is particularly beneficial in cases where photodynamic therapy fails or is contraindicated due to tumour location or recurrence. RT's ability to target deeper vascular layers without significant collateral damage makes it ideal for choroidal lesions near the fovea or optic nerve.

Thus, the role of radiation in modulating the tumour microenvironment—not just tumour size—forms the cornerstone of its therapeutic utility in choroidal haemangiomas.

16.3 Role of Radiation Therapy (RT)

Radiation therapy is indicated for visually threatening or symptomatic choroidal haemangiomas, particularly when [2]:

- There is persistent or recurrent subretinal fluid.
- Lesions are not responsive to PDT, TTT, or anti-VEGF therapy.
- Tumours are located close to the macula or optic disc.
- Other modalities are contraindicated due to systemic or ocular comorbidities.

Advantages of RT

- Deep tissue penetration without the need for direct access
- Precision delivery minimizing toxicity.
- Globe- and vision-preserving outcomes

Plaque Brachytherapy Performed using isotopes like Ru-106 or I-125, is the most used method. It allows targeted high-dose delivery while sparing adjacent normal tissues. Studies report resolution of exudation and visual improvement in 60–80% of patients. Image 16.3 shows applicator illustration used for plaque brachytherapy [4].

Proton Beam Therapy (PBT), with its Bragg peak property, enables high-dose delivery conforming to the tumour shape with minimal exit dose, ideal for posterior pole lesions. PBT has demonstrated excellent tumour control and low toxicity in large retrospective cohorts.

External Beam Radiotherapy (EBRT), including stereotactic radiotherapy, is another option. CyberKnife and Gamma Knife offer noninvasive, outpatient-based precision RT suitable for select patients.

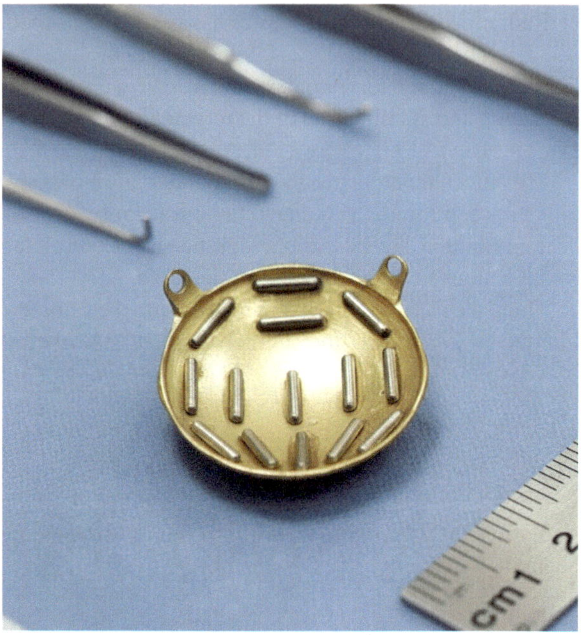

Image 16.3 Schematic representation of episcleral plaque brachytherapy applicator with I^{125} seeds

Patient selection is crucial. Candidates for RT include:

- Tumours >3 mm in thickness or >6 mm in diameter
- Lesions causing symptomatic serous retinal detachment
- Failed response to or contraindication for PDT or TTT

Limitations and Challenges

- Delayed onset of response; visual recovery may take months.
- Radiation-related toxicities, though rare, can include radiation retinopathy, optic neuropathy, and cataracts.
- Access to specialized techniques like PBT may be limited.

Overall, RT remains a valuable tool in the multimodal approach to managing choroidal haemangiomas, especially for recalcitrant or centrally located tumours.

16.4 Radiation Techniques

Plaque Brachytherapy Involves surgical placement of a radioactive plaque over the sclera adjacent to the tumor. Immobilization is achieved with conjunctival sutures. Treatment duration ranges from 2 to 5 days. Preoperative ultrasound aids in tumour localization and dosimetry [4].

Proton Beam Therapy Immobilization is ensured with a customized head frame. CT- or MRI-based planning is used to delineate tumour extent. Doses typically range between 20 and 30 Gy (RBE) in 4–5 fractions. Eye tracking systems may be employed to manage ocular motion [5].

Stereotactic Radiotherapy (SRS/SRT) Systems like CyberKnife use real-time image guidance. Doses of 16–20 Gy in 1–3 fractions have been effective. Immobilization uses thermoplastic masks with bite blocks or eye fixation targets [6].

Dose and Fractionation
- Plaque brachytherapy: 40–60 Gy to the apex
- PBT: 20–30 Gy in 4–5 fractions
- SRS: 16–20 Gy in 1–3 fractions [7, 8]
- IMRT: 20 Gy in 10 fractions [9]

Normal Tissue Constraints Dose to optic nerve <10–12 Gy, lens <5–8 Gy, and retina <30 Gy to minimize retinopathy.

Special Considerations Eye motion during therapy can impact dosimetric accuracy. Use of retrobulbar anaesthesia or ocular fixation methods can improve targeting precision.

16.5 Toxicity Profile and Strategies to Minimize Risks

Radiation therapy for choroidal haemangiomas is generally well tolerated. Common toxicities include:

- *Radiation retinopathy*: May present months to years post-therapy; managed with intravitreal anti-VEGF injections.
- *Optic neuropathy*: Risk increases with proximity and higher dose; dose constraint adherence critical.
- *Cataracts*: Especially with anterior segment dose >8 Gy; modern techniques help minimize exposure.
- *Dry eye and keratitis*: Rare, associated with EBRT.

Minimization Strategies
- Precise dosimetry and image-guided therapy
- Conformal techniques like PBT or SRT for posterior lesions
- Regular follow-up with ophthalmologic exams and OCT to detect early changes
- Use of shielding and strict dose constraints during planning

16.6 Review of Literature

Multiple retrospective series have demonstrated the efficacy of RT:

- *Shields et al.* reported 85% resolution of subretinal fluid and visual stabilization in 78% of patients with I-125 brachytherapy [10].
- *Kocsis et al.*: This retrospective review analysed 15 patients with DCH treated with custom-designed I-125 plaque, yielding significant outcomes. 73% of patients saw complete resolution of subretinal fluid within 9 months, while tumour thickness reduced by 47% over an average follow-up of 27 months. Visual acuity improved or remained stable for 69% of patients, with minimal radiotherapy side effects observed. Plaque brachytherapy proved effective for local treatment without DCH recurrence [11].
- *Proton therapy studies* from Harvard and France noted tumour control rates exceeding 95% with minimal complications.
- *CyberKnife studies* showed resolution of exudation with improved or stable vision in majority of patients [12].
- Long-term data confirms sustained tumour control and acceptable toxicity profiles, particularly when modern planning and delivery techniques are used.

16.7 Future Directions

Advancements in radiation delivery such as adaptive radiotherapy and eye-tracking-based SRS promise enhanced precision. *Proton arc therapy* is under exploration to further conform dose [13].

AI and Radiomics may assist in tumuor characterization and response prediction, aiding personalized treatment.

Research Gaps include optimal dose-fractionation, head-to-head comparison with PDT, and long-term toxicity surveillance.

Emerging Indications RT may be considered earlier in management, particularly for macula-threatening lesions or in settings where PDT is ineffective.

16.8 Conclusion

Radiation therapy represents a safe and effective option for managing symptomatic choroidal haemangiomas, especially in cases unresponsive to conventional therapy or involving critical visual structures. Techniques such as plaque brachytherapy and proton therapy offer precise, globe-sparing treatment with promising outcomes. With advances in imaging, delivery systems, and personalized approaches, radiation therapy is poised to expand its role in benign ocular tumours. Collaborative, multidisciplinary evaluation and individualized treatment planning remain crucial for optimal results.

References

1. Karimi S, Nourinia R, Mashayekhi A. Circumscribed choroidal hemangioma. J Ophthalmic Vis Res. 2015;10(3):320.
2. Finger PT. Radiation therapy for exudative choroidal hemangioma. Indian J Ophthalmol. 2019;67(5):579–81.
3. Witschel H, Font RL. Hemangioma of the choroid. A clinicopathologic study of 71 cases and a review of the literature. Surv Ophthalmol. 1976;20(6):415–31.
4. Chao AN, Shields CL, Shields JA, Krema H. Plaque radiotherapy for choroidal hemangioma with total retinal detachment and iris neovascularization. Retina. 2001;21(6):682–4.
5. Levy-Gabriel C, Lumbroso-Le Rouic L, Plancher C, Dendale R, Delacroix S, Asselain B, Habrand JL, Desjardins L. Long-term results of low-dose proton beam therapy for circumscribed choroidal hemangiomas. Retina. 2009;29(2):170–5.
6. Yarovaya V, Golanov A, Yarovoy A, Kostjuchenko V, Loginov R, Lestrovaya A. Gamma Knife radiosurgery in eyes with diffuse choroidal hemangioma (Sturge-Weber syndrome) as a rescue treatment. J Radiosurg SBRT. 2022;8
7. Augsburger JJ, Freire J, Bradyb LW. Radiation therapy for choroidal and retinal Hemangiomas[1]. Radiother Ocular Dis. 1997;30:265–80.
8. Kim YT, Kang SW, Lee JI. Gamma knife radiosurgery for choroidal hemangioma. Int J Radiat Oncol Biol Phys. 2011;81(5):1399–404.
9. Ufondu A, Oakey Z, Puthussery JC, Cherian S, Singh AD. Diffuse choroidal hemangioma: IMRT versus episcleral plaque brachytherapy. Taiwan J Ophthalmol. 2025;15(1):109–13.
10. Mashayekhi A, Shields CL. Circumscribed choroidal hemangioma. Curr Opin Ophthalmol. 2003;14(3):142–9.
11. Kocsis J, Komarnicky LT, Emrich J, Shields C. Management of diffuse choroidal hemangioma with plaque brachytherapy. Int J Radiat Oncol Biol Phys. 2019;105(1):E632.
12. Kaliki S, Shields CL. Recent trends in ocular oncology. Oman J Ophthalmol. 2011;4(3):103–4.
13. Puthussery JC, Ufondu A, Cherian S, Singh AD. Diffuse choroidal hemangioma: ophthalmic outcomes following intensity-modulated radiation therapy. Taiwan J Ophthalmol. 2025;15(1):103–8.

17 Pseudotumor Orbitae

Sobhana Vallabhaneni

17.1 Introduction

Pseudotumor orbitae is a spectrum of non-specific non-cancerous inflammatory processes of the orbit. It was first described by Birch-Hirschfeld, a renowned German pathologist, in 1905 under "idiopathic orbital inflammatory syndrome" or "nonspecific orbital inflammation." In 1954, Umiker et al. changed the name to "inflammatory pseudotumor" as the presentation and findings closely resembled a malignant tumor [1].

It is more prevalent in the adult population and less commonly seen in children. The mean age at diagnosis is 44 years (range 4–80 years) [2]. There is no gender or ethnic predilection seen in orbital pseudotumor. Onset is usually insidious, progressing gradually over weeks to months [3]. NSOI accounts for ~10% of all orbital tumors and is the third most common ophthalmologic disease of the orbit, following Graves ophthalmopathy and orbital lymphoma [3]. Etiology is still unknown, hence the name idiopathic orbital inflammatory syndrome, but may be attributed to infections, autoimmune conditions, or improper wound healing [4]. There is some association between orbital pseudotumor and Group B *Streptococcus* infection, causing Streptococcal pharyngitis, and *Borrelia burgdorferi* infections.

17.2 Role of Radiation in Benign Diseases

The role of radiation in the management of benign disease differs significantly from the management of malignancies. Within the benign diseases, the effect of radiation has a different pathophysiology for different conditions [5].

S. Vallabhaneni (✉)
Radiation Oncology, Max Superspeciality Hospital, Saket, New Delhi, India

K. Sood Sharma (ed.), *Radiation Therapy for Benign Disorders*,
https://doi.org/10.1007/978-981-95-6635-8_17

Radiation can exert its effects on benign conditions in one of the following ways or a combination of these [5]:

1. Antiproliferative effects of radiation, e.g., heterotopic ossificans (doses >10 Gy).
2. Anti-inflammatory and analgesic effects, e.g.,: osteoarthritis, ankylosing spondylitis (doses 2–6 Gy).
3. Functional radiation effects modulating responses of the autonomic nervous system or interfering with gene activation processes (doses <2 Gy).

In the management of pseudotumor orbitae, radiation exerts an anti-inflammatory effect. The initial effect of radiation is a stress response that will then trigger a chain of events to regulate the inflammatory response [5].

17.3 Clinical Manifestations and Diagnosis

Inflammation seen in NSOI can be localized or diffuse. In localized NSOI, can affect extraocular muscles, lacrimal glands, sclera, uvea, superior orbital fissure or cavernous sinus. Involvement of orbital fatty tissues makes it a diffuse process [6]. The presentation may be heterogeneous and varied, making diagnosis very difficult. It may range from orbital myositis, dacryoadenitis, scleritis, uveitis to Tolosa-Hunt syndrome. Tolosa-Hunt syndrome is characterized by episodic orbital pain due to involvement of III, IV, or VI cranial nerves in the cavernous sinus due to any cause. The most common presenting symptom in a patient with pseudotumor orbitae is proptosis, followed by a palpable mass, eyelid swelling, and restricted eye movements [2]. A typical patient of NSOI presents with pain, erythema, edema, chemosis, and a distinct sensitivity to corticosteroid treatment with responses reported as early as 1–2 days. However, both the presentation and response to steroids are significantly variable and are not considered for establishing a diagnosis of pseudotumor orbitae [7].

Orbital pseudotumor is a diagnosis of exclusion. Before concluding it as NSOI, it is of critical importance to rule out all the other known causes, as an orbital malignant tumor might also have a similar presentation. The diagnostic investigation of choice is magnetic resonance imaging (MRI). The most common radiologic finding is mass within the orbit (50%), dacryoadenitis (29%), myositis (8%), perineuritis (4%), eyelid pseudotumor (4%), and diffuse orbital inflammation (4%) [3]. Biopsy for histopathological confirmation is not done routinely as the risks of the procedure outweigh the benefits. Biopsy is preferred in specific conditions, such as multiple recurrences or unresponsive to standard therapy [8].

Histologically, there is a pleomorphic cellular infiltrate admixed with fibrous tissue reaction. There is a vast heterogeneity in the presentation, ranging from granulomatous inflammation to non-granulomatous inflammation, fibrosis, or a combination of all these [8]. The presence of granulomatous infiltrate needs to be differentiated from sarcoidosis or Wegener's granulomatosis.

Many times, the distinction between orbital pseudotumor and lymphoproliferative disorders of the eye cannot be made with histology alone and might need additional investigations like immunophenotyping and molecular analyses for better characterization of the condition [8]. Hence, the diagnosis of pseudotumor orbitae is made after thorough history, examination, and a battery of investigations and after ruling out the common and malignant ophthalmic conditions [7].

Systemic manifestations are often seen associated with orbital pseudotumor, including other autoimmune conditions like rheumatoid arthritis, systemic lupus erythematous, Crohn's disease, and giant cell myocarditis. Cases of giant cell myocarditis and orbital myositis are reported in the literature. It is important to differentiate it from more serious conditions like orbital rhabdomyosarcoma, Ewing's sarcoma, chronic recurrent multifocal osteomyelitis (CROM) and SAPHO (synovitis, acne, pustulosis, hyperostosis, osteitis) [4, 7]. There is co-existing sinusitis in 17.2% of cases, the majority being maxillary sinusitis in a study that speculated sinusitis as a cause for pseudotumor orbitae [2].

17.4 Treatment

17.4.1 First-Line Treatment

A systematic approach and comprehensive treatment plan will help in the management of this rare ophthalmologic condition [9].

In case of mild inflammation in NSOI, observation is a reasonable option as a few of them resolve spontaneously. Additional therapy is needed if there is no resolution within 6 months or if there is worsening of symptoms. Swamy et al. identified a maintained remission in only 20.8% [2] of patients at 6 months in their study of 24 patients with mild NSOI [10].

Similarly, Mannor et al. observed that NSAIDs can be used for mild NSOI for as long as 3 weeks if clinical improvement is noted [11].

Gold standard treatment for NSOI is corticosteroids, with greater than 75% showing tremendous responses within 24–48 h of administration [7, 12]. They are usually reserved for moderate to severe cases or those cases that do not respond to conservative management. They are highly efficacious due to their dual anti-inflammatory and immunosuppressive effects. A corticosteroid-responsive orbital tumor is more likely to be a pseudotumor [7]. It is recommended for an extended taper, as shorter tapering schedules are associated with early relapses. Doses range between 1 and 1.5 mg/kg or 50 and 100 mg/day for 1–2 weeks. It is extremely important to follow prophylaxis for gastroesophageal reflux disease (GERD), insomnia, mood changes, etc., during a prolonged steroid course [12].

Corticosteroids showed significant responses in the acute relief of symptoms in pseudotumor orbit in ~75% of the patients, but the response lasted only in 30–35% of the patients. Hence, low-dose radiation was used to consolidate and maintain the response.

17.4.2 Role of Radiation

In a retrospective review of 65 patients (90 eyes) over 10 years by Yuen et al., systemic steroids with slow taper proved to be the first line of treatment for pseudotumor orbitae. While 64% of patients showed complete relief in symptoms, 37% of patients had recurrence after a period of quiescence or had refractory symptoms despite the use of first-line therapy [12].

In this study, the majority of the cases were constituted by dacryoadenitis, followed by isolated myositis [12]. This study elucidated the need for searching alternative options to systemic steroids for the management of pseudotumor orbitae.

External beam radiation is reserved for cases refractory or intolerant to steroid therapy. The literature shows variable response of pseudotumor orbitae with the use of radiation, ranging between 50% and 100% in some studies. Radiation dose utilized is also highly variable, but all the studies used low-dose radiation ranging in between 20 and 30 Gy.

In one of the earliest studies on NSOI by Sergott et al. in 1981, 19 patients (21 orbits) were treated with low-dose supervoltage radiation of 10–20 Gy. All the patients were either not eligible to receive steroids or had progression during the tapering of steroids. At a mean follow-up of 25 months, greater than 90% of patients were free of any recurrences [13].

In a study by Orcutt et al. in 1983, 22 patients (24 orbits) were treated with radiation, and all of them, except 1 patient, were treated with a C0–60 unit. One other patient was treated with 250 kV X-rays. All the patients received 25 Gy in 12 fractions at 2.08 Gy/fraction over 16 days. The cornea was shielded using a 1.5 cm diameter lead disc in all the patients. A total of 18 patients (19 orbits) received steroids before radiation. Anterior and lateral wedged fields were used in treatment with a corneal shield in the anterior field for extraconal orbital pseudotumor. Intraconal orbital pseudotumor was treated with a single lateral field or a wedged superolateral or an inferolateral field [14].

Full response with complete recovery and no residual signs was seen in 46% (11 orbits). Partial response, termed as adequate by the patients with some residual, was seen in 29% (7 orbits). In total, 25% (6 orbits) had no response to radiation. Responses were seen as early as 3.2 months in a large number of patients. Full and partial responses were durable until a median of 22.3 months (1–50 months). There were no complications seen except for progression of a preexisting cataract in one of the patients [14].

A retrospective review of pseudotumor orbitae with low-dose radiation, mean 20 Gy, showed 81% of patients who had complete or partial response, while 18% had no long-term control after radiation. This study concluded that radiation is an effective option for the management of acute symptoms and achieving long-term control in pseudotumor orbitae [15].

A total of 20 patients with orbital pseudotumor between 1971 and 2012 were treated with definitive low-dose radiotherapy. At a median follow-up of 8 years,

75% of patients had symptomatic improvement, 40% showed complete response, and 35% showed a partial response. Major toxicities observed were cataracts and dry eye. Local control rates at 5 years and 10 years were 63% and 53%, respectively. Therefore, they concluded that radiation is well tolerated and results in long-term control in a majority of the patients and a durable local control in greater than 50% of the patients [16].

Low-dose radiation ranging between 4-36Gy (median dose 21Gy) delivered to 241 patients with pseudotumor orbitae from 1978 to 2018 using conventional fractionation showed varying response rates between 74% and 100% and a median recurrence rate of 10% in a systematic review by Fionda et al including a total of 19 studies [17].

These studies suggest that radiation can be used for the treatment of pseudotumor orbitae in those patients who have relapsed or have a refractory disease after the use of steroids and those who have medical contraindications to prolonged use of steroids, like diabetes mellitus or peptic ulcer disease. Doses ranging between 4 and 36 Gy with conventional fractionation were used in the literature, with local control between 67% and 100%. There was no dose-response relationship that could be established, but understanding the etiology as inflammation, low doses would be sufficient to achieve a response and maintain a durable control. There is evidence to suggest alternate histologies of pseudotumor, like sclerosing, granulomatous or necrotizing, or a malignant etiology if a presumed orbital pseudotumor does not respond to radiation doses greater than 30 Gy [18].

17.4.3 Radiation Technique

Patients are immobilized with a head mask. 3D treatment planning is done in this position. There is evidence for the use of both megavoltage photons and electrons for treatment. The technique to be used depends on the location of the tumor to provide uniform coverage of the involved orbit while sparing the uninvolved globe and orbit. The ipsilateral lens is shielded with a lead block. Wedge pair technique with photons or a single angled lateral field can be used for retrobulbar lesions. Angled lateral field helps in preventing irradiation of the opposite lens [19].

Linear accelerators can help in the delivery of asymmetric beams from different angles, achieving the target dose and efficiently sparing the surrounding organs at risk. Target volume delineation plays an important role in radiation delivery using intensity-modulated radiotherapy (IMRT) or volumetric modulated arc therapy (VMAT).

MRI post-contrast T1-weighted images are registered with the planning CT, and gross tumor volume (GTV) is delineated. A 3 mm margin is added to the GTV to develop a clinical target volume (CTV). An additional 3 mm margin is added to the CTV to account for set-up uncertainties to form the planning target volume. The mean lens doses using these techniques were 5.4 Gy [20].

17.4.4 Toxicities

The acute or chronic toxicities of using radiation in benign conditions like pseudotumor orbitae are insignificant. Acute toxicities can be seen in the form of dry eyes with dose to lacrimal glands exceeding 25–30 Gy, conjunctivitis, and erythema of skin. They are self-limiting and resolve after completion of radiotherapy. Due to the low doses of radiation used, long-term toxicities are highly unlikely. Cataracts are the only anticipated long-term complication with lens doses exceeding Dmax 9–11.5 Gy. The optic nerve and retina have a tolerance of >50 Gy with conventional fractionation and, hence, are not affected by low-dose anti-inflammatory doses of radiation. There exists ~1% theoretical risk of developing radiation-induced second malignancies in the long term; however, none have been reported until now in the literature [19].

17.4.5 Alternate Treatment Options

There are small case series and retrospective data available in the literature that have shown the use of immunosuppressants like calcineurin inhibitors (cyclosporine, tacrolimus), cytotoxic agents like azathioprine, cyclophosphamide, and methotrexate, specific biologic agents like adalimumab, infliximab, rituximab, etc., and intravenous immunoglobulins (IVIG) for the management of NSOI with very limited or negligible immediate or long-term benefit.

A specific clinicopathologic entity named idiopathic sclerosing inflammation of the orbit can lead to significant ocular morbidity due to primary, chronic, and immunologic-mediated fibrosis. It exhibits a poor response to steroids and external beam radiation. In one of the studies by Rootman et al., including 16 patients with this histology, early and aggressive immunotherapy is recommended to achieve some control [21].

17.4.6 Surgery

Surgical resection is not the primary treatment of choice in patients with orbital pseudotumor due to its diffuse nature and involvement of vital structures. The only indication of surgery with exenteration in a histologically confirmed case of orbital pseudotumor is incessant pain or blindness that has failed all other treatment options.

17.5 Conclusion

Orbital pseudotumor is a rare non-neoplastic inflammatory condition of the orbit due to autoimmunity, infections or fibrous overgrowth. Corticosteroids with prolonged taper are the gold standard of treatment, providing excellent symptomatic relief but poor local control over the long term. Low-dose anti-inflammatory radiotherapy with doses in between 20 Gy and 30 Gy has been shown to provide excellent symptomatic relief in 75% of the patients and maintain local control in over half of the patients at 10 years. Sequelae of radiation are negligible, and it is well tolerated. Pseudotumors of the orbit that do not respond to radiation can be attributed either to extensive growth of fibrotic tissue due to a long history of symptoms in the patient or to a different orbital pathology. Surgery is avoided due to cosmetic outcomes and the presence of critical structures. Lesions that do not respond to radiation are treated with cytotoxic agents like methotrexate or specific monoclonal antibodies like adalimumab, however, with limited efficacy.

References

1. Umiker WO, Iverson LC. Post inflammatory tumor of the lung: report of four cases simulating xanthoma, fibroma, or plasma cell granuloma. J Thorac Surg. 1954;28:55–62.
2. Yan J, Wu Z, Li Y. A clinical analysis of idiopathic orbital inflammatory pseudotumor. Yan Ke Xue Bao. 2000;16(3):208–13.
3. Chaudhry IA, Shamsi FA, Arat YO, Riley FC. Orbital pseudotumor: distinct diagnostic features and management. Middle East Afr J Ophthalmol. 2008;15(1):17–27. https://doi.org/10.4103/0974-9233.53370.
4. Mombaerts I, Goldschmeding R, Schlingemann RO, Koornneef L. What is orbital pseudotumor? Surv Ophthalmol. 1996;41:66–78. https://doi.org/10.1016/s0039-6257(97)81996-0.
5. Trott K-R, Kamprad F-H, Hildebrandt G. Radiobiological principles. In: Seegenschmeidt M, Makoshi H, Trott K, Brady L, editors. Radiotherapy for non-malignant disorders: contemporary concepts and clinical results. Springer; 2008, Ch. 1.
6. Chundury A, Espinoza G, Chundury R, Phelps P, et al. Non-specific orbital inflammation. American Academy of Ophthalmology; 2025.
7. Harris GJ. Idiopathic orbital inflammation: a pathogenic construct and treatment strategy: the 2005 ASOPRS foundation lecture. Ophthalmic Plast Reconstr Surg. 2006;22(2):79–86. https://doi.org/10.1097/01.iop.0000203734.52333.93.
8. Jacobs D, Galetta S. Diagnosis and management of orbital pseudotumor. Curr Opin Ophthalmol. 2002;13(6):347–51. https://doi.org/10.1097/00055735-200212000-00001.
9. Gordon LK. Diagnostic dilemmas in orbital inflammatory disease. Ocul Immunol Inflamm. 2003;11(1):3–15. https://doi.org/10.1076/ocii.11.1.3.15577.
10. Swamy BN, McClusky P, Nemet A, Crouch R, Martin P, Benger R, Ghabriel R, Wakefiled D. Idiopathic orbital inflammatory syndrome: clinical features and treatment outcomes. Br J Ophthalmol. 2007;91:1667–70.
11. Mannor GE, Rose GE, Moseley IF, et al. Outcome of orbital myositis: clinical features associated with recurrence. Ophthalmology. 1997;104:409–14.
12. Yuen SJ, Rubin PA. Idiopathic orbital inflammation: distribution, clinical features, and treatment outcome. Arch Ophthalmol. 2003;121:491–9. https://doi.org/10.1001/archopht.121.4.491.
13. Sergott RC, Glaser JS, Charyulu K. Radiotherapy for idiopathic inflammatory orbital pseudotumor. Indications and results. Arch Ophthalmol. 1981;99(5):853–6. https://doi.org/10.1001/archopht.1981.03930010853013.
14. Orcutt JC, Garner A, Henk JM, Wright JE. Treatment of idiopathic inflammatory orbital pseudotumours by radiotherapy. Br J Ophthalmol. 1983;67(9):570–4. https://doi.org/10.1136/bjo.67.9.570.
15. Matthiesen C, Bogardus C Jr, Thompson JS, Farris B, Hildebrand L, Wilkes B, Syzek E, Algan O, Ahmad S, Herman T. The efficacy of radiotherapy in the treatment of orbital pseudotumor. Int J Radiat Oncol Biol Phys. 2011;79(5):1496–502. https://doi.org/10.1016/j.ijrobp.2009.12.071.

16. Mokhtech M, Nurkic S, Morris CG, Mendenhall NP, Mendenhall WM. Radiotherapy for orbital Pseudotumor: the university of Florida experience. Cancer Investig. 2018;36(6):330–7.
17. Fionda B, Pagliara MM, Lancellotta V, Sammarco MG, Casà C, Savino G, et al. The role of radiotherapy in orbital pseudotumor: a systematic review of literature. Ocul Immunol Inflamm. 2022;30(5):1162–7. https://doi.org/10.1080/09273948.2020.1871493.
18. Yamashita K, Kobayashi S, Kando M, Ishikura H, Shibuya Y, Hayasaka S. Elevated anti-neutrophilic cytoplasmic antibody titer in a patient with atypical orbital pseudotumor. Ophthalomologica. 1995;209:172–5.
19. Notter M, Greven KM. Pseudotumor Orbitae. In: Seegenschmeidt M, Makoshi H, Trott K, Brady L, editors. Radiotherapy for non-malignant disorders: contemporary concepts and clinical results. Springer; 2008, Ch. 27.
20. Ma Y, Chen H-Y, Huang F-J, Pang XL, Zheng J, He F, et al. Outcomes of volumetric modulated arc therapy for refractory corticosteroid-resistant orbital inflammatory disease. Adv Radiat Oncol. 2025;10:101811. https://doi.org/10.1016/j.adro.2025.101811.
21. Rootman J, McCarthy M, White V, Harris G, Kennerdell J. Idiopathic sclerosing inflammation of the orbit. A distinct clinicopathologic entity. Ophthalmology. 1994;101(3):570–84. https://doi.org/10.1016/s0161-6420(94)31298-x.

Grave's Ophthalmopathy

18

Akash Bellige, Sarthak Tandon, and Munish Gairola

18.1 Background

Graves' ophthalmopathy (GO), also known as Graves' orbitopathy or thyroid eye disease, is the most common orbital disorder encountered in adults. It occurs in approximately 25–50% of patients with Graves' disease [1]. It is characterized by autoimmune-mediated inflammation causing lymphocytic infiltration of the orbital tissues, which affects the musculature of the orbits, leading to periorbital edema, conjunctival redness, eyelid retraction, proptosis (exophthalmos), restrictive strabismus, and exposure keratopathy, and can rarely progress to compressive optic neuropathy [2]. Although typically associated with hyperthyroidism, GO can also present in euthyroid or hypothyroid patients.

The clinical course of GO is often biphasic, beginning with an active, inflammatory phase followed by a quiescent, fibrotic phase. Symptoms range from mild discomfort to severe manifestations such as diplopia, exposure keratopathy, and compressive optic neuropathy. Risk factors influencing disease severity include smoking, older age, male sex, and poorly controlled thyroid function [1, 3]. It can substantially impact patients' visual function and quality of life, causing double vision, ocular pain, and cosmetic disfigurement. The overall prevalence of orbital involvement among Graves' disease patients is up to 40%, though most cases are mild; approximately 6% develop moderate-to-severe GO and about 0.5% develop sight-threatening complications such as dysthyroid optic neuropathy. [3, 4]

The pathogenesis of GO involves autoimmunity against the thyroid-stimulating hormone receptor (TSHR) and insulin-like growth factor-1 receptor (IGF-1R), which are expressed on orbital fibroblasts. The subsequent activation of T lymphocytes, cytokine release, and fibroblast differentiation into adipocytes or

A. Bellige · S. Tandon (✉) · M. Gairola
Department of Radiation Oncology, Rajiv Gandhi Cancer Institute and Research Centre, Delhi, India

K. Sood Sharma (ed.), *Radiation Therapy for Benign Disorders*,
https://doi.org/10.1007/978-981-95-6635-8_18

myofibroblasts contributes to tissue remodeling, glycosaminoglycan deposition, edema, and fibrosis [4, 5].

Optimal care of GO patients is inherently multidisciplinary. Endocrinologist ensure achieving euthyroid status, and ophthalmologists on the other hand assess and manage local eye symptoms. While high-dose corticosteroids remain the cornerstone of initial treatment, a significant subset of patients demonstrate suboptimal or transient responses. Orbital decompression surgery is typically reserved for chronic, vision-threatening cases [6]. In this context, RT has evolved as a valuable therapeutic option—particularly in patients with active, moderate-to-severe GO who are refractory to or intolerant of medical therapy [7].

Given its anti-inflammatory and immunomodulatory properties, RT holds promise as a non-invasive adjunct in the multidisciplinary management of GO. With advancements in radiation techniques, such as intensity-modulated radiotherapy (IMRT) with better delivery systems and arch therapy (VMAT—volumetric modulated arc therapy), concerns regarding radiation-induced toxicity have been significantly mitigated, enabling safer and more effective treatment delivery.

18.2 Pathogenesis

Graves' ophthalmopathy (GO) arises from an autoimmune process directed against antigens shared by the thyroid and orbital tissues which is characterized by the presence of circulating thyroid-stimulating antibodies (TSAb) that contribute to both hyperthyroidism and the pathogenesis of GO. The prevailing immune response in GD and GO is predominantly a T helper (Th)1 response, which is crucial during the active phase of the disease. This response is mediated by Th1 chemokines and their receptor (C-X-C) R3, highlighting the importance of these immune pathways in the disease's progression [8]. The pathophysiology of GO involves a multifactorial interplay of immune mechanisms, particularly focusing on the role of $CD34^+$ orbital fibroblasts (OF) as primary targets of autoimmune attack, which subsequently proliferate and differentiate into adipocytes and myofibroblasts in the orbit. In the early stages of the disease, OF exhibit low expression of TSH receptors and are stimulated by cytokines released from activated infiltrating T cells, rather than by Graves' IgG. As the disease progresses, differentiated OF can produce glycosaminoglycans (such as hyaluronan), which draw fluid into orbital tissues, causing edema and swelling [9]. This suggests that the immune response is not solely directed against TSH receptors but may also involve other autoantigens. Recent studies have shifted attention toward the insulin-like growth factor-1 receptor (IGF-1R) as a significant autoantigen in GO. While the presence of IGF-1R stimulating antibodies in serum remains contentious, their expression on T and B lymphocytes may contribute to the ongoing autoimmune response against orbital fibroblasts [10]. This evolving understanding of the immune mechanisms involved in GO has opened avenues for novel therapeutic strategies, including the use of monoclonal antibodies targeting specific cytokines and receptors implicated in the disease. A key feature of GO pathogenesis is that active inflammation is time-limited—over time, the chronic phase is dominated by fibrosis rather than active cell proliferation. This distinction has therapeutic implications: anti-inflammatory therapies (steroids, radiotherapy, biologics) are most effective in the active phase, whereas fibrotic changes in the chronic phase may only be correctable by surgery. The understanding of these mechanisms has led to therapies targeting various points in the inflammatory cascade.

Current treatment modalities for GO, such as corticosteroids and intravenous immunoglobulins, aim to reduce inflammation and orbital congestion, yet they often fall short of providing long-term remission [11]. Radiotherapy, when combined with systemic glucocorticoids, has been shown to enhance treatment efficacy while minimizing corticosteroid dependence. The combination of RT and steroids is particularly effective in patients with refractory GO, allowing for the cessation of corticosteroids in many cases. The introduction of targeted therapies, such as teprotumumab, which blocks IGF-1R, has shown promising results in clinical trials, indicating a potential shift toward more effective management of GO. In conclusion, the pathogenesis of Graves' ophthalmopathy is characterized by a complex interplay of immune responses, particularly involving Th1 pathways, TSH receptors, and IGF-1R. Further research is essential to elucidate these mechanisms and develop more effective targeted therapies for patients suffering from this debilitating condition.

18.3 Role of Radiation Therapy

Orbital radiotherapy (ORT) has emerged as a pivotal second-line treatment for moderate-to-severe and active GO, particularly following the failure of glucocorticoids. First utilized in the 1930s, this modality has gained traction since the 1980s, with studies indicating its effectiveness in reducing soft tissue involvement in 70–80% of patients and improving ocular mobility in 30–80% of cases [12].

Rationale ORT is employed in GO for its ability to disrupt the auto-immune inflammatory process. Ionizing radiation induces DNA double-strand breaks and apoptotic cell death in highly radiosensitive cells, particularly the inflammatory T lymphocytes, B cells, and macrophages infiltrating the orbit, as well as proliferating orbital fibroblasts [13]. By depleting these cells and dampening cytokine-driven inflammation (including modulating inflammatory mediators like nitric oxide), radiotherapy can halt disease progression and allow swollen tissues to regress. In effect, radiotherapy serves as a *targeted immunosuppressive* therapy confined to the orbit. This is especially valuable in GO because the orbit is a closed bony compartment where even a moderate degree of inflammation can cause significant symptoms [14].

The European Group on Graves' Orbitopathy recognizes orbital radiotherapy as a viable option when combined with glucocorticoids, although optimal dosing regimens remain to be fully established. The most commonly employed regimen consists of 20 Gy delivered in ten fractions of 2 Gy, although advancements in radiotherapy techniques, such as intensity-modulated radiation therapy, may enhance organ sparing compared to traditional methods [12]. ORT has emerged as a valuable treatment modality for managing GO, particularly in cases resistant to corticosteroids or when surgical intervention is not immediately feasible. This is particularly beneficial for patients with active disease, as it can halt disease progression and improve quality of life [15, 16]. Wong et al. conducted a systematic review and meta-analysis that evaluated the efficacy of RT with a total dose of 20 Gy in treating GO. Their findings indicated that RT, particularly when combined with glucocorticoids, significantly improved clinical outcomes, including diplopia grade, visual acuity, and ocular motility [17]. The study highlighted that the overall response rates were notably higher for patients receiving a radiation dose of 20 Gy along with glucocorticoids compared to those receiving glucocorticoids alone, suggesting a synergistic effect that enhances treatment efficacy. Predictors of response to RT include the severity of extra-ocular muscle (EOM) enlargement and EOM limitation at baseline. Patients with higher clinical activity score (CAS) and greater EOM involvement are more likely to benefit from RT [18, 19]. Conversely, smoking and persistent vision loss at 4 month post-RT have been identified as negative predictors of response, increasing the likelihood of requiring salvage decompressive surgery [20]. Hong et al. investigated the role of smoking as a predictive factor in the response to intravenous methylprednisolone therapy in patients with active moderate-to-severe GO [21]. Their study highlighted the correlation between smoking and treatment outcomes, suggesting that lifestyle factors may influence the effectiveness of therapeutic interventions.

Clinical Indications The consensus among specialists is that radiotherapy is indicated for moderate-to-severe, active Graves' ophthalmopathy, particularly when orbital inflammation and extraocular muscle involvement are prominent. Current multidisciplinary guidelines (ATA/ETA Consensus 2022) recommend radiotherapy as a preferred treatment in active moderate-to-severe TED when progressive diplopia or restrictive myopathy is the principal feature. In practice, this means patients with appreciable diplopia, impaired ocular motility, and an active CAS typically ≥ 3 or 4/7 are candidates for orbital radiotherapy. Radiotherapy is commonly used in conjunction with systemic corticosteroids, either concurrently or sequentially, to maximize the anti-inflammatory effect. The synergistic benefit of combining radiotherapy with glucocorticoids is well documented: combined therapy yields higher response rates than radiotherapy alone, and it allows tapering steroids faster while maintaining disease control. [22, 23]

The optimal timing of RT in the treatment of GO remains a topic of debate. Early intervention during the active phase of the disease is generally recommended, as delayed treatment may reduce the likelihood of significant improvement. A study comparing early- and late-active phase groups found that RT was effective in both groups, but early intervention was associated with greater improvements in EOM limitation and CAS [18]. Radiotherapy is particularly indicated for patients with moderate-to-severe active GO who are refractory to or intolerant of corticosteroids.

It is also a suitable alternative for patients who cannot tolerate steroids due to contraindications or side effects [24]. Likewise, radiotherapy does not significantly reduce established fibrosis or fat expansion; thus, it cannot reverse fixed proptosis or fibrotic strabismus, which often require surgical solutions. Employing RT in late phase may delay or avoid the need for surgical decompression in some cases [20, 23]. Xing et al. conducted a comprehensive review of the literature surrounding RT for GO, emphasizing the need for standardized protocols and response scoring systems [25]. They noted that despite the widespread use of RT, the optimal timing and dosage remain contentious. Their findings advocate for a more structured approach to evaluating treatment responses, which could facilitate better comparisons across studies and improve clinical guidelines. In conclusion, the role of radiation therapy in Graves' ophthalmopathy is supported by a growing body of evidence that underscores its efficacy in symptom management and the importance of response scoring in evaluating treatment outcomes.

In sight-threatening GO—i.e., dysthyroid optic neuropathy (DON) due to apical nerve compression—the first-line treatment is urgent IV glucocorticoids and/or orbital decompression surgery. ORT may be used as an adjunct to prevent relapse or as a second-line measure in optic neuropathy once urgent measures are in place [2]. Some clinicians administer orbital radiotherapy after high-dose steroids in DON to reduce the chance of reactivation of inflammation as steroids are weaned, especially if surgical decompression is not done. Additionally, radiotherapy can be considered for severe corneal exposure in GO to reduce inflammation and chemosis contributing to exposure. However, if vision is acutely threatened, radiotherapy alone is insufficient.

Caution An important precaution is in diabetic patients, particularly those with diabetic retinopathy. Radiation can exacerbate microvascular damage in the retina. ORT should be used cautiously or avoided in patients with significant diabetic or hypertensive retinopathy because of the risk of inducing or worsening retinal vascular injury. Patients with mild diabetes who require ORT are closely monitored, and tight glycemic and blood pressure control is recommended to mitigate this risk [14]. Also, one must ensure the patient's thyroid function is stable and that any necessary orbital imaging has been done to confirm the diagnosis and rule out other causes of orbital inflammation. Additionally, theoretically, there is slightly increased risk of malignancy secondary to exposure to radiotherapy especially in young patients $\leq$35 years [26].

18.4 Radiation Technique

Delivering ORT for Graves' ophthalmopathy requires meticulous planning to balance efficacy with safety. The target of treatment is the retrobulbar orbital contents, encompassing the extraocular muscles and orbital fat. Key organs-at-risk (OARs) include the eyes (especially the lenses), the retinae, optic nerves, and the pituitary and brain structures behind the orbits. Historically, radiation therapy for GO has utilized lateral opposing fields (LOF) or three-dimensional conformal radiotherapy (3DCRT). However, the advent of IMRT has revolutionized treatment planning by allowing for more precise targeting of the affected tissues while sparing surrounding OARs. A study by Liu et al. highlights the effectiveness of IMRT in treating moderate to severe active thyroid-associated ophthalmopathy (TAO) [27]. The study demonstrated significant improvements in clinical activity scores (CAS) at 12-month post-treatment, indicating that IMRT not only alleviates symptoms but also enhances patient quality of life. The findings underscore the importance of advanced radiation techniques in managing GO, particularly for patients who do not respond adequately to corticosteroids. In a comparative analysis of VMAT and IMRT for GO, Wang et al. evaluated dosimetric parameters in a cohort of 19 patients. The study found that while both techniques are feasible, IMRT provided superior homogeneity in dose distribution and better protection for critical structures such as the optic nerves and lenses. Specifically, the homogeneity index (HI) was significantly better in IMRT plans compared to VMAT, suggesting that IMRT may offer a more consistent therapeutic dose across the target volume [28].

Beige et al. discussed the historical context of orbital radiotherapy, noting that while the technique has evolved, there remains a lack of standardized guidelines for its application in GO [29]. This is particularly relevant in the context of GO, where precise dosing is crucial to minimize complications and maximize therapeutic outcomes. The planning of ORT for GO patients is complex and requires a thorough understanding of the disease's pathophysiology.

The radiotherapy planning parameters for ORT are summarized in Table 18.1.

Simulation and Immobilization Patients are usually simulated in the supine position with a thermoplastic mask or other immobilization to minimize movement and ensure reproducibility. A CT simulation scan of the orbits is obtained. The eyes may be in primary gaze; sometimes patients are instructed to gaze slightly upward or a fixed direction during setup to position the orbital tissues consistently relative to the beams. Radiopaque markers can be placed on the lateral canthus to help localize the outer orbit on simulation films. Orbital contours are delineated on the planning CT—typically the clinical target volume (CTV) includes the posterior two-thirds of the orbit (to cover the extraocular muscle bellies and orbital fat) while intentionally excluding the anterior globe and cornea to spare the lens and anterior chamber. The lens of each eye is contoured to minimize its dose. Other OARs contoured may include the optic nerves and chiasm, brainstem, and temporal lobes, though these are usually well outside the low-dose orbit fields.

Field Design The classical approach for orbital radiotherapy uses lateral parallel-opposed fields to treat each orbit. Traditionally, each orbit is treated with a direct lateral or slight anterior oblique beam so that the beam axis passes through the orbit and exits posteriorly, thereby avoiding significant exposure to the contralateral eye. In bilateral cases, each eye is treated with its own lateral beam rather than opposing beams through the head, to avoid irradiating through the brain or opposite eye. To protect the anterior structures, a beam block or shield for the lens can be used. The

Table 18.1 Summary of planning aspects for orbital radiotherapy

Aspect	Details
Target volume	Retrobulbar orbital contents—Extraocular muscles and orbital fat (posterior 2/3 of the orbit)
Organs-at-risk (OARs)	Lenses, retinae, optic nerves, optic chiasm, brainstem, pituitary, contralateral eye
Simulation and immobilization	Supine position with thermoplastic mask; CT scan with primary or upward gaze; radiopaque markers for localization
Dose and fractionation	Standard: 20 Gy in 10 fractions; alternative: 20 Gy in 12 fractions to reduce lens dose. Doses >20 Gy not recommended due to increased toxicity
Laterality	Usually bilateral; unilateral in rare cases, with careful consideration of risks to uninvolved eye
Plan evaluation	Dose constraints: Lens <8–10 Gy; apex 20 Gy; retina and optic nerves within tolerance. Plan checked with image guidance (kV, CBCT, port films)
Efficacy	Improves CAS, reduces inflammation and diplopia; minimal effect on proptosis
Safety and toxicity	Low toxicity with proper shielding; mild acute effects; cataracts rare with modern techniques

Abbreviations: *CT* Computed Tomography, *kV* kilovolt, *CBCT* Cone Beam Computed Tomography, *CAS* Clinically Activity Score

field is generally shaped to cover the bony orbit outline on the lateral view, with the anterior margin at the orbital rim (blocking the anterior eye), the posterior margin at least 5 mm beyond the back of the orbit, the superior/inferior margins a few millimeters beyond the orbital roof and floor. Due to orbital geometry, a small wedge or tilting of the couch/gantry can help align the field if needed. (Fig. 18.1).

IMRT/VMAT (Figs. 18.2 and 18.3) allows multiple beam angles or arc delivery, which can create a more conformal dose and further reduce dose to the OARs. IMRT can produce a concave isodose curve to avoid the cornea and lens, while still encompassing the posterior orbit. Proton therapy is another modality that can be considered, which in principle, could treat the orbit from lateral or oblique angles with little spill to deeper brain tissues, which might be advantageous in younger patients or those requiring repeat irradiation. However, proton therapy's advantage for GO is debatable because the lens and retina are within the orbit (in-field), and protons will still deposit dose there as needed to cover the target.

Thus, while proton RT can reduce integral dose to the skull and brain, careful photon IMRT is generally sufficient in most GO cases.

Dose and Fractionation The standard radiotherapy regimen for Graves' ophthalmopathy is 20 Gy in 10 fractions (2 Gy per fraction once daily, over 2 weeks). Many historical studies employed 20 Gy, and it remains widely used. Some variations exist—for instance, 20 Gy delivered in 12 fractions (~1.67 Gy/fraction) can be used to slightly reduce the per-fraction dose to the lens, potentially lessening cataract risk. Total doses in the range of 16–24 Gy have been reported, but there is no evi-

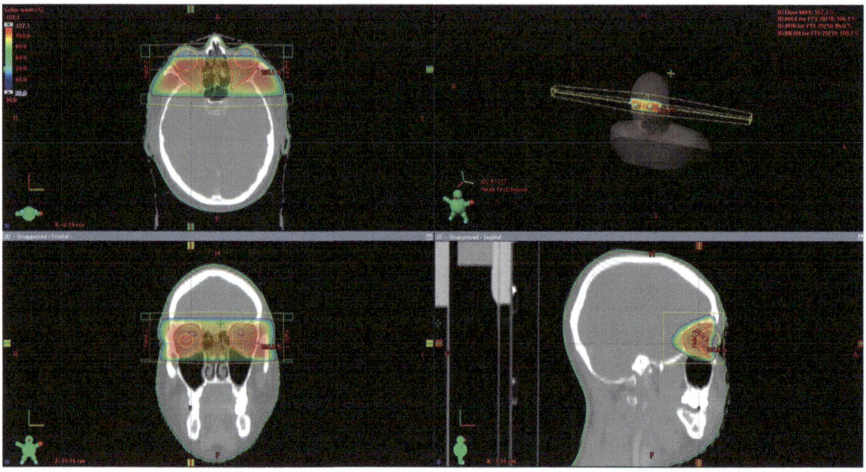

Fig. 18.1 Axial, frontal, and sagittal CT sections and bird's eye view of 50% dose colorwash to bilateral orbits by parallel opposed fields

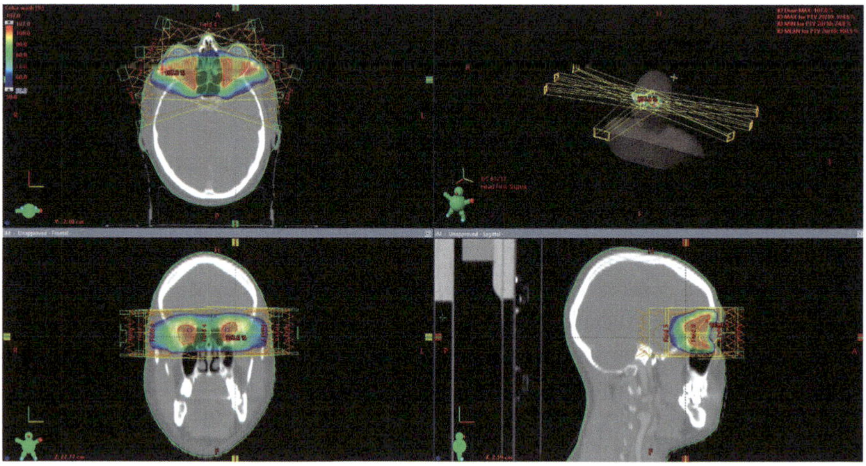

Fig. 18.2 Axial, frontal, and sagittal CT sections and bird's eye view of 50% dose colorwash to bilateral orbits by IMRT

dence that higher doses improve outcomes in GO; indeed, doses above 20 Gy likely only increase toxicity without additional benefit. The therapeutic mechanism does not require very high doses, and even lower doses (e.g. 10–12 Gy) have shown some efficacy in other inflammatory conditions; however, 20 Gy in fractions remains the most evidence-backed schedule [7]. Both orbits are often treated, as GO is usually bilateral. If one eye is clinically uninvolved, some clinicians still treat both orbits to pre-empt disease in the fellow eye. This should be decided on a case-by-case basis, weighing the risk to the uninvolved eye's lens against potential future benefit.

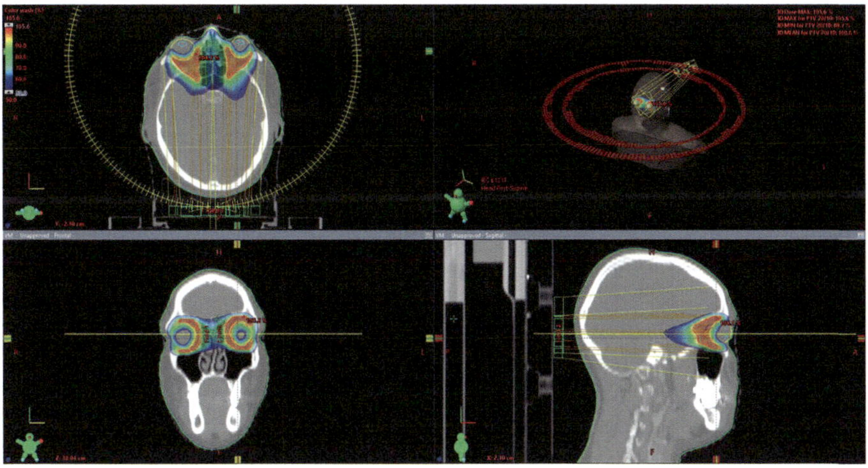

Fig. 18.3 Axial, frontal, and sagittal CT sections and bird's eye view of 50% dose colorwash to bilateral orbits by VMAT

Plan Evaluation and Verification During planning, dose–volume constraints are set for critical structures. A common goal is to keep the lens dose <8–10 Gy if possible. In practice, with 20 Gy to the orbit, the lens often gets a scattered dose of a few Gy; careful beam blocking can limit direct lens exposure to only 10–20% of the prescription dose or less. The optic nerve and retina are usually well within tolerance at 20 Gy. Thus, a plan that covers the orbit to 100% (20 Gy) will typically give the orbital apex 20 Gy, which is safe, especially since the retina/nerve tolerate this dose without late effects. Patients are monitored during treatment and setup accuracy is ensured via port films or image guidance (kV X-rays or cone-beam CT if available).

In summary, orbital radiotherapy is delivered using carefully tailored lateral fields or modern IMRT to confine dose to the orbit. The technique strives to maximize dose to the retrobulbar tissues while minimizing exposure of the anterior eye and adjacent brain. With a standard regimen of ~20 Gy in 10 fractions, this technique achieves the desired immunomodulatory effect in the orbit and well tolerated by patients.

18.5 Toxicity Profile and Strategies to Minimize Risk

Radiotherapy for Graves' ophthalmopathy is generally well tolerated, owing to the modest total dose and fractionated delivery.

Acute Effects Transient worsening of orbital inflammation, temporary flare in redness, swelling, or even proptosis is not uncommon during treatment. Symptoms like ocular irritation, periorbital edema, and chemosis can transiently worsen [16]. Mild erythema of the skin and dryness or grittiness in the eyes from lacrimal gland irradiation is common [23]. Epilation of the eyebrow or temple region can occur, but this is usually temporary given the low doses. To mitigate acute inflammation, it is standard practice to co-administer corticosteroids, if not already on them, during radiotherapy. A low-to-moderate dose prednisone taper can mask the radiation-induced flare and provide symptomatic relief. Lubricating eye drops and cool compresses can help manage irritation. Close follow-up is needed to ensure that any visual symptoms during treatment are promptly addressed, distinguishing tumor flare from any rare complication.

Chronic Effects The most notable late toxicity of orbital radiotherapy is radiation-induced cataract. The lens of the eye is highly sensitive to radiation; doses above ~5–10 Gy significantly increase the risk of cataract formation months to years later. Fortunately, by using lens blocking/shielding techniques, one can reduce the dose to the lens to well under 10 Gy in most cases. Clinical series have shown that using lens shielding to keep lens dose ≤10 Gy results in only a small incidence of late cataracts, and those that do occur can be managed with outpatient lens surgery. Radiation retinopathy is a concern typically at higher doses (≥30 Gy to the retina), so at 20 Gy it is very uncommon. However, in diabetic patients, even moderate radiation doses can synergistically worsen microangiopathy. There are case reports of radiation precipitating proliferative retinopathy in diabetics, which is why this is a relative contraindication. For non-diabetics, studies indicate no meaningful risk of retinopathy or optic neuropathy at orbital doses—"within the dose range recommended for Graves' ophthalmopathy, late radiation effects on the retina or optic nerve should be nonexistent" [7]. Chronic dry eye from reduced tear production is mostly tolerated well, with some requiring regular artificial tears. Radiation-induced neuropathy of the optic nerve and damage to the extraocular muscles is unlikely.

The safety profile of RT is further supported by studies showing no increased risk of secondary malignancies or radiation retinopathy, even with long-term follow-up [16, 30]. However, in younger patients (<35 years old), the lifetime risk is higher simply because of their longer remaining lifespan and more active cell division; this underpins the guideline to generally avoid radiotherapy in young adults unless absolutely necessary.

To mitigate risks:

- Avoid radiotherapy in patients with inactive disease (no benefit) and in those with significant diabetic retinopathy (higher harm).
- Shield the lens aggressively in planning.
- Use fractionation to allow sublethal damage repair in normal tissues, especially lens/retina.
- Monitor ocular health long term: schedule slit-lamp exams at baseline and periodically after radiotherapy to catch cataract formation early. Cataracts, if they occur, are treatable with surgery.

- Encourage smoking cessation and control of diabetes, as these factors compound radiation injury.

18.6 Review of Literature and Case Studies

Orbital RT has been a treatment modality for Graves' ophthalmopathy since the 1940s. Initial case series suggested benefits, and modern randomized controlled trials (RCTs) have since refined its role. RT is particularly effective in improving extraocular muscle function and reducing diplopia, though its effects on proptosis are limited.

One of the earliest pivotal studies by Bartalena et al. in the 1980s showed that combining RT (20 Gy) with systemic steroids resulted in better outcomes than steroids alone [31]. The Mourits et al. RCT confirmed the efficacy of RT over placebo, especially for ocular motility [32]. Another RCT by Prummel et al. demonstrated benefits even in mild GO cases [33]. These trials confirmed RT's specific efficacy for muscle-related symptoms like diplopia, rather than for proptosis or eyelid changes.

18.6.1 Radiotherapy vs Other Treatments

- RT vs Steroids: A meta-analysis by Wei et al. (2008) concluded that RT and steroids offer comparable benefits [22]. Steroids may act faster on soft tissue inflammation, while RT offers steady improvement, particularly on muscle involvement.
- Combination Therapy: Most studies, including a Cochrane review and a trial by Marcocci et al., support combining RT with steroids, showing significantly better outcomes (reduced relapse, better motility) [23, 34].
- RT with Immunosuppressants: The CIRTED trial (2018) evaluated RT with azathioprine in steroid-treated patients. It found limited additional benefit from RT when steroids were prolonged and high dose, though trial limitations and dropout rates temper conclusions [35].

18.6.2 Clinical Outcomes and Timing

RT primarily improves diplopia and extraocular muscle function, with little effect on proptosis or chronic lid retraction. These benefits are gradual, often manifesting 2–6 months post-treatment. Long-term data show that many patients maintain stable disease post-RT, though some may require subsequent surgery [36–38].

18.6.3 Controversies and Considerations

- Variability in Results: Some studies showed no short-term benefits, possibly due to lack of steroid cover and short follow-up [32].
- Optimal Timing: While early treatment in active disease may prevent fibrosis, no trial has directly compared early vs delayed RT.
- Monotherapy vs Combined Treatment: RT alone is modestly effective, especially in mild GO, but combination with steroids is generally preferred.
- Biologic Therapies: Newer agents like teprotumumab offer promising results, especially for proptosis, but cost and availability limit their widespread use [39]. RT remains relevant due to its accessibility and established safety profile.

18.6.4 Special Scenarios and Guidelines

Case reports suggest RT may be effective even in long-standing or refractory cases, including re-irradiation in select patients. Current guidelines (EUGOGO 2021, ATA/ETA 2022, AAO 2022) endorse RT as part of multimodal therapy for moderate-to-severe active GO, particularly for those with diplopia or steroid intolerance [2, 40–42].

In conclusion, orbital radiotherapy is a validated and effective treatment for moderate-to-severe active Graves' ophthalmopathy, especially for improving motility and diplopia. Best results are achieved when RT is used during the active inflammatory phase and in combination with systemic therapy. Despite the advent of new biologics, RT continues to play a crucial role in multidisciplinary GO management.

18.7 Future Directions

The management of Graves' ophthalmopathy is evolving with new therapies and technologies that may refine the role of ORT. The most significant development is the introduction of *teprotumumab in two major RCTs* that showed dramatic results in reducing proptosis and inflammation, leading to its FDA approval in 2020 [2, 39, 43]. While it offers outcomes RT cannot match, especially in proptosis, its high cost and side effects limit accessibility. As a result, RT may remain a preferred option for patients with motility issues or those unable to access biologics.

Other *immunomodulatory agents* like rituximab, tocilizumab, and sirolimus are being studied, with the potential to serve as steroid-sparing agents that could be used alongside RT.

Technological advances in radiotherapy, including proton therapy, IMRT refinements, and image-guided techniques, offer better targeting with reduced toxicity—especially valuable for young or re-treatment patients. Adaptive radiotherapy and MRI-based planning may further improve precision.

Improved imaging could help better assess disease activity and predict RT response, aiding in patient selection. *Radiobiological research* is exploring how RT affects immune pathways, potentially leading to the use of radiosensitizers or ocular radioprotectors [13] [14].

The possibility of *safe re-irradiation protocols* for recurrent cases is under exploration, based on emerging evidence from case reports [30].

Future care will be increasingly *personalized* and *multidisciplinary*, integrating RT with systemic therapies and surgery, guided by biomarkers and predictive tools.

In summary, while new therapies are reshaping GO treatment, radiotherapy will retain a valuable role—especially for patients with predominant muscle involvement or limited access to biologics—as part of a tailored, multi-modality approach.

18.8 Conclusion

Orbital radiotherapy remains a proven, evidence-based treatment for moderate-to-severe active Graves' ophthalmopathy (GO), especially in patients with diplopia, orbital pain, and inflammation who are refractory to or intolerant of corticosteroids. While surgical intervention may still be necessary in some cases, RT can delay or avoid the need for surgery in many patients. Typically delivered as 20 Gy in 10 fractions, radiotherapy improves extraocular muscle function and orbital congestion in about 50–66% of patients. Ideal candidates are those in the active inflammatory phase of GO with restrictive myopathy or optic nerve involvement. Radiotherapy is best used in coordination with endocrinologists and ophthalmologists. Effects develop gradually over 2–6 months and serve to stabilize disease, often allowing for later surgical correction of residual issues like proptosis. Modern techniques like IMRT with meticulous lens shielding minimize side effects, with cataracts now being rare. Key principles in the management of GO with radiotherapy include using radiotherapy only for active inflammatory phase, confirming inflammation through clinical activity scores and imaging, and ensuring close multidisciplinary follow-up.

In conclusion, orbital radiotherapy is an essential tool in the multidisciplinary care of GO, offering localized disease control with minimal toxicity and a durable impact when properly selected and executed.

References

1. Hiromatsu Y, Eguchi H, Tani J, Kasaoka M, Teshima Y. Graves' ophthalmopathy: epidemiology and natural history. Intern Med. 2014;53(5):353–60.
2. Burch HB, Perros P, Bednarczuk T, Cooper DS, Dolman PJ, Leung AM, et al. Management of thyroid eye disease: a consensus statement by the American Thyroid Association and the European thyroid association. Eur Thyroid J. 2022;11(6):e220189.
3. Chin YH, Ng CH, Lee MH, Koh JWH, Kiew J, Yang SP, et al. Prevalence of thyroid eye disease in graves' disease: a meta-analysis and systematic review. Clin Endocrinol. 2020;93(4):363–74.

4. Ippolito S, Cusini C, Lasalvia P, Gianfagna F, Veronesi G, Gallo D, et al. Change in newly diagnosed graves' disease phenotype between the twentieth and the twenty-first centuries: meta-analysis and meta-regression. J Endocrinol Investig. 2021;44(8):1707–18.
5. Taylor PN, Zhang L, Lee RWJ, Muller I, Ezra DG, Dayan CM, et al. New insights into the pathogenesis and nonsurgical management of Graves orbitopathy. Nat Rev Endocrinol. 2020;16(2):104–16.
6. Wakelkamp IMMJ, Baldeschi L, Saeed P, Mourits MP, Prummel MF, Wiersinga WM. Surgical or medical decompression as a first-line treatment of optic neuropathy in graves' ophthalmopathy? A randomized controlled trial. Clin Endocrinol. 2005;63(3):323–8.
7. Smitt MC, Donaldson SS. Radiation therapy for benign disease of the orbit. Semin Radiat Oncol. 1999;9(2):179–89.
8. Antonelli A, Fallahi P, Elia G, Ragusa F, Paparo SR, Ruffilli I, et al. Graves' disease: clinical manifestations, immune pathogenesis (cytokines and chemokines) and therapy. Best Pract Res Clin Endocrinol Metab. 2020;34(1):101388.
9. Moledina M, Damato EM, Lee V. The changing landscape of thyroid eye disease: current clinical advances and future outlook. Eye. 2024;38(8):1425–37.
10. Fallahi P, Ferrari SM, Elia G, Ragusa F, Paparo SR, Patrizio A, et al. Cytokines as targets of novel therapies for Graves' ophthalmopathy. Front Endocrinol. 2021;12:654473.
11. Wiersinga WM. Autoimmunity in Graves' ophthalmopathy: the result of an unfortunate marriage between TSH receptors and IGF-1 receptors? J Clin Endocrinol Metabol. 2011;96(8):2386–94.
12. Zhou X, Zhou D, Wang J, Chen G. Treatment strategies for Graves' ophthalmopathy: a network meta-analysis. Br J Ophthalmol. 2020;104(4):551–6.
13. Grudzenski S, Raths A, Conrad S, Rübe CE, Löbrich M. Inducible response required for repair of low-dose radiation damage in human fibroblasts. Proc Natl Acad Sci USA. 2010;107(32):14205–10.
14. Dolman PJ, Rath S. Orbital radiotherapy for thyroid eye disease. Curr Opin Ophthalmol. 2012;23(5):427–32.
15. Ravishankar B, Madhvi BV, Tyagi T, Srivastava V, Kuppusamy A, Prithviraj B, et al. Role of radiotherapy in thyroid-related ophthalmopathy: a case series. J Curr Oncol. 2022;5(2):111–8.
16. Li YJ, Luo Y, He WM, Li P, Wang F. Clinical outcomes of graves' ophthalmopathy treated with intensity modulated radiation therapy. Radiat Oncol. 2017;12(1):171.
17. Wong NTY, Yuen KFK, Aljufairi FMAA, Lai KKH, Hu Z, Chan KKW, et al. Magnetic resonance imaging parameters on lacrimal gland in thyroid eye disease: a systematic review and meta-analysis. BMC Ophthalmol. 2023;23(1):347.
18. Choi JH, Lee JK. Efficacy of orbital radiotherapy in moderate-to-severe active graves' orbitopathy including long-lasting disease: a retrospective analysis. Radiat Oncol. 2020;15(1):220.
19. Kim BY, Mok JO, Kang SK, Jang SY, Jung CH, Kim CH. The relationship between serum adipocytokines and Graves' ophthalmopathy: a hospital-based study. Endocr J. 2016;63(5):425–30.
20. Prabhu RS, Liebman L, Wojno T, Hayek B, Hall WA, Crocker I. Clinical outcomes of radiotherapy as initial local therapy for Graves' ophthalmopathy and predictors of the need for post-radiotherapy decompressive surgery. Radiat Oncol. 2012;7(1):95.
21. Hong JH, Choi KH, Kim JS, Yang SW, Kim YS. Radiation therapy for Graves' ophthalmopathy: when is the optimal timing of treatment and evaluation. Pract Radiat Oncol. 2025;15(3):e221–9.
22. Wei RL, Cheng JW, Cai JP. The use of orbital radiotherapy for Graves' ophthalmopathy: quantitative review of the evidence. Ophthalmologica. 2008;222(1):27–31.
23. Nicosia L, Reverberi C, Agolli L, Marinelli L, De Sanctis V, Minniti G, et al. Orbital radiotherapy plus concomitant steroids in moderate-to-severe graves' ophthalmopathy: good results after long-term follow-up. Int J Endocrinol Metab. 2019;17(1):e84427.
24. Grassi P, Strianese D, Piscopo R, Pacelli R, Bonavolontà G. Radiotherapy for the treatment of thyroid eye disease—a prospective comparison: is orbital radiotherapy a suitable alternative to steroids? Ir J Med Sci. 2017;186(3):647–52.

25. Xing L, Ye L, Zhu W, Shen L, Huang F, Jiao Q, et al. Smoking was associated with poor response to intravenous steroids therapy in Graves' ophthalmopathy. Br J Ophthalmol. 2015;99(12):1686.
26. Tanda ML, Bartalena L. Efficacy and safety of orbital radiotherapy for Graves' orbitopathy. J Clin Endocrinol Metabol. 2012;97(11):3857–65.
27. Liu W, Zhang L, Dai G, Zhang X, Li G, Yi Z. Deep neural network with structural similarity difference and orientation-based loss for position error classification in the radiotherapy of graves' ophthalmopathy patients. IEEE J Biomed Health Inform. 2022;26(6):2606–14.
28. Wang SC, Wu J, Xie XQ, Liu XL, Luo Y, Wang F, et al. Comparison of IMRT and VMAT radiotherapy planning for Graves' ophthalmopathy based on dosimetric parameters analysis. Eur Rev Med Pharmacol Sci. 2020;24(7):3898–906.
29. Beige A, Boustani J, Bouillet B, Truc G. Management of Graves' ophthalmopathy by radiotherapy: a literature review. Cancer/Radiothérapie. 2024;28(3):282–9.
30. Matthiesen CL, Thompson J, Wilkes B, Farris B, Hildebrand L, Herman T, et al. The efficacy of radiation therapy in the treatment of graves' Orbitopathy. Int J Radiat Oncol Biol Phys. 2010;78(3):S560.
31. Bartalena L, Marcocci C, Bogazzi F, Manetti L, Tanda ML, Dell'Unto E, et al. Relation between therapy for hyperthyroidism and the course of Graves' ophthalmopathy. N Engl J Med. 1998;338(2):73–8.
32. Mourits MP, van Kempen-Harteveld ML, García MB, Koppeschaar HP, Tick L, Terwee CB. Radiotherapy for Graves' orbitopathy: randomised placebo-controlled study. Lancet. 2000;355(9214):1505–9.
33. Prummel MF, Terwee CB, Gerding MN, Baldeschi L, Mourits MP, Blank L, et al. A randomized controlled trial of orbital radiotherapy versus sham irradiation in patients with mild Graves' ophthalmopathy. J Clin Endocrinol Metab. 2004;89(1):15–20.
34. Marcocci C, Bartalena L, Tanda ML, Manetti L, Dell'Unto E, Rocchi R, et al. Comparison of the effectiveness and tolerability of intravenous or oral glucocorticoids associated with orbital radiotherapy in the management of severe Graves' ophthalmopathy: results of a prospective, single-blind, randomized study. J Clin Endocrinol Metab. 2001;86(8):3562–7.
35. Rajendram R, Taylor PN, Wilson VJ, Harris N, Morris OC, Tomlinson M, et al. Combined immunosuppression and radiotherapy in thyroid eye disease (CIRTED): a multicentre, 2 × 2 factorial, double-blind, randomised controlled trial. Lancet Diabetes Endocrinol. 2018;6(4):299–309.
36. Sisti E, Menconi F, Leo M, Profilo MA, Mautone T, Mazzi B, et al. Long-term outcome of Graves' orbitopathy following high-dose intravenous glucocorticoids and orbital radiotherapy. J Endocrinol Investig. 2015;38(6):661–8.
37. Stiebel-Kalish H, Robenshtok E, Hasanreisoglu M, Ezrachi D, Shimon I, Leibovici L. Treatment modalities for graves' ophthalmopathy: systematic review and metaanalysis. J Clin Endocrinol Metab. 2009;94(8):2708–16.
38. Marquez SD, Lum BL, McDougall IR, Katkuri S, Levin PS, MacManus M, et al. Long-term results of irradiation for patients with progressive Graves' ophthalmopathy. Int J Radiation Oncol Biol Phys. 2001;51(3):766–74.
39. Smith TJ, Kahaly GJ, Ezra DG, Fleming JC, Dailey RA, Tang RA, et al. Teprotumumab for thyroid-associated ophthalmopathy. N Engl J Med. 2017;376(18):1748–61.
40. Bartalena L, Kahaly GJ, Baldeschi L, Dayan CM, Eckstein A, Marcocci C, et al. The 2021 European group on Graves' orbitopathy (EUGOGO) clinical practice guidelines for the medical management of Graves' orbitopathy. Eur J Endocrinol. 2021;185(4):G43–67.
41. Kahaly GJ, Bartalena L, Hegedüs L, Leenhardt L, Poppe K, Pearce SH. 2018 European Thyroid Association Guideline for the management of Graves' hyperthyroidism. Eur Thyroid J. 2018;7(4):167–86.
42. Hoang TD, Stocker DJ, Chou EL, Burch HB. 2022 update on clinical management of Graves Disease and Thyroid eye disease. Endocrinol Metab Clin N Am. 2022;51(2):287–304.
43. Douglas RS, Kahaly GJ, Patel A, Sile S, Thompson EHZ, Perdok R, et al. Teprotumumab for the treatment of active thyroid eye disease. N Engl J Med. 2020;382(4):341–52.

Desmoid Tumors

19

Gagan Saini, Rashmi Shukla, and Vivek Verma

19.1 Introduction

Desmoid tumors (aggressive fibromatosis) represent a rare yet clinically challenging group of soft tissue neoplasms. Although these tumors lack metastatic potential, their locally invasive nature results in significant morbidity. Originating from musculoaponeurotic structures, desmoid tumors are characterized by an unpredictable clinical course—from periods of indolence to relentless local progression. The term "desmoid" (from the Greek desmos, meaning tendon-like) reflects the tumor's fibrous morphology. The annual incidence is approximately 2–4 cases per million, accounting for less than 3% of all soft tissue tumors, with most cases occurring in the third and fourth decades of life and a slight female predominance [1–3].

Over recent decades, the management of desmoid tumors has evolved from primarily surgical excision to a more nuanced, multidisciplinary approach. Advances in imaging, molecular diagnostics, systemic therapies, and precision radiation have provided radiation oncologists with an expanding arsenal to achieve excellent disease control while minimizing toxicity. This chapter critically examines the molecular mechanisms, clinical perspectives, and treatment advancements—including state-of-the-art radiotherapy techniques—to inform both trainees and practicing radiation oncologists.

G. Saini (✉) · R. Shukla
Department of Radiation Oncology, Yashoda Medicity, Shakti Khand 2, Indirapuram, Ghaziabad, Uttar Pradesh, India

V. Verma
Department of Ortho Oncology and Joint Reconstruction, Max Vaishali and Patparganj. Vaishali & Patparganj, Delhi, India

K. Sood Sharma (ed.), *Radiation Therapy for Benign Disorders*,
https://doi.org/10.1007/978-981-95-6635-8_19

19.2 Epidemiology and Etiology

Desmoid tumors present either sporadically or in association with familial adenomatous polyposis (FAP), especially within the context of Gardner syndrome. In sporadic cases, mutations in the CTNNB1 gene—encoding β-catenin—are common, leading to its aberrant stabilization and nuclear accumulation. In contrast, FAP-associated desmoids are typically linked to truncating mutations in the APC gene [4, 5]. In addition, estrogen plays a role in tumor pathogenesis; for example, hormonal manipulation has shown benefits in certain cases [6]. Risk factors include previous surgical trauma, pregnancy-related hormonal changes, genetic predisposition, and estrogen exposure [7]. In FAP patients, desmoids most frequently arise in the intra-abdominal region (particularly the mesentery) and can precipitate life-threatening complications such as bowel obstruction and ischemia [8].

19.3 Advanced Molecular Mechanisms in Desmoid Tumorigenesis

19.3.1 The Wnt/β-Catenin Pathway and Beyond

At the molecular level, the Wnt/β-catenin signaling pathway is central to desmoid tumorigenesis. In sporadic desmoids, mutations in exon 3 of CTNNB1 impede β-catenin degradation, promoting its nuclear translocation and the activation of proliferation-related target genes. In FAP-associated tumors, mutations in the APC gene similarly result in β-catenin stabilization [9].

Recent evidence suggests that specific CTNNB1 mutation subtypes (for example, S45F versus T41A) may differentially influence tumor behavior, recurrence risk, and therapy responsiveness. Beyond these genetic alterations, emerging data implicate other signaling pathways—including transforming growth factor-beta (TGF-β) and fibroblast growth factors (FGFs)—as well as epigenetic modifications in modulating tumor growth. The tumor microenvironment, characterized by extracellular matrix remodeling and angiogenic factors, further contributes to desmoid proliferation. These insights have the potential to inform the development of novel radiosensitizing agents and to integrate molecular diagnostics with precision radiotherapy [10, 11].

19.4 Epigenetic Modulation and the Tumor Microenvironment

Non-genetic factors such as altered methylation patterns and histone modifications also appear to impact β-catenin transcriptional regulation and the downstream effectors that drive tumor progression. The interplay of activated fibroblasts, inflammatory mediators, and matrix metalloproteinases creates a supportive microenvironment. This nuanced understanding may eventually lead to combined modality treatments where agents that modulate the tumor microenvironment are used alongside tailored radiation protocols—optimizing local control and preserving quality of life.

For the radiation oncologist, such molecular insights are essential both in the selection of patients for radiotherapy and in guiding potential combinations with systemic agents aimed at improving radiosensitivity.

19.5 Clinical Perspectives and Diagnostic Considerations

19.5.1 Clinical Presentation and Challenges

The clinical manifestations of desmoid tumors depend largely on their anatomical location. Patients may present with:

Abdominal wall tumors: Often detected as firm, painless masses.
Intra-abdominal tumors: These can present with vague abdominal discomfort or complications such as bowel obstruction.
Extra-abdominal tumors: Commonly located in the shoulder or limb girdle, these may cause pain, functional impairment, or neurovascular compromise.

Given the heterogeneity in presentation, management must be highly individualized. Even lesions that are asymptomatic at presentation may eventually compromise adjacent structures, underscoring the need for a proactive, yet measured, treatment approach [10].

19.5.2 Diagnostic Workup and Imaging Advances

Magnetic resonance imaging (MRI) remains the modality of choice because of its superior soft tissue contrast and its ability to precisely delineate tumor margins. Characteristic features include a heterogeneous hyperintense signal on T2-weighted images and variable enhancement on post-contrast T1-weighted sequences [11]. Computed tomography (CT) may be employed as an adjunct—especially for evaluating intra-abdominal lesions, calcifications, or for treatment planning. Emerging functional imaging modalities, such as positron emission tomography (PET) with fibroblast activation protein (FAP)-targeted tracers, promise to further refine tumor delineation and may soon play a role in optimizing radiotherapy target volumes.

Histologic confirmation via core needle biopsy is essential, not only for definitive diagnosis but also for molecular testing (e.g., for CTNNB1 or APC mutations). Minimally invasive biopsy techniques are advocated to prevent tumor seeding and to avoid complicating subsequent management [10].

19.6 Treatment Strategies: A Multimodal Approach

The management of desmoid tumors requires a multidisciplinary strategy that takes into account tumor location, size, growth rate, patient symptoms, and overall functional status.

19.6.1 Active Surveillance

Active surveillance ("watchful waiting") is now widely accepted as the first-line approach for many patients with asymptomatic or indolent disease. Multiple studies have documented spontaneous stabilization—and in some cases regression—in up to 50% of patients. Close imaging surveillance every 3–6 months helps to promptly identify changes in tumor biology that may necessitate intervention [12–14].

19.6.2 Surgical Management

Historically, complete surgical resection with negative margins (R0) was the gold standard; however, high local recurrence rates (up to 40% even after macroscopically complete excision) and the potential for functional compromise have prompted a shift toward more conservative surgical approaches. Current practice favors surgery only when symptomatic relief or immediate functional benefit is required. In cases with positive margins (R1), adjuvant treatment options—including radiation therapy—are considered based on overall tumor behavior [15, 16].

19.6.3 Systemic Therapies

Systemic treatment is reserved for unresectable, multifocal, or progressive tumors. The therapeutic repertoire includes

- NSAIDs and anti-estrogen agents (e.g., tamoxifen): These have been shown to slow or stabilize disease progression in some cases [17].
- Tyrosine kinase inhibitors (TKIs): Agents such as sorafenib and pazopanib have demonstrated activity in refractory desmoid tumors [18].
- Traditional chemotherapy regimens: Low-dose methotrexate/vinblastine or doxorubicin-based treatments are considered for aggressive, symptomatic cases [19].

Combining systemic therapies with radiotherapy is an area of active investigation; such combinations may enhance radiosensitivity and improve local control, particularly in rapidly progressive tumors.

19.7 Radiation Therapy in Desmoid Tumors

Radiation therapy (RT) has emerged as a vital modality in the management of desmoid tumors—especially for patients with unresectable, recurrent, or functionally compromising tumors—as well as in the setting of positive surgical margins. Advances in RT planning and delivery have enabled clinicians to achieve high local control rates while mitigating toxicity.

19.7.1 Indications for Radiation Therapy

RT is indicated for:

Unresectable tumors in critical or anatomically complex regions: tumors in the head and neck, pelvis, or deep abdominal locations where surgical resection is problematic.
Recurrent disease following surgery: RT is used to control local recurrences after prior surgical treatment.
Postoperative cases with close or positive margins: When additional surgery might lead to significant morbidity, RT can serve as an effective adjuvant.
Poor surgical candidates: Patients with significant comorbidities may be better managed with RT [20, 21].

19.7.2 Radiotherapy Dose and Technique

Optimal RT dosing is tailored to individual patient and tumor characteristics:

Definitive RT: Doses typically range from 50 to 56 Gy in 1.8–2 Gy fractions over 5 to 6 weeks.
Adjuvant RT: Doses of 50–54 Gy in 1.8–2 Gy fractions over 5 weeks are typically prescribed for cases with close or positive margins.

Evidence suggests that doses below 50 Gy may be insufficient, particularly for bulky or rapidly progressing tumors. Modern RT techniques are therefore crucial to maximize the therapeutic ratio.

19.7.3 Intensity-Modulated Radiation Therapy (IMRT)

IMRT has revolutionized the delivery of radiation by allowing highly conformal dose distributions. For desmoid tumors that often lie in proximity to critical structures (such as bowel loops or neural tissues), IMRT can specifically target the gross tumor volume (GTV) plus an appropriate clinical target volume (CTV) margin (typically 4–5 cm, adjusted for anatomical boundaries) while sparing adjacent normal tissues. The planning target volume (PTV) is then derived by adding a 5–10 mm margin to the CTV, accounting for treatment uncertainties [22]. The PTV is determined by the type of the immobilization employed as well as the treating institutional protocol.

19.7.4 Image-Guided Radiation Therapy (IGRT)

IGRT further refines RT accuracy by using imaging modalities (e.g., cone-beam CT or kV orthogonal imaging) immediately before or during treatment sessions to verify and adjust patient positioning. This is especially important in the management of desmoid tumors in the abdomen or pelvis, where internal organ motion and postoperative changes can significantly alter target positioning [23].

19.7.5 Proton Therapy and Particle Beam Radiotherapy

Proton therapy leverages the Bragg peak phenomenon to deposit high doses within the target while dramatically reducing the exit dose to surrounding tissues. This approach is particularly attractive for younger patients—and for those with recurrent tumors—because it minimizes the risk of long-term toxicity and secondary malignancies [24].

19.7.6 MR-Guided Adaptive Radiation Therapy (MRgRT)

MR-guided adaptive radiation therapy (MRgRT) represents one of the most exciting technological advances in the field. MRgRT provides real-time soft tissue visualization during treatment, thereby permitting adaptive modifications in response to anatomical shifts during each session. This capability may allow for more precise dose delivery with reduced margins, thus lowering toxicity without compromising local control [25].

19.7.7 Stereotactic Body Radiation Therapy (SBRT)

Although considered investigational for desmoid tumors, SBRT offers the prospect of delivering high-dose radiation in a limited number of fractions with submillimeter precision. Early studies in select patients with small, well-localized tumors indicate favorable outcomes, though long-term data regarding efficacy and late toxicity are still evolving [26].

19.8 Outcomes and Efficacy

Multiple studies have documented excellent local control with RT. For instance, a 5-year local control rate exceeding 80% has been reported in patients treated definitively with RT [27]. Comparable outcomes have been observed with adjuvant RT, supporting its role as a stand-alone therapeutic modality in many scenarios. Notably, tumor responses may be delayed, with stabilization or gradual regression observed over several months after treatment initiation. Although complete radiologic responses are uncommon, substantial clinical benefit can be realized without them [22, 27].

19.9 Toxicity and Late Effects

Acute RT-related side effects are generally mild and depend on the treatment site. Nonetheless, late toxicities remain an important consideration and may include:

Fibrosis and joint stiffness: particularly in tumors involving the extremities.
Dermatologic changes, such as skin induration or ulceration, when treating superficial lesions.
Bowel toxicity: Meticulous attention to dose–volume constraints is required during abdominal irradiation.
Secondary malignancies: Although rare, the risk is heightened in young patients or in re-irradiation scenarios [28].

19.10 Re-irradiation Strategies

Re-irradiation for recurrent desmoid tumors is complex. Decisions regarding re-treatment involve a careful evaluation of cumulative doses, tissue tolerance, and advanced planning strategies such as dose de-escalation or hyperfractionation. Adaptive planning and rigorous monitoring are essential to minimize the risk of additive toxicity, especially in previously irradiated regions [24, 29, 30].

19.11 Future Directions and Research Opportunities

The field of desmoid tumor management continues to evolve, driven by advances in molecular biology and radiation technology. Promising areas of future research include:

19.11.1 Radiogenomics and Personalized Radiotherapy

Emerging data linking specific genetic mutations (such as certain CTNNB1 subtypes) to radiotherapy outcomes may soon enable individualized adjustments in dose and fractionation schemes. Radiogenomics thus promises to enhance local control while reducing toxicity by tailoring treatment plans to each tumor's unique biology.

19.11.2 Combined Modality Therapy

Ongoing clinical trials are examining the benefits of combining RT with systemic agents. Preliminary data suggest that the integration of TKIs or hormonal agents with RT may produce synergistic antitumor effects—enhancing radiosensitivity and promoting apoptosis in desmoid cells.

19.11.3 Technological Innovations in Radiation Delivery

Advancements such as MRgRT and SBRT are geared toward further refining the balance between tumor control and normal tissue sparing. Future studies will likely focus on long-term safety outcomes and quality-of-life impacts associated with these advanced modalities.

19.11.4 Molecular Imaging and Theranostics

Incorporating molecular imaging techniques—such as PET imaging with novel fibroblast activation protein–targeted tracers—might enable dose painting strategies where escalated doses are delivered to biologically aggressive regions of the tumor, thereby optimizing the therapeutic ratio.

19.11.5 Collaborative Clinical Trials

Given the relative rarity of desmoid tumors, international collaboration and multicentric clinical trials are essential to generating high-quality evidence. Such efforts will be instrumental in establishing standardized treatment guidelines and integrating new molecular and imaging biomarkers into clinical practice.

For the practicing radiation oncologist and trainees, ongoing engagement with emerging research and participation in multidisciplinary tumor boards will be key to incorporating these advancements into routine patient care.

19.12 Conclusion

Desmoid tumors, despite their benign histology, present significant challenges due to their locally aggressive behavior and high recurrence rates. Progress in understanding their molecular underpinnings—chiefly alterations in the β-catenin pathway—has paved the way for innovations in therapy. In the realm of radiation oncology, there has been a transformative shift from conventional techniques to advanced modalities (such as IMRT, IGRT, MRgRT, and proton therapy) that permit precise, conformal treatment with minimized toxicity.

A tailored, multidisciplinary approach that judiciously balances surgical resection, active surveillance, systemic therapy, and advanced radiation delivery offers the best prospect for durable local control and improved patient outcomes. As ongoing research continues to elucidate molecular drivers and optimize radiation techniques, the integration of these innovations into clinical practice will remain paramount for both trainees and established radiation oncologists.

References

1. Kasper B, et al. Desmoid tumors: clinical features and treatment options for advanced disease. Oncologist. 2011;16(5):682–93.
2. Reitamo JJ, et al. The Desmoid tumor: analysis of 105 cases. Am J Surg. 1982;143(5):500–5.
3. Shields CJ, et al. Desmoid Tumours. Eur J Surg Oncol. 2001;27(8):701–6.
4. Surgailis D, et al. Pathogenesis and emerging therapies in desmoid tumors. Cancers (Basel). 2021;13(2):286.
5. Alman BA, et al. Increased beta-catenin protein and somatic APC mutations in sporadic aggressive fibromatoses (Desmoid tumors). Am J Pathol. 1997;151(2):329–34.
6. Mace J, et al. Response of extra-abdominal Desmoid tumors to therapy with tamoxifen and Sulindac: results of a prospective study. Cancer. 2002;95(11):2373–9.
7. Weiss SW, et al. Soft tissue tumors. Mosby-Year Book; 1986.
8. Church J, et al. Desmoid tumors in familial adenomatous polyposis. Dis Colon Rectum. 2005;48(3):559–64.
9. Tejpar S, et al. Clinical and biological analysis of Desmoid tumors associated with familial adenomatous polyposis. Gastroenterology. 1999;117(4):844–54.
10. Fiore M, et al. Desmoid-type fibromatosis: evolving treatment standards. Surg Oncol Clin N Am. 2009;18(2):567–82.
11. van Broekhoven DL, et al. Prognostic value of CTNNB1 gene mutation in primary sporadic aggressive fibromatosis. Ann Surg Oncol. 2015;22(5):1464–70.
12. Kasraeian S, et al. Management of Desmoid tumors: a retrospective review of 154 cases. Am Surg. 2011;77(3):325–31.
13. Bonvalot S, et al. Spontaneous regression of primary abdominal wall desmoid tumors: more common than previously thought. Ann Surg Oncol. 2013;20(13):4096–102.
14. Colombo C, et al. Management of desmoid-type fibromatosis: a new approach. Eur J Cancer. 2022;167:137–45.
15. Wilcken N, Tattersall MH. Management of Desmoid Tumours. Eur J Cancer. 1991;27(4):454–6.
16. Gronchi A, et al. Outcome of surgery for primary and recurrent desmoid-type fibromatosis. Ann Surg Oncol. 2003;10(9):1172–7.
17. Hansmann A, et al. High-dose tamoxifen and sulindac as first-line treatment for Desmoid tumors. Cancer. 2004;100(3):612–20.

18. Gounder MM, et al. Sorafenib for advanced and refractory desmoid tumors. N Engl J Med. 2018;379(25):2417–28.
19. Azzarelli A, et al. Low-dose chemotherapy with methotrexate and vinblastine for patients with advanced aggressive fibromatosis. Cancer. 2001;92(5):1259–64.
20. Alman BA, et al. The Management of desmoid tumours: a joint global consensus-based guideline approach for adult and paediatric patients. Eur J Cancer. 2020;127:96–107.
21. Gluck I, et al. Radiation therapy for desmoid tumors: the Princess Margaret hospital experience. Int J Radiat Oncol Biol Phys. 1999;44(4):1007–13.
22. Keus RB, et al. The role of radiotherapy in the management of Desmoid Tumors. Radiother Oncol. 2013;106(1):138–42.
23. Garton et al. (2020). Advances in image-guided radiotherapy for soft tissue tumors. J Radiat Oncol., [Details Pending].
24. Hong TS, et al. Proton beam therapy for unresectable intra-abdominal desmoid tumors. Int J Radiat Oncol Biol Phys. 2012;83(2):571–6.
25. Boeke S, et al. Clinical implementation of MR-guided radiotherapy: experience of a single institution. J Radiat Res. 2021;62(1):84–90.
26. Ulaner GA, et al. Stereotactic body radiation therapy (SBRT) for the treatment of desmoid tumors. Radiat Oncol. 2016;11:86.
27. Nuyttens JJ, et al. Surgery versus radiation therapy for patients with aggressive fibromatosis or desmoid tumors: a comparative review of 22 articles. Cancer. 2000;88(7):1517–23.
28. Merchant TE, et al. Late effects of radiation therapy on pediatric patients with CNS tumors: clinical and imaging findings. J Neuro-Oncol. 2005;75(3):279–86.
29. Salas S, et al. Prognostic factors influencing progression-free survival determined from a series of sporadic desmoid tumors: a wait-and-see policy according to tumor presentation. J Clin Oncol. 2011;29(26):3553–9.
30. Riesterer O, et al. 26th annual SASRO meeting. Strahlenther Onkol. 2023;2(199):208–50.

Peyronie's Disease

20

David K Simson, Shaifali Mahajan,
and Jaskaran Singh Sethi

20.1 Background

20.1.1 Brief Overview

Peyronie's disease (PD) is a benign condition characterised by fibrotic plaque formation on the penile shaft [1]. The plaque replaces the normally elastic fibres of the tunica albuginea and presents as a palpable induration, often associated with penile pain, deformity, erectile dysfunction (ED), and interference with sexual intercourse [2, 3]. The condition was first documented in 1561 through correspondence between anatomists Andreas Vesalius and Gabriele Falloppio and also independently described by Falloppio himself [4]. However, it was first clinically described by François Gigot de la Peyronie, surgeon to King Louis XV of France, in 1743 [5].

20.1.2 Epidemiology and Prevalence

PD likely has a higher true prevalence than reported, due to its subclinical and stigmatised nature [6]. Lindsay et al. reported 389 cases per 100,000 men in Rochester, Minnesota [7]. Schwarzer's German study showed a 3% prevalence overall, increasing with age—from 1.5% in men aged 30–39 to 6.5% in those over 70 years [3]. Among men attending prostate cancer screening, 8.9% had palpable plaques [8]. PD

D. K. Simson (✉)
Department of Radiation Oncology, Auckland City Hospital, Auckland, New Zealand
e-mail: DSimson@adhb.govt.nz

S. MahajanJ. S. Sethi
Department of Radiation Oncology, Rajiv Gandhi Cancer Institute and Research Centre, New Delhi, India

K. Sood Sharma (ed.), *Radiation Therapy for Benign Disorders*,
https://doi.org/10.1007/978-981-95-6635-8_20

is most common in men over 40 and is associated with diabetes, hypertension, smoking, Dupuytren's contracture, and prostatectomy [2, 3, 8–11].

20.1.3 Historical Context and Evolution of Treatment Approaches

Historically, treatment for PD has mirrored prevailing medical beliefs [5]. Early remedies included mercury, iodides, vitamin E, potassium para-aminobenzoate (Potaba), tamoxifen, and colchicine [12–16]. Intralesional injections—initially steroids, later verapamil and collagenase—gained popularity in the mid-twentieth century [17–19]. Surgical techniques, from Nesbit's procedure to plaque excision with grafting, became mainstays for severe deformities [20, 21]. With the evolution of technology, non-invasive options such as histamine iontophoresis and shockwave therapy have also emerged [22, 23]. Radiation therapy (RT) was introduced in the early 1900s, initially with radium and later external beam radiotherapy (EBRT) techniques, based on its potential anti-inflammatory effects [24–28].

20.2 Role of RT

20.2.1 Rationale

RT has been explored for PD based on its potent anti-inflammatory and antifibrotic properties at low doses [29]. Low-dose radiotherapy (LDRT) modulates several pathways central to the pathogenesis of PD [30]. It suppresses pro-inflammatory cytokines (TNF-α, IL-1β), reduces endothelial adhesion molecule expression, and inhibits macrophage and fibroblast activation [31].

One key mediator of these effects is nitric oxide (NO), whose production is upregulated through the induction of endothelial nitric oxide synthase (eNOS) following LDRT [31, 32]. NO reduces leukocyte-endothelium interaction, downregulates TGF-β-driven collagen synthesis, and may help maintain penile vascular function. These actions collectively reduce inflammation, limit fibrotic remodelling, and may slow plaque progression.

20.2.2 Indications for Radiation Therapy

RT is not a first-line treatment for PD, but it has been selectively used, especially in the early inflammatory phase, primarily to manage persistent penile pain. RT is most commonly considered during the acute phase of PD—usually within 12–18 months from symptom onset—when inflammation and pain are prominent and progressive plaque formation is ongoing, but penile deformity is not yet stabilised [30]. It is typically reserved for patients who have failed to respond to oral therapies such as vitamin E, pentoxifylline, tamoxifen, or Potaba, which are often used as initial conservative approaches [30]. RT may also be considered after unsuccessful intralesional therapies, including verapamil, interferon-α2b, or collagenase *Clostridium histolyticum*, particularly if pain persists or progresses [30]. Additionally, RT may serve as a non-invasive alternative in patients who are unsuitable for or decline surgery, provided their erectile function is preserved and curvature is not the dominant symptom [33]. However, it is not recommended in the chronic, stable phase of PD or for correcting curvature, where surgical options are more effective [30].

20.2.3 Benefits of RT Compared to Alternative Treatments

RT offers a non-invasive approach to PD, with studies showing significant pain relief in most patients [33, 34]. Similar to extracorporeal shockwave therapy (ESWT), which can reduce Peyronie's pain but does not improve curvature, RT focuses on symptom relief—often exceeding the minimal efficacy of oral agents (e.g., vitamin E, Potaba, colchicine) that have shown little impact on pain or deformity [35, 36]. While surgery and intralesional collagenase injections aim to straighten the penis, low-dose RT yields only limited improvement in penile curvature (~20–50% of cases) [33, 34]. Nonetheless, early RT may stabilise disease progression, halting plaque enlargement in ~78% of cases [34]. In contrast to intralesional injections (e.g., verapamil, collagenase), which require repeated treatments and carry local risks (e.g., haematoma or rare corporal rupture), RT is painless and well-tolerated, typically causing only transient skin erythema [34, 37, 38]. It is also much less invasive than surgery—while surgery remains the most effective option for severe curvature, it carries substantial risks (postoperative ED in up to 50% and penile shortening in ~40% of cases) [37]. RT's safety profile is favourable at therapeutic doses (no serious long-term adverse events observed up to ~32 Gy), making it an appealing option for patients prioritising pain control and tolerability over maximal curvature correction [34].

20.2.4 Patient Selection

RT for PD is generally reserved for select older patients during the acute phase, particularly those with persistent painful erections refractory to conservative therapies [34]. Younger patients are typically not offered RT due to long-term risk considerations (potential radiation-induced fibrosis or malignancy) and concern for adverse effects on future erectile function [30, 34]. RT is delivered as low-dose superficial EBRT (total ~10–30 Gy in fractions) with the primary goal of pain relief. It is primarily indicated in the early inflammatory phase, when pain is present. By the chronic phase (stable plaque without pain), radiation has little role, as pain usually resolves spontaneously [30]. RT is considered a second-line option after failure of other treatments and is avoided in men who are surgical candidates (e.g. those with severe stable deformity), as well as in those with significant baseline ED. Contraindications include prior radiation exposure to the region and comorbid conditions that could increase radiation toxicity (such as systemic connective tissue disorders or severe diabetes/vascular disease). Historically, LDRT provided pain relief in most patients (many series report ~50–90% reduction in pain) but yielded only modest improvements in curvature, with a substantial proportion still requiring surgical correction later [30, 33]. Recent series have confirmed that superficial RT can significantly alleviate pain (about 71% of patients report improvement) and may stabilise or slightly reduce plaque/curvature in early-stage PD, with minimal acute side effects [34]. However, RT does not reverse established fibrosis or restore lost erectile function, and there is a theoretical risk of exacerbating fibrosis via cytokine upregulation [39]. Given these limitations, contemporary guidelines advise against routine use of radiation in PD, reserving it only for rare cases of refractory pain in the active phase [35].

20.2.5 Limitations and Challenges

RT for PD offers at best a modest improvement in penile curvature, with negligible effect on chronic stable plaques [37]. Long-term safety concerns, including radiation-induced fibrosis, ED, and radiation toxicity, further limit its use [30]. Moreover, no standardised RT protocols exist, and treatment response is difficult to assess objectively [30]. RT is typically limited to the acute phase of the disease and is generally avoided in patients with significant comorbidities or if surgical intervention is planned [37]. Historically, inconsistent outcomes in older studies and the emergence of more effective alternative treatments have led to a decline in the use of RT [30, 37].

20.3 Radiation

20.3.1 Overview of Radiotherapy Techniques

Historically, orthovoltage X-rays were used to treat PD, later replaced mainly by superficial electron-beam therapy via linear accelerators (LA) [33, 40, 41]. Occasional brachytherapy (BT) attempts have been reported, but EBRT remained the primary modality [41, 42]. Typical regimens delivered total doses of ~10–30 Gy in multiple fractions [41]. Shallow-penetration modalities like orthovoltage and low-energy electrons confine dose to the tunica albuginea plaque (penetration ~1–1.5 cm), whereas megavoltage photons penetrate more deeply (often requiring bolus to treat superficial lesions) and risk unnecessary exposure of deeper tissues [34].

20.3.2 Techniques, Dosage, Setup and Delivery

In the study conducted by Gunilla Pietsch, superficial radiation therapy was delivered using a Siemens Dermopan II unit, following informed consent and established protocols [34]. The treatment utilised 50 kV photons at a tube current of 25 mA, incorporating a 2 mm Cellon filter along with a 1 mm aluminium filter to minimise adverse effects. Radiation was administered through a 4 cm diameter applicator with a focus-to-skin distance of 15 cm, yielding a half-value depth of 15 mm. Each treatment cycle comprised two consecutive daily fractions of 4 Gy, followed by an 8-week break. This regimen was repeated four times over 24 weeks, resulting in a cumulative radiation dose of 32 Gy.

In a 2006 study, Marcus Niewald reported on the outcomes of radiotherapy in PD, employing both cobalt units and LA units [43]. The RT technique was tailored according to the location of the plaque. For plaques located in the distal two-thirds of the penis (65 of 101 patients, 64%), the penis was inserted into a slit tube and held upright using a clamp. This setup facilitated lateral opposing fields using Co-60 gamma rays or 4–6 MV photon beams from an LA. The tube served dual purposes—as both a fixation device and a bolus, mitigating dose build-up effects. A lead shield was used for testicular protection when feasible. For plaques near the abdominal wall (36% of cases), upright positioning was not possible; instead, the penis was laid flat with a 1 cm silicone mat serving as a bolus. Treatment in these cases was delivered using direct electron beams (5–8 MeV), with a 1 cm polyethylene shield for testicular protection. All patients received daily fractions of 2 Gy. Most patients were treated to a total dose of 30 Gy ($n = 72$) or 36 Gy ($n = 25$), with a few receiving doses of 32–34 Gy or 38–40 Gy. No treatments were discontinued due to side effects.

In a separate study, Luca Incrocci investigated LDRT for PD using two distinct treatment regimens. Orthovoltage radiotherapy was administered to 123 patients (69%) using a median photon energy of 250 kV (range: 120–250 kV), delivering a total dose of 13.5 Gy in 3 weekly fractions of 1.5 Gy. This course was repeated twice more, with 3–4 week intervals between each cycle. The remaining 56 patients (31%) received electron beam therapy with a median energy of 10 MeV (range: 4–14 MeV), applying a total dose of 12 Gy in six daily fractions of 2 Gy, with bolus material used to ensure adequate surface dosing. The treatment targeted the plaque area with generous margins, often encompassing the whole penile shaft while sparing the glans. The median treated surface area was 48 cm^2 (range: 12–120 cm^2). A single radiation field was employed, and a 5-mm lead shield was consistently used to protect the testicles, scrotum, and suprapubic region.

In a 2008 European survey conducted by Luca Incrocci, RT practices for PD were evaluated across multiple institutions [41]. The reported fraction doses ranged from 0.5 to 8 Gy, with a mean of 2.4 Gy; most centres ($n = 43$) administered 2 Gy per fraction. Total doses varied between 3 and 30 Gy, with an average of 17 Gy, and 29 centres delivered a total dose of 20 Gy. The number of treatment sessions per week ranged from 1 to 5, with a mean of 4 sessions; the majority ($n = 39$) treated patients five times per week. In terms of technology, 32 institutions used orthovoltage equipment (50–300 kV), three employed megavoltage photon beams (4 or 6 MV), and 44 used electron beams (4–13 MeV). Additionally, two centres utilised either low-dose-rate (LDR) or high-dose-rate (HDR) BT, and two others operated cobalt units.

20.3.2.1 Role of BT

Historically, BT was explored as a treatment for PD, though it is no longer in routine clinical use. In a 1996 study by Koren et al., RT was delivered via a localised iridium-192 (^{192}Ir) mould technique [42]. This involved a tubular Plexiglas cylinder (moulage) designed to encase the pars pendula of the penis, with eight iridium needles positioned evenly around the cylindrical wall. The device was anchored to the os pubis, and lead shielding was used to protect the testes. Two moulage sizes—22 mm and 25 mm in diameter—were selected based on the patient's penile girth. The iridium needles were inserted at the patient's bedside, and radiation was delivered over 11.6–39.1 h (median 24.1 h). After treatment, the mould was removed and patients were discharged. While technically innovative for its time, this approach has since been abandoned in favour of more standardised and less invasive EBRT techniques.

20.4 Toxicity Profile and Strategies to Minimise Risks

20.4.1 Acute Side Effects

RT for PD is generally well tolerated with no significant RT-related morbidity in most patients. Acute effects are primarily limited to mild skin reactions (erythema, dryness) and very infrequent urinary irritation [43]. Radiation dermatitis presenting as transient skin erythema of the penile shaft is common, with a reported incidence of approximately 27–39% [34, 43]. Approximately 9–10% of patients report transient skin dryness or desquamation [34]. These reactions are typically mild and self-limited. Four percent of the patients experience mild urethritis as an acute side effect [43]. These resolve spontaneously or may need NSAID support. A transient pain "Flare" or worsening of penile pain during or immediately after RT is not commonly reported. Between 50% and 71% of patients experience a reduction in pain during therapy [33, 43].

20.4.2 Chronic Side Effects

Long-term erectile function can be affected. In a 9-year follow-up study, roughly half of the men reported new or worsened erection problems [44]. Only about 54% had erections rigid enough for intercourse at long-term follow-up [44]. Ionising radiation can stimulate fibrogenic cytokine pathways—for example, an upregulation of TGF-β1 and other profibrotic signals in irradiated plaque fibroblasts [39].

This raises the possibility of radiation-induced plaque fibrosis or tunical scarring, which could theoretically cause ED via vascular damage.

Mulhall et al., reported chronic skin changes such as telangiectasias of the penis which were observed in approximately 12% of patients on long-term follow-up [39]. This appears as small red spider-vein–like lesions in the irradiated penile skin. Atrophic skin changes (thinning or fibrosis of the skin in the treated area) were reported in ~10% of their cohort of patients [39]. This manifests as a loss of elasticity or softness of the penile skin over time. A minority of patients (about 5 in number, ~6%) experienced paraesthesia in the form of persistent numbness or tingling in the treated area of the penis after RT [39].

In a series with ~4 years of follow-up, about 7% of the patients experienced continued progression of fibrosis despite RT [45]. Thus, while RT essentially stabilises the disease, a small percentage of patients may still see progression of penile fibrosis post-therapy. No cases of radiation-induced second malignancy have been reported. A patient series observed no malignant transformation at any time during treatment or follow-up [46]. Another systematic review noted no incidence of long-term complications in some studies and concluded that the risk of secondary cancer with penile LDRT is negligible [47].

20.4.3 Risk Mitigation Strategies and Management of Toxicities

Risk mitigation starts with careful treatment planning and shielding of adjacent structures (e.g., gonads) to minimise unnecessary dose [46]. Field setups using superficial X-rays or electrons, combined with lead shields, can limit deep tissue exposure and reduce skin and urethral toxicity [46]. The use of modern RT techniques and strict dose constraints for the surrounding normal tissues can be beneficial.

Topical corticosteroids (e.g., mometasone) have been shown to reduce the severity of radiation dermatitis and improve patient comfort [45]. Patients are advised to use emollient moisturisers to maintain skin hydration and integrity throughout therapy [48]. If mild radiation urethritis (dysuria) occurs, increasing oral fluid intake (while avoiding bladder irritants) can alleviate symptoms [49]. Short-term analgesics (e.g., NSAIDs) can be used for transient pain flares. Patient education on skin care, adequate hydration, and prompt reporting of side effects to ensure timely management.

20.5 Clinical Outcomes

Early studies on RT for PD have yielded mixed outcomes. In a 1975 analysis, Furlow et al. observed that patients treated with orthovoltage RT had similar long-term outcomes to untreated patients, with the primary benefit being a faster symptomatic improvement by a few months [50]. Likewise, a 1980 retrospective series of 56 cases noted that many PD cases improve or stabilise spontaneously over time, complicating the assessment of RT's true benefit [46]. Nonetheless, these early reports hinted that RT might transiently reduce PD-related symptoms, even if it did not alter the eventual natural history of the disease.

Subsequent case series in the 1990s and the 2000s suggested that LDRT could safely provide symptomatic relief, especially for penile pain. Rodrigues et al. (1995) treated 38 PD patients with orthovoltage X-rays (total 9 Gy in 5 fractions, with an optional additional 9 Gy for partial responders). They reported that overall, 76% experienced pain relief, 48% had reduced curvature, and 60% reported improved sexual function, with no radiation-induced morbidity noted [28]. Incrocci et al. (2000) published a larger retrospective series of 179 patients treated with 12–13.5 Gy. At ~3 months post-RT, 83% had diminished or resolved pain, 23% noted improvement in curvature, and no significant RT-related complications were observed. In that series, roughly one-third of patients ultimately still required surgery for persistent deformity, and a long-term follow-up survey found about half had ED. However, this was attributed to PD's progression or ageing rather than the radiation itself [33]. Niewald et al. (2006) likewise reported that among 101 patients (median 5-year follow-up) treated with 30–36 Gy, about 50% experienced pain relief and 47% saw improvement in penile deviation, with only mild, transient side effects (dermatitis in 28 patients, mild urethritis in 4) and no long-term complications noted [43]. These case studies collectively indicate that RT, typically delivered in low doses, can alleviate acute-phase symptoms of PD in a significant subset of patients while producing minimal acute toxicity.

More recent studies have reinforced the benefits of RT for PD, particularly for pain, while also highlighting the variability in outcomes. The European survey, as discussed above, found that only ~19% of radiation oncology centres were offering RT for PD, reflecting its limited adoption. Those centres reported pain reduction in about 80% of treated cases and very infrequent side effects; however, practices varied widely, and no standardised protocol existed [41]. In a 2018 retrospective study of 83 patients, it was reported that after a mean 52-month follow-up, 71% of patients experienced substantial pain relief, and 78% had no further disease progression. Nearly half (49%) noted an improvement in curvature, and ~42% reported a decrease in plaque hardness. Patient satisfaction in that cohort was high (median 8/10), and aside from transient skin erythema (38.6%) and dryness (9.6%), no severe adverse effects or radiation-induced malignancies occurred with total doses up to 32 Gy [34].

However, improvements in penile curvature and plaque size have been inconsistent across studies, ranging from modest gains to no significant change, and the outcomes for sexual function remain difficult to interpret without controlled comparisons between the two groups. Importantly, all existing studies have been uncontrolled (mostly retrospective or case series), lacking placebo comparison and uniform criteria for success [45]. This makes it challenging to distinguish the effects of RT from the variable natural course of PD or concurrent therapies in some reports. Expert opinion has become more cautious regarding the role of RT in PD. Mulhall et al. (2012) conducted a comprehensive review and concluded that due to the absence of robust efficacy data and concerns about potential radiation injury to erectile tissues, RT should not be used for managing PD [30].

Consistent with these cautionary findings, the American Urological Association's 2015 guidelines issued a moderate recommendation against the use of RT for PD, citing the unproven benefit and potential risks of exposing patients to radiation [35]. Thus, while historical and contemporary case series suggest that RT can provide meaningful symptomatic relief (especially pain reduction) in PD, the lack of high-quality evidence and the availability of other treatments have relegated RT to an off-label, last-resort option. Currently, most experts and guidelines discourage its use, emphasising that its role is limited in the modern management of PD.

20.6 Future Directions

Modern RT have greatly improved precision. Image-guided intensity-modulated radiotherapy (IMRT) now allows highly conformal dose delivery to the plaque while sparing adjacent tissues [51]. Theoretically, proton beam therapy can further limit collateral dose via the Bragg peak, reducing radiation to healthy structures.

RT is increasingly being used in non-malignant conditions (about 20% of RT cases in Germany) [51]. Fibroproliferative disorders like Dupuytren's contracture—analogous to Peyronie's—show high control rates with LDRT, fuelling interest in similar use for PD [51]. Prospective research is needed to establish the role of RT in PD. Future trials should compare modern RT (e.g. IMRT or proton therapy) to standard treatments (such as intralesional therapy or surgery) in appropriate patients, with objective endpoints including pain relief, curvature changes, and sexual function over long-term follow-up. Ultimately, such studies will determine if RT can be safely and effectively integrated into the management of PD [51].

With modern techniques and better patient selection, re-evaluation of RT for PD is a future possibility, ideally in the context of controlled clinical studies.

20.6.1 Personalized Medicine and Artificial Intelligence (AI)

Personalised treatment planning will likely enhance RT outcomes in PD. Advanced imaging techniques (such as ultrasound and MRI) can delineate each patient's plaque for tailored targeting, and dosing can be adjusted to individual tolerances. AI is poised to aid these efforts: in oncology, AI-driven systems can analyse images and generate patient-specific dose plans that improve treatment success [52]. Similar AI tools could optimise RT by identifying an optimal dose that maximises plaque resolution while minimising exposure to healthy tissue.

20.7 Conclusion

PD is a benign condition characterised by fibrotic plaque formation on the penile shaft with significant physical and psychological implications. RT, though historically explored, has remained a controversial modality, primarily due to variable outcomes and concerns over long-term safety. However, evidence from case series suggests that LDRT can provide effective pain relief in the acute phase, stabilise plaque progression in selected patients, and is generally well-tolerated with minimal acute toxicity.

Despite its potential, RT for PD remains underutilised due to a lack of high-quality, controlled trials, and ongoing concerns about its long-term impact on erectile function. Current guidelines advise against routine use but acknowledge its selective utility in refractory, pain-predominant cases during the early inflammatory phase. Moving forward, robust prospective studies comparing RT with standard interventions are essential to clearly define its role. With careful patient selection and technical advances, RT may yet find a valuable niche in the evolving therapeutic landscape of PD.

References

1. Hellstrom WJ, Bivalacqua TJ. Peyronie's disease: etiology, medical, and surgical therapy. J Androl. 2000;21(3):347–54.
2. Carrieri MP, Serraino D, Palmiotto F, Nucci G, Sasso F. A case-control study on risk factors for Peyronie's disease. J Clin Epidemiol. 1998;51(6):511–5.
3. Schwarzer U, Sommer F, Klotz T, Braun M, Reifenrath B, Engelmann U. The prevalence of Peyronie's disease: results of a large survey. BJU Int. 2001;88(7):727–30.
4. Falloppio G. Gabrielis Falloppii medici Mutinensis Observationes anatomicae ad Petrum Mannam medicum Cremonensem. Venetiis: Apud Marcum Antonium Ulmum; 1561.
5. Dunsmuir WD, Kirby RS. Francois de LaPeyronie (1978-1747): the man and the disease he described. Br J Urol. 1996;78(4):613–22.
6. Sommer F, Schwarzer U, Wassmer G, Bloch W, Braun M, Klotz T, et al. Epidemiology of Peyronie's disease. Int J Impot Res. 2002;14(5):379–83.
7. Lindsay MB, Schain DM, Grambsch P, Benson RC, Beard CM, Kurland LT. The incidence of Peyronie's disease in Rochester, Minnesota, 1950 through 1984. J Urol. 1991;146(4):1007–9.
8. Mulhall JP, Creech SD, Boorjian SA, Ghaly S, Kim ED, Moty A, et al. Subjective and objective analysis of the prevalence of Peyronie's disease in a population of men presenting for prostate cancer screening. J Urol. 2004;171(6 Pt 1):2350–3.
9. Tal R, Hall MS, Alex B, Choi J, Mulhall JP. Peyronie's disease in teenagers. J Sex Med. 2012;9(1):302–8.
10. Deveci S, Hopps CV, O'Brien K, Parker M, Guhring P, Mulhall JP. Defining the clinical characteristics of Peyronie's disease in young men. J Sex Med. 2007;4(2):485–90.
11. Arafa M, Eid H, El-Badry A, Ezz-Eldine K, Shamloul R. The prevalence of Peyronie's disease in diabetic patients with erectile dysfunction. Int J Impot Res. 2007;19(2):213–7.
12. Curling TB. Impotency. Diseases of the testis, spermatic cord and scrotum. London: J & A Churchill; 1878. p. 460–5.
13. Scardino PL, Scott WW. The use of tocopherols in the treatment of Peyronie's disease. Ann N Y Acad Sci. 1949;52:390–3.

14. Zarafonetis CJD, Horrax TM. Treatment of Peyronie's disease with potassium p-amino benzoate (POTABA). J Urol. 1959;81:770–2.
15. Akkus E, Carrier S, Rehman J, Breza J, Kadioglu A, Lue TF. Is colchicine effective in Peyronie's disease? A pilot study. Urology. 1994;44(2):291–5.
16. Ralph DJ, Brooks MD, Bottazzo GF, Pryor JP. The treatment of Peyronie's disease with tamoxifen. Br J Urol. 1992;70(6):648–51.
17. Teasley GH. Peyronie's disease; a new approach. J Urol. 1954;71(5):611–4.
18. Levine LA, Merrick PF, Lee RC. Intralesional verapamil injection for the treatment of Peyronie's disease. J Urol. 1994;151(6):1522–4.
19. Gelbard MK, James K, Riach P, Dorey F. Collagenase versus placebo in the treatment of Peyronie's disease: a double-blind study. J Urol. 1993;149(1):56–8.
20. Nesbit RM. Congenital curvature of the phallus: report of three cases with description of corrective operation. Trans Am Assoc Genitourin Surg. 1964;56:20–2.
21. Devine CJ Jr, Horton CE. Surgical treatment of Peyronie's disease with a dermal graff. J Urol. 1974;111(1):44–9.
22. Di Mauro M, Russo GI, Della Camera PA, Di Maida F, Cito G, Mondaini N, et al. Extracorporeal shock wave therapy in Peyronie's disease: clinical efficacy and safety from a single-arm observational study. World J Mens Health. 2019;37(3):339–46.
23. Whalen WH. A new concept in the treatment of Peyronie's disease. J Urol. 1960;83:851–2.
24. Kumer L. Ueber die Radium Behandlung der Induratio Penis Plastica. Dermatologische Wochenschrift Leipzig V Hamb. 1922;125:673–7.
25. Dahl O. The treatment of plastic induration of the penis (Peyronie's disease). Acta Radiol (Stockh). 1954;41(3):290–301.
26. Duggan HE. Effect of X-ray therapy on patients with Peyronie's disease. J Urol. 1964;91:572–3.
27. Viljoen IM, Goedhals L, Doman MJ. Peyronie's disease--a perspective on the disease and the long-term results of radiotherapy. S Afr Med J. 1993;83(1):19–20.
28. Rodrigues CI, Njo KH, Karim AB. Results of radiotherapy and vitamin E in the treatment of Peyronie's disease. Int J Radiat Oncol Biol Phys. 1995;31(3):571–6.
29. Incrocci L. Radiotherapeutic treatment of Peyronie s disease. Expert Rev Pharmacoecon Outcomes Res. 2004;4(2):235–42.
30. Mulhall JP, Hall M, Broderick GA, Incrocci L. Radiation therapy in Peyronie's disease. J Sex Med. 2012;9(5):1435–41.
31. Rödel F, Keilholz L, Herrmann M, Sauer R, Hildebrandt G. Radiobiological mechanisms in inflammatory diseases of low-dose radiation therapy. Int J Radiat Biol. 2007;83(6):357–66.
32. Trott K-R, Kamprad F. Radiobiological mechanisms of anti-inflammatory radiotherapy. Radiother Oncol. 1999;51(3):197–203.
33. Incrocci L, Wijnmaalen A, Slob AK, Hop WC, Levendag PC. Low-dose radiotherapy in 179 patients with Peyronie's disease: treatment outcome and current sexual functioning. Int J Radiat Oncol Biol Phys. 2000;47(5):1353–6.
34. Pietsch G, Anzeneder T, Bruckbauer H, Zirbs M, Gutermuth J, Hofmann H, et al. Superficial radiation therapy in peyronie's disease: an effective and well-tolerated therapy. Adv Radiat Oncol. 2018;3(4):548–51.
35. Nehra A, Alterowitz R, Culkin DJ, Faraday MM, Hakim LS, Heidelbaugh JJ, et al. Peyronie's disease: AUA guideline. J Urol. 2015;194(3):745–53.
36. Barrett-Harlow B, Wang R. Oral therapy for Peyronie's disease, does it work? Transl Androl Urol. 2016;5(3):296–302.
37. Sandean DP, Lotfollahzadeh S. Peyronie disease. Treasure Island (FL): StatPearls Publishing; 2025.
38. Lizza E. Peyronie disease treatment & management: emedicine. medscape; 2023 [updated Jan 28, 2023]. Available from: https://emedicine.medscape.com/article/456574-treatment#:~:text=In%20general%2C%20the%20oral%20and,blinded%20placebo%20control%20remains%20unclear.
39. Mulhall JP, Branch J, Lubrano T, Shankey TV. Radiation increases fibrogenic cytokine expression by Peyronie's disease fibroblasts. J Urol. 2003;170(1):281–4.

40. Carson CC 3rd, Coughlin PW. Radiation therapy for Peyronie's disease: is there a place? J Urol. 1985;134(4):684–6.
41. Incrocci L, Hop WC, Seegenschmiedt HM. Radiotherapy for Peyronie's disease: a European survey. Acta Oncol. 2008;47(6):1110–2.
42. Koren H, Alth G, Schenk GM, Jindra RH. Induratio penis plastica: effectivity of low-dose radiotherapy at different clinical stages. Urol Res. 1996;24(4):245–8.
43. Niewald M, Wenzlawowicz KV, Fleckenstein J, Wisser L, Derouet H, Rübe C. Results of radiotherapy for Peyronie's disease. Int J Radiat Oncol Biol Phys. 2006;64(1):258–62.
44. Lue TF, Giuliano F, Montorsi F, Rosen RC, Andersson KE, Althof S, et al. Summary of the recommendations on sexual dysfunctions in men. J Sex Med. 2004;1(1):6–23.
45. Hayat S, Brunckhorst O, Alnajjar HM, Cakir OO, Muneer A, Ahmed K. A systematic review of non-surgical management in Peyronie's disease. Int J Impot Res. 2023;35(6):523–32.
46. Mira JG, Chahbazian CM, del Regato JA. The value of radiotherapy for Peyronie's disease: presentation of 56 new case studies and review of the literature. Int J Radiat Oncol Biol Phys. 1980;6(2):161–6.
47. Jutkowitz E, Rieke K, Caputo EL, Yan SX, Rudolph J, Mai HJ, et al. VA evidence-based synthesis program reports. Radiation therapy for benign conditions: a systematic review. Washington, DC: Department of Veterans Affairs (US); 2024.
48. Chan RJ, Webster J, Chung B, Marquart L, Ahmed M, Garantziotis S. Prevention and treatment of acute radiation-induced skin reactions: a systematic review and meta-analysis of randomized controlled trials. BMC Cancer. 2014;14:53.
49. Salvo N, Barnes E, van Draanen J, Stacey E, Mitera G, Breen D, et al. Prophylaxis and management of acute radiation-induced skin reactions: a systematic review of the literature. Curr Oncol. 2010;17(4):94–112.
50. Furlow WL, Swenson HE Jr, Lee RE. Peyronie's disease: a study of its natural history and treatment with orthovoltage radiotherapy. J Urol. 1975;114(1):69–71.
51. Nardone V, D'Ippolito E, Grassi R, Sangiovanni A, Gagliardi F, De Marco G, et al. Non-oncological radiotherapy: a review of modern approaches. J Pers Med. 2022;12(10):1677.
52. Bibault JE, Giraud P, Burgun A. Big data and machine learning in radiation oncology: state of the art and future prospects. Cancer Lett. 2016;382(1):110–7.

Radiotherapy in Dupuytren's Contracture: Current Evidence and Future Directions

21

Sankalp Singh

21.1 Introduction

Dupuytren's contracture, also known as 'Viking disease', Morbus Dupuytren, or Dupuytren's Disease (DD), is a chronic fibroproliferative connective tissue disorder which affects the palmar fascia of the hands. It is characterized by the progressive development of fibrous nodules and cords that cause flexion contractures of fingers, most commonly affecting the fourth and fifth phalanges of the hand (the ring and little fingers). This progressive contracture leads to disability and impaired hand functions like holding and grabbing, significantly affecting daily activities. The origin of these contractures was correctly identified to be from the palmar fascia by the British surgeon Henry Cline in 1777, who also performed successful surgery for the same. However, the disease is named after the Frenchman Guillaume Dupuytren, who described it and the corrective surgery in 1833 in a *Lancet* publication [1–4].

DD is estimated to affect 8.2% (95% confidence interval (CI), 5.7–11.7%) of the global population though variable prevalence rates are reported in different geographic regions. The incidence is higher in populations of Northern European ancestry, with the disease affecting 4–6% of all whites, but prevalence has been reported from the African and Asian continents as well. It affects men 2–3 times more commonly than women, and incidence rates rise after 40 years of age. Besides genetic predisposition, the presence of type I or type II diabetes, hypercholesterolaemia, human immunodeficiency virus (HIV) infection and environmental factors like smoking and alcohol are known risk factors. Exposure of hands to repetitive mechanical stress like vibrations and hand trauma, particularly surgical trauma, is also associated with development of DD [3, 5–7].

S. Singh (✉)
Department of Radiation Oncology, Army Hospital (Research & Referral), Delhi, India

K. Sood Sharma (ed.), *Radiation Therapy for Benign Disorders*,
https://doi.org/10.1007/978-981-95-6635-8_21

Management strategies range from conservative observation to invasive surgery, depending on disease stage and severity. Surgical excision (fasciectomy, dermofasciectomy) remains the mainstay for correcting contractures but carries risks such as recurrence and neurovascular injury. Physical therapy, corticosteroids, minimally invasive interventions like needle fasciotomy and collagenase injections have emerged but have limitations in durability and availability [3, 5, 8].

Radiotherapy (RT) has proven to be an effective, non-invasive treatment modality especially targeting early-stage disease to prevent progression by modulating fibroblast activity. While RT has been used since the mid-twentieth century for DD, its precise role continues to evolve with accumulating evidence and advances in radiation techniques [2, 8].

21.2 Relevant Anatomy

A. Structure of palmar fascia: The palmar aponeurosis is a dense fibrous sheet beneath the skin, continuous proximally with the palmaris longus tendon and dividing distally into pretendinous bands that connect to flexor tendons (see Fig. 21.1).
B. Pathological changes in Dupuytren's contracture: The main involved region is the pretendinous cords in the palm and digital cords extending into fingers. DD thickens and contracts these pretendinous cords causing finger contractures, mainly at proximal interphalangeal (PIP) and metacarpophalangeal (MCP) joints and rarely at distal interphalangeal (DIP) joints as well. Early disease

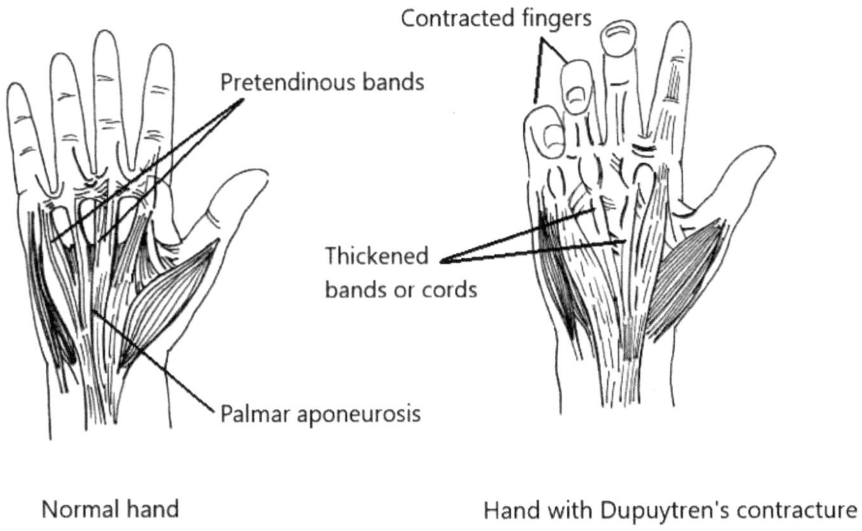

Fig. 21.1 Classical deformity and relevant anatomy of Dupuytren's contracture. (Illustrator—Dr Shashank B. Karvekar)

manifests as palmar nodules and skin thickening (Tubiana Stage 0-1), while advanced stages involve the thickened cords reaching the periosteum leading to established flexion deformities (Stages 2-4) causing the affected fingers to curl (see Fig. 21.1) [1, 5, 9, 10]. Tables 21.1 and 21.2 show the original and revised Tubiana clinical staging for DD [11, 12]. The revised staging system incorporates the original Tubiana staging criteria and adds scoring for additional clinical parameters, making it more comprehensive, and surrounding neurovascular bundles, tendons, and skin must be spared during treatment.

Table 21.1 Original Tubiana classification [12]

Stage	Deformity
0	No lesion
N	Palmar nodule without presence of contracture
1	TFD between 0° and 45°
2	TFD between 45° and 90°
3	TFD between 90° and 135°
4	TFD greater than 135°

TFD total flexion deformity

Table 21.2 Revised Tubiana classification [11]

Criteria	Score
Surgical procedures	Total no of operations for left and right hand
Recurrence	Total no of recurrences for left and right hand
Number of digits affected	Total for left and right hand
Number of nodules	Total for left and right hand (palmar/digital)
Number of pits	Total for left and right hand
Garrod's pads	1
Peyronies' disease	1
Lederhoses' disease	1
Bilateral/unilateral disease	Unilateral 1, bilateral 2
Stage 1 = TFD of each digit	1
Stage 2 = TFD	2
Stage 3 = TFD	3
Stage 4 = TFD	4

21.3 Pathophysiology

DD is fundamentally a disorder of aberrant fibroblast and myofibroblast activity within the palmar fascia, manifesting clinically as fibrotic thickening and contracture formation. The pathogenesis involves microangiopathic ischemia of the palmar fascia, triggered by factors such as smoking, diabetes, and aging. This ischemia increases free radical production, which promotes fibroblast proliferation, cytokine release (notably IL-1), and perivascular tissue damage, inducing a reparative fibroblast response. Aberrant immune responses further contribute, with autoantibodies against elastin and collagen activating immune cells like macrophages that secrete growth factors, causing endothelial proliferation, microvascular occlusion, and hypoxia, which enhances fibroblast growth via free oxygen radicals.

At the cellular level, DD is characterized by proliferation of fibroblasts and myofibroblasts and abnormal extracellular matrix remodelling. Activated fibroblasts produce excess collagen type III, while contractile myofibroblasts expressing alpha-smooth muscle actin cause palmar fascia thickening and contracture. Molecularly, several growth factors—transforming growth factor beta (TGF-β), fibroblast growth factor (FGF), platelet-derived growth factor, epidermal growth factor, and connective tissue growth factor—and inflammatory cytokines like IL-1 drive this uncontrolled fibrosis process, leading to characteristic hand deformities in DD. Genetic predisposition and association with other fibromatoses such as Ledderhose disease (plantar), Peyronie disease (penile), and Garrod nodes (dorsal PIP joints) further contribute [3, 5, 8, 9].

This integrated pathogenic process highlights how genetic, vascular, immunological, cellular, and molecular factors collectively drive the fibroproliferative changes in Dupuytren's disease.

Treatment Modalities A wide variety of treatment options for different stages and with differing advantages are commonly utilized for DD. Key modalities are summarized in Table 21.3 and described in detail below.

A. *Non-operative Management*—In latent or very early-stage disease without contracture, conservative approaches include:
   - *Active Surveillance*: In the majority of affected individuals, DD is known to remain stable in early-stages without progression for many years. In a population study from Netherlands, only 21.5% of DD patients were reported to progress over 7 years of surveillance. For patients with stable, painless, early-stage Dupuytren disease who exhibit minimal contracture and no functional limitations, observation is a suitable option. Individuals with mild symptoms can be followed-up every 6–12 months. These follow-up appointments enable the evaluation of contracture progression, the assessment of any functional impairments, and the discussion of potential surgical referrals [5, 13, 14].

Table 21.3 Summary of treatment modalities in Dupuytren's contracture

Modality	Indications	Advantages	Limitations/ Complications
Observation	Early/asymptomatic disease	Non-invasive	Disease progression possible
Splinting/Physical Therapy	Early disease	Symptomatic relief	No proven effect on progression
Corticosteroid injections	Early inflammatory phase	May reduce nodules	Side effects, limited efficacy
Percutaneous Needle Fasciotomy	Established cords	Minimally invasive, quick recovery	High recurrence (~80% in 3–5 years)
Collagenase Injection	Established cords	Non-surgical, good short-term efficacy	Cost, allergic reactions, recurrence (~35%)
Surgical Fasciectomy	Contractures impairing function	Durable correction	Risk of nerve injury, recurrence (30–50%)
Radiotherapy	Early-stage/ precontracture	Non-invasive, outpatient	Requires early diagnosis, controversial

- *Physical Therapy and Splinting*: Use of physical therapy approaches like stretching, range of motion (ROM) exercises, heat application, and use of a custom splint are used to maintain finger extension and hand mobility. However, the benefits are limited, and there is limited evidence. Occupational therapy may help patients to learn adaptive techniques and use assistive devices to improve their daily functional abilities. Physical therapy is often employed in post-operative period after surgical correction of the contracture to help patients regain range of motion and function [5, 13].
- *Intralesional Corticosteroids*: Corticosteroid injections are occasionally used by administration directly into Dupuytren's nodules, to potentially inhibit the inflammation and retard growth of the disease but have shown only limited effectiveness. While steroid injections have been reported to slow the progression of the disease and reduce nodule size, the results are inconsistent and broader utilization is hindered by possibility of complications such as skin thinning, depigmentation, and tendon rupture [8, 13, 15, 16].
- *Other Medications*: Several other medications like vitamin E, allopurinol, botulinum toxin, and biologic agents like the tumour necrosis factor inhibitor adalimumab have been tested in the treatment of Dupuytren's disease, but none have yet demonstrated consistent clinical efficacy, and their use remains experimental or limited to research settings [3, 8].

B. *Minimally Invasive Procedures*

- *Percutaneous Needle Fasciotomy (PNF)*: This technique involves multiple needle punctures to mechanically manipulate and disrupt the cords, offering rapid relief within 24 h. The procedure can be carried out using a regular 25-gauge needle on a 10 ml syringe under minimal local anaesthesia. Despite ease of procedure and low morbidity, PNF is associated with high recurrence rates of up to 85% within 5 years and is less effective for severe or multiple cord involvement [1, 17, 18].

- *Collagenase Clostridium Histolyticum (CCH) Injection*: This enzymatic approach uses collagenase from *Clostridium histolyticum* (CCH) injected directly into the cords to selectively dissolve cord collagen by breakdown of peptide bonds, allowing finger extension and release of contracture. It has received regulatory approvals for use in adults with DD with palpable cords and has demonstrated good initial efficacy with quicker functional recovery than surgery. The CORD I and CORD II randomized studies showed that CCH injections were able to reduce contractures in a significantly larger proportion of patients (44–64%) compared to placebo. While CCH is proving to be an effective and minimally invasive technique for late-stage DD, it's limitations include cost, availability, allergic reactions, localized swelling, pain and bruising, and concerns about recurrence rates which range from 35% at 3 years to 80% at 7 years [3, 19–22].

C. *Surgical Treatment*—Surgery remains the gold standard for contractures limiting hand function, especially at later disease stages. The aim of surgery is to remove diseased tissue to prevent disease progression, repair deformity, and restore functional movements of the hand. The patient should be counselled about the potential morbidity of surgery and should realize that surgery may not be curative.

- *Limited Fasciectomy*: Fasciectomy entails the precise removal of the abnormal fascia, including the thickened cords and nodules, while ensuring the tendons and neurovascular bundle remain intact, thus allowing for the correction of the flexion contracture. Fasciectomy can be performed in a segmental, limited, or total manner. Segmental fasciectomy involves excising a portion of the cord (1 cm) at each incision site, leaving the intervening sections of the affected fascia untouched. Limited or selective fasciectomy entails removing the visibly diseased fascia from the palm and finger, whereas total fasciectomy involves excising all fascia from the palm and digits. Limited fasciectomy is the most commonly employed procedure and leads to successful outcomes in 80–90% cases. Complication rates range between 15% and 24% and include nerve damage, infections, wound breakdown, and stiffness necessitating rehabilitation. Recurrence rates can be high despite successful surgery and range from 30% to 50% at 3 years [1, 3, 23–25].
- *Dermofasciectomy*: Dermofasciectomy is recommended in cases of disease recurrence after a limited fasciectomy and for aggressive disease presentations in younger individuals. It involves removing the diseased fascia, along with the skin and subcutaneous fat above it, and then applying a skin graft. Both the surgery and the recovery period are prolonged and postoperative splinting and physiotherapy are advised for correction of extension deficits and preventing postoperative contractures. The procedure is associated with complication rates of 12% and a recurrence rate of 8.4% in 6 years has been reported [3, 25].

D. *Role of Radiotherapy*

Radiotherapy (RT) is recommended for use in early, non-contractured stages of DD (<10° deformity) aiming to inhibit fibroblast proliferation and fibrosis before irreversible contractures develop. It is administered as a non-invasive, outpatient procedure with minimal discomfort, making it an attractive option for patients unsuitable or unwilling to undergo surgery and for prevention of early-stage DD [5, 8, 10].

Furthermore, RT is being explored as an adjuvant therapy following surgery to minimize the chance of recurrence by targeting any remaining proliferative fibroblasts in the surgical bed.

Mechanism of Action The main rationale for RT in DD is its ability to modulate cellular proliferation and fibrotic activity through radiobiological mechanisms of low-dose radiotherapy (LDRT) (Fig. 21.2).

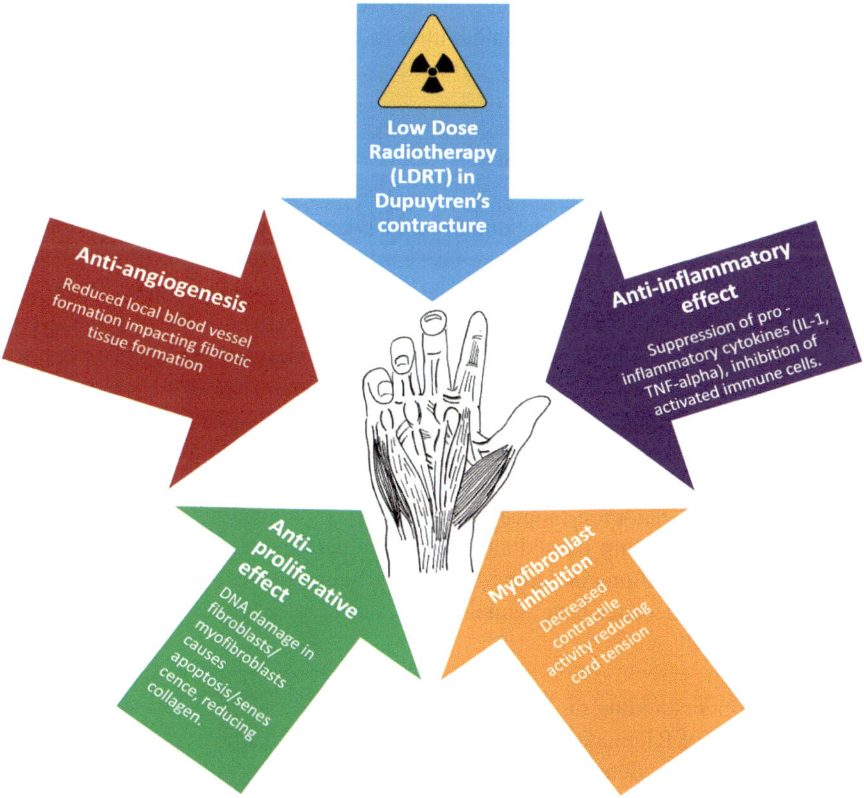

Fig. 21.2 Mechanism of action of radiotherapy in Dupuytren's Disease. (Illustrator—Dr. Shashank B. Karvekar)

- *Anti-proliferative effect*: RT induces DNA single and double-strand breaks primarily in actively dividing fibroblasts and myofibroblasts, leading to apoptosis or senescence and thus reduced collagen production.
- *Anti-inflammatory effects*: LDRT suppresses secretion of pro-inflammatory cytokines like Il-1 and TNF-α, which also contribute to fibrogenic signalling. RT also has inhibitory and apoptotic effect on the activated immune and inflammatory cells which further contribute to its clinical effect. Activation of nitric oxide synthetase and generation of free radicals also interferes with activation and progression of the inflammatory response.
- *Myofibroblast inhibition*: RT reduces contractile cell activity responsible for mechanical tension in cords.
- *Anti-angiogenesis*: RT diminishes local angiogenesis, which may impact fibrotic tissue maintenance.

These combined effects make RT uniquely suited to early, active fibroproliferative disease phases where targeted fibroblasts predominate but before mature fibrosis and contractures establish [2, 26, 27].

Because RT typically targets superficial tissues where DD lesions reside, techniques exploiting low-penetration modalities (e.g., electron beams) are ideal, maximizing diseased tissue dose while sparing deeper structures [10, 28].

21.4 Historical Perspective

RT for DD was first reported around the mid-twentieth century as use of superficial X-rays to halt fibroproliferative processes in various benign fibrotic conditions was popularized. Earliest published reports were by Finney (1955) and Wasserburger (1956) who reported good long-term outcomes for more than half the treated patients. Subsequent case series and observational studies reported varying regression and stabilization rates ranging from 21% to 81% and 19% to 98% respectively for DD treated with RT. However, the techniques and methodology used in the studies varied widely, lacking standardized dosing or validated outcome measures [27, 29, 30].

Concerns over radiation-induced carcinogenesis, coupled with the rise of surgical techniques providing immediate contracture correction, led to a decline in RT use for benign conditions including DD during the mid-to-late twentieth century.

The last three decades have witnessed a resurgence in RT for benign fibromatoses due to:

- Greater understanding of differential radiosensitivity of fibroblast subsets.
- Refinement of RT modalities (electron beam therapy, orthovoltage).
- Accumulating evidence demonstrating low malignancy risk with low-dose RT.

This renaissance has positioned RT as a valuable, non-invasive tool predominantly for early-stage DD management [26, 31].

21.5 Current Available Evidence

21.5.1 Single-Arm Cohort Studies

In 1996, Keilholz et al. published a retrospective study from Germany, evaluating the role of RT in early-stage DD in 96 patients (142 hands) treated with orthovoltage RT as two courses of 5 × 3 Gy fractions (total 30 Gy) separated by a 6-week interval. Objective reduction of symptomatic cords and nodules occurred in 75% patients with 87% reporting subjective symptom relief. At a mean follow-up of 6 years, 77% had no disease progression; 23% progressed either inside (14%) or outside (9%) the RT field. RT-related toxicity was low with no major adverse effects. This study suggested that RT could be an effective early intervention to control progression of DD, delaying or preventing the need for surgical treatment [32].

In a similar study by Adamietz et al. published in 2001, results were reported for 99 patients (176 hands) at a mean follow-up of 10 years. DD remained stable in the majority of early stage cases (Stage N - 84%, Stage N/I 67%) and progressed in the majority of later stages (Stage I - 65%, Stage II - 83%) [33].

Betz et al. (2010) in an analysis of 135 patients (208 hands) of DD treated with 120 kV orthovoltage RT with 13 years of median follow-up reported that across all stages, 66% patients reported symptomatic relief, with the DD remaining clinically stable in 59%, improving in 10% and progressing to contractures in 31%. The stabilization/regression rates were higher in early stages (stage N-87%, stage N/1-70%), while the progression rates increased in the later stages (stage I – 62%, stage II – 86%). Despite the long follow-up, no RT-induced malignancy was reported, and only minor late skin-related adverse effects were seen in one third of the patients [9].

Zirbs et al. described their experience with treatment of 206 patients (297 hands) treated with 50 kV orthovoltage RT to a total dose of 32 Gy in four courses of 2 fractions of 4 Gy separated by 8 weeks. No further disease progression was recorded in 80% patients, and 45% patients had regression of symptoms at a median follow-up of 40 months. The majority of patients were satisfied with the therapy [34].

A study from the United States of America of 33 patients of palmar-plantar fibromatoses in which 45 hands were irradiated with en-face electrons reported that 83% treated sites (including 4 re-irradiated ones) achieved local control of 83%. There was improvement in pre-treatment symptoms in 81% sites and 94% patients reported the treatment outcome as successful [35].

In a retrospective study from Poland, results of RT for 117 patients of DD treated with 21 Gy in 7 fractions of 3 Gy each were reported. During follow-up (mean 6.6 months), 57.5% patients were observed to have an improvement in the condition, 35% had stable disease while 7.5% had disease progression. Only 12.5% had minor skin-related adverse effects like erythema and dryness [36].

21.5.2 Randomized Controlled Trials (RCTs)

Seegenchmiedt et al. were the first to utilize an RCT to compare the effectivity of two different RT regimens in the treatment of early-stage DD. While one group of 63 patients (95 hands) was randomized to receive a total dose of 30 Gy in 10 fractions in 2 courses (5 fractions of 3 Gy each) 8 weeks apart, the other group of 66 patients (103 hands) received a total dose of 21 Gy in 7 fractions of 3 Gy over 2 weeks. At the end of 1 year, there was no difference in the objective or subjective outcomes of both regimens and both were found to be equally effective. No difference was also found in the RT-associated adverse effects experienced by the two groups all of which were skin-related [27].

Subsequently in 2012, the authors reported results of a longer follow-up (05 years) including those of a control group that did not receive RT and were kept under observation alone. 52% of the observed group experienced disease progression compared to 22% in 21 Gy arm and 16% in 30 Gy arm. Surgery due to disease progression was required in 30% of control hands but only 12% and 8% in the 21 and 30 Gy RT groups, respectively. All these differences were statistically significant in favour of RT. A higher proportion of regression or stability in nodules and cords, extension deficit and better symptom scores, and patient satisfaction was recorded in the RT groups compared to controls. Mild skin toxicity in the acute stage occurred in 28% of irradiated sites and was slightly more in the 21 Gy group. Chronic skin effects were mild and similar in both RT dose groups [37].

21.5.3 Radiotherapy as an Adjuvant Therapy

The role of RT in DD is limited to its use in early stages for halting progression. However, even some early studies have suggested its use in advanced stages in combination with other modalities to reduce the chances of recurrence though there is little to no evidence available to support this indication [25, 29].

The first clinical study reporting on the safety and efficacy of adjuvant RT in patients of DD after interventions carried out to release contractures was reported by Schaffer et al. in 2022. Interventions for contracture release included needle fasciotomy (NF), collagenase injection (CI), or limited fasciectomy (LF). RT was delivered either early (2–12 weeks) or late (4 months or more) after the interventions. At 1 year of mean follow-up, functional stability between 57% and 90% was reported in the various sub-groups. Cosmetic and functional outcome were reported by patients to be excellent to satisfactory in 75% cases. Forty percent patients suffered long-term dryness of skin; however, there was no incidences of wound healing complications or post-intervention infections [38].

The Dupuytren's disease Evaluation of Preventative or Adjuvant Radiation Therapy (DEPART) study is an ongoing, multi-centric, RCT designed to assess the reduction in progression of DD with the use of RT alone in the early stages as well as in combination with local therapies in the later stages [39].

Burgess et al. recently reported on the adverse effects of the DEPART trial. Only 44.1% of the mild and 25% of the moderate-to-severe adverse effects were attributable to RT. Nearly all RT-related side effects were mild and self-limiting, with reduced sweating the only adverse effect persisting for the complete follow-up period of 4 years, reflecting the safety and tolerability of adjuvant RT [40].

21.5.4 Technical Case Reports

A recent dosimetric comparison of 6 MeV electron beams with superficial RT using 90 kV photons by Meredith et al. reported a more precise dosimetry tailored to lesion depth and anatomy with the 6-MeV electron beams used with a bolus providing a more superior CTV coverage than the superficial RT [28].

21.6 Systematic Reviews and Meta-analyses

In a systematic analysis of 26 studies on non-surgical treatment options of DD, ten studies were analysed to assess the effect of RT. Studies suggested that RT was able to cause regression of nodules and prevent disease progression, but the quality of the available evidence was low [41].

Kadhum et al. in a systematic review evaluated six studies which included 770 hands affected by DD, almost all early-stage (0 or 1) treated mostly with RT doses of 30 Gy in 10 fractions. Overall, disease regression rates ranged between 0% and 56% while stability rates were reported between 14% and 98%. Progression of disease varied widely from 2% to 86%, a likely result of heterogeneity in patient selection and follow-up. Importantly, there were no cases of radiation-induced malignancy reported; salvage surgery in cases of progression post-RT was successful without any wound complications [2].

A comprehensive review of evidence published by the US Department of Veterans Affairs in 2024 on use of RT for DD concluded that RT was able to stabilize or regress disease stage, nodules, and symptoms in most patients, and overall patients were satisfied with the results of treatment. Erythema, skin atrophy, and other skin-related side effects were the most commonly reported adverse effect [42].

Table 21.4 lists major studies on role of RT in DD, while Table 21.5 summarizes the results and derivations from the available evidence.

Table 21.4 Summary of important studies in the field of radiotherapy for Dupuytren's Disease from the last three decades

Study	Design	Sample size	RT technique	Dose	Follow-up	Stabilization/ Regression rates	Symptomatic improvement	Adverse effects
Keilholz et al. [32]	Retro spective	96 patients (142 hands)	120 kV Ortho voltage RT	30 Gy (2 courses of 5 × 3 Gy) 6 weeks gap	Mean 6 years	77%	87%	Acute: Erythema, dry desquamation, swelling (grade 1 or 2)—43% Late: Dry skin, mild atrophy, fibrosis, telangiectasia (grade 1)—77%
Adamietz et al. [33]	Retro spective	99 patients (176 hands)	120 kV Ortho voltage RT	30 Gy (2 courses of 5 × 3 Gy) 6–8 weeks gap	Median 10 years	Stage N 84% Stage N/I 67%	NR	Late: Anhidrosis—25% Skin atrophy—8.5%
Betz et al. [9]	Retro spective	135 patients (208 hands)	120 kV Ortho voltage RT	30 Gy (2 courses of 5 × 3 Gy) 6–8 weeks gap	Median 13 years	Stage N 87% Stage N/I 70%	66%	Late skin effects—32% (Mild)
Zirbs et al. [34]	Retro spective	206 patients (297 hands)	50-kV super-ficial RT	32 Gy (4 courses of 2 × 4 Gy) 8-week interval	Median 3 years & 3 months	80%	Reduction in 21.6% nodules & cords. Very good satisfaction with RT	Acute: Erythema—20.4%, Skin dryness—39.8%, Desquamtion—3.8% Chronic: Dryness—20%, skin atrophy—3%, anhidrosis—4%, teleangiectasia—3%, desquamation—2%, sensory affection—2%

Schuster et al. [35]	Retro spective	33 patients (45 hands)	6–12 MeV electrons	30 Gy (2 courses of 5 × 3 Gy), 6–8 weeks gap OR 21 Gy (7 × 3 Gy)	Median 31 months	83% (including 4 patients reirradiated for recurrence)	81%	Acute: 39% (mild erythema, dryness, dry desquamation, edema, tenderness, and fatigue) Late: Mild dryness, weakness, reduced nail health, and hyperpigmentation.
Latusek et al. [36]	Retro spective	117 patients	Superficial RT	21 Gy (7 × 3 Gy), 2 series with a break in-between	Mean 4.8 months	92.5%	NR	Acute: Erythema—7.5%, exfoliation2.5%, dry skin—2.5%
Seegenschmiedt et al. [37]	RCT	Control: 122 Gp A: 293 Gp B: 245	120 kV Ortho voltage RT	Control: Observation Gp A: 30 Gy (2 courses of 5 × 3 Gy), 6–8 weeks gap Gp B: 21 Gy (7 × 3 Gy)	Median 104 months	Control: 38% Gp A: 80% Gp B: 76%	Control: 8% Gp A: 26% Gp B: 21%	Acute—28% (Gp A: 26%, Gp B: 32%; Grade 1 or 2—erythema, desquamation, local swelling) Late—14% (Gp A: 11.5%, Gp B: 16%; Dryness, desquamation, mild skin atrophy, subcutaneous fibrosis)

Table 21.5 Summary of derivations and results about the role of RT in DD based on the available evidence

Role of radiotherapy in DD	RT is effective in preventing progression of early-stage DD with acceptable side effects. It is superior to observation alone, especially in early stages (N and NI). RT may delay or reduce the need for surgery. RT as an adjuvant to contracture-release procedures is safe and its effectivity in reducing recurrences is under evaluation.
Outcomes and results	
Efficacy	RT in early-stage DD shows disease control rates ranging between 69% and 93%. Symptomatic improvements in pain, tenderness, and pruritus are reported in 45–87% of treated patients. Progression rates are significantly reduced compared to observational management. The majority of patients are satisfied with treatment with RT. Post-RT salvage surgical interventions remain feasible without added surgical risks.
Recurrence and long-term follow-up	Long-term durability of RT effects is documented in cohorts followed up to 10–15 years. Recurrence, when it occurs, tends to be less severe and slower than natural disease progression. Patient hand function and quality of life generally improve or stabilize after RT.
Possible adverse effects and reported percentages Though considered safe, RT carries potential acute and chronic toxicities	
Acute toxicities (during and within weeks after RT)	Mild erythema or skin redness reported in 20–43% of patients. Adverse effects skin dryness, desquamation or swelling which are mild and temporary. Effects are self-limiting and resolve with conservative skin care.
Late toxicities (months to years post-treatment)	Skin atrophy, dryness, telangiectasia, or subcutaneous fibrosis in up to 10–30% of cases. Reduced sweating or altered skin texture may develop but rarely impact function. No RT-induced malignancies have been observed in studies with medium-term follow-up of up to 13 years, though ongoing surveillance remains prudent. The balance of mild, mostly transient side effects with efficacy supports RT's favourable risk-benefit ratio

21.7 Patient Selection

Based on a review of the available literature, the Royal College of Radiologists, UK, recommended through their 2023 consensus guidelines that RT can be used as an effective treatment of early stage (stage N/1) DD where there is either no contracture or a contracture of up to 10 degrees. DD is known to remain static in a high proportion of patients for several years; therefore, RT should ideally be offered only to patients who have progressed in the past 6–12 months (Royal College of Radiologists, 2023).

Thus, the ideal candidates for treatment by RT for Dupuytren's disease are those with early-stage disease and those who face a risk of rapid progression. As the course of DD can be unpredictable, regular assessment and recording of disease status is encouraged by using photographs, hand-grip strength assessment and deformity measurements using goniometers. Patients with more advanced deformities who select RT over surgical therapy should be counselled about the low probability of improvement in their condition. Similarly, use of adjuvant RT after surgery or other invasive procedures should be limited to clinical trial settings as of now.

The latest National Institute for Health and Care Excellence (NICE) guidelines of the UK for the use of RT in DD recommend that while use of RT in treatment of DD is safe, due to the limited evidence available, patients should be made aware of the uncertainty of effectiveness of RT and the unpredictable nature of the disease. The patient should also be informed about the theoretical risk of RT-induced malignancy [43]. Just for reference, the increased risk of getting fatal skin cancer from RT treatment of DD is very minimal and has been calculated to be only 0.02% higher than the baseline [44].

21.8 Techniques and Radiation Dose Schedules

RT techniques optimize dose delivery to superficial fibrotic nodules and cords while sparing neurovascular bundles and deeper tissues.

21.8.1 Radiation Modalities

Orthovoltage and superficial X-rays have been traditionally used in the treatment of DD due to the low depth of treatment required and the popularity and availability of the equipment in Germany and other parts of Europe. However, recent evidence suggests that electron beam therapy (6–9 MeV) is a preferable option due to controlled dose penetration (1–2 cm depth), uniform dose distribution, and minimal exit dose allowing superior and more conformal CTV coverage. Use of a standard 1 cm or a customized bolus material over the skin ensures adequate skin surface dosing, essential for targeting superficial lesions [10, 28]. Orthovoltage X-rays continue to be used in older centres and with older protocols.

21.8.2 Treatment Planning

The patient is ideally seated comfortably next to the treatment machine with their hand placed on the couch with the palmar surface facing up. A thermoplastic mould, vaculock mattress or other suitable immobilization device is used for reproducibility of the treatment position. The palpable nodules and cords on the palm are demarcated with a black marker pen.

21.8.3 Treatment Volume

Traditionally the treatment volume includes the palpable nodules and cords with margins of 1 cm in the medial and lateral planes and 1–2 cm proximal and distal margins to cover the subclinical disease. Given the small possibility of out-of-field recurrence and improved local control with complete over limited fasciectomy, some radiation oncologists prefer treating the entire palm, though it would likely be associated with higher adverse effects.

Given the benign nature of disease and the small target volume, CT-based treatment should be preferred despite the fairly straightforward clinical treatment set-up. The goal of treatment planning is for the 90% isodose curve to cover the palmar aponeurosis and reach up to the periosteum of the bones of the palm and fingers. Avoidance of radiation hotspots over neurovascular bundles and joints should be ensured when possible [10, 28, 45].

21.8.4 Dose and Fractionation

The standard and preferred regimen consists of a total dose of 30 Gy, divided into 10 fractions of 3 Gy each, delivered 5 days/week over 2 weeks. The 2 weeks of treatment are often separated by an interval of 6–8 weeks to maximize fibroblast inhibitory effects. And minimize toxicity to skin and subcutaneous tissues.

Alternatively, a regimen of 21 Gy in 7 fractions of 3 Gy each over 2 weeks can also be used when a longer treatment course is inconvenient but is associated with higher acute and chronic side effects [10, 28, 45].

21.9 Future Directions and Research

- Standardized clinical trials: Further prospective, randomized, controlled, multi-centre trials with standardized outcome measures and long-term follow-up are needed to:
  - Generate high-quality evidence of efficacy of RT in DD
  - Optimize dosing and fractionation regimens
  - Compare efficacy versus minimally invasive treatments and surgery
  - Long-term safety including malignancy risk
  - Evaluate efficacy of RT as adjuvant therapy after contracture-release treatment
  - Ongoing trials such as the DEPART study of Netherlands and the pilot study from University of Minnesota seek to answer these questions.
- Technological Improvements:
  - Use of intensity-modulated or image-guided RT to minimize collateral tissue damage.
  - Use of image-guided surface or interstitial brachytherapy in reirradiation scenario.

- Molecular targeted RT:
  - Mechanistic studies to elucidate RT effects on fibroblast signalling.
  - Use of radiosensitizers or antifibrotic combination therapies to enhance RT response.
- Broader Clinical Applications:
  - Expansion of RT indications to other fibromatoses like Ledderhose disease and Peyronie's disease.
  - Potential roles in other non-malignant proliferative and inflammatory disorders.

21.10 Conclusion

Dupuytren's contracture remains a challenging fibroproliferative disorder with multifactorial pathogenesis and unpredictable progression. The accumulated international data suggest that radiotherapy can be an effective and safe, non-invasive treatment option for early-stage disease, capable of halting fibroblast proliferation and delaying progression before irreversible contractures occur. Multiple studies demonstrate favourable outcomes with radiotherapy in disease stabilization, symptom relief, and patient satisfaction, with minimal toxicity and no proven increase in malignancy risk. Nevertheless, the current evidence base is predominantly derived from observational cohorts and single-centre experiences. Consequently, well-designed multicentric randomized controlled trials are necessary to define optimal dose schedules, long-term safety, and comparative efficacy against other non-surgical modalities. Integration of modern radiation technologies, combined with molecular insights into fibroblast signalling, holds promise for more precise and individualized therapy. In the evolving landscape of benign radiotherapy, Dupuytren's disease exemplifies how early intervention and multidisciplinary management can restore function, improve quality of life, and set new standards for non-invasive fibromatosis care.

References

1. Ghaznawi K, Krug D, Kovács G. Radiotherapy for benign conditions: Dupuytren's and Peyronie's disease. In: Halperin EC, Wazer DE, Perez CA, Brady LW, editors. Perez and Brady's principles and practice of radiation oncology. 7th ed. Wolters Kluwer Health; 2018. p. 6663–5.
2. Kadhum M, Smock E, Khan A, Fleming A. Radiotherapy in Dupuytren's disease: a systematic review of the evidence. J Hand Surg Eur Vol. 2017;42(7):689–92. https://doi.org/10.1177/1753193417695996.
3. Sarkar M, Kashyap N, Madabhavi I. Dupuytren's disease: a review. Chin J Plast Reconstr Surg. 2024;6(3):142–8. https://doi.org/10.1016/j.cjprs.2024.08.002.
4. Verheyden CN. The history of Dupuytren's contracture. Clin Plast Surg. 1983;10(4):619–25.
5. Kovacs E. Dupuytren contracture: practice essentials, background, pathophysiology, 2023. https://emedicine.medscape.com/article/329414-overview#a1. Accessed 16 Oct 2025.

6. Novo J, Gao D, Seth I, Rozen WM. Incidence of Dupuytren's disease following hand trauma: a systematic review. J Hand Surg Eur Vol. 2025;1:17531934251360545. https://doi.org/10.1177/17531934251360545.
7. Salari N, Heydari M, Hassanabadi M, et al. The worldwide prevalence of the Dupuytren disease: a comprehensive systematic review and meta-analysis. J Orthop Surg. 2020;15(1):495. https://doi.org/10.1186/s13018-020-01999-7.
8. Nanchahal J, Chan JKK. Treatments for early-stage Dupuytren's disease: an evidence-based approach. J Hand Surg Eur Vol. 2023;48(3):191–8. https://doi.org/10.1177/17531934221131373.
9. Betz N, Ott OJ, Adamietz B, Sauer R, Fietkau R, Keilholz L. Radiotherapy in early-stage Dupuytren's contracture. Long-term results after 13 years. Strahlenther Onkol. 2010;186(2):82–90. https://doi.org/10.1007/s00066-010-2063-z.
10. Yunes MJ. Radiation therapy for Dupuytren contracture. Pract Radiat Oncol. 2025;15(3):248–52. https://doi.org/10.1016/j.prro.2024.11.010.
11. Hindocha S, Stanley JK, Watson JS, Bayat A. Revised Tubiana's staging system for assessment of disease severity in Dupuytren's disease—preliminary clinical findings. Hand. 2008;3(2):80–6. https://doi.org/10.1007/s11552-007-9071-1.
12. Tubiana R, Michon J, Thomine JM. Scheme for the assessment of deformities in Dupuytren's disease. Surg Clin North Am. 1968;48(5):979–84. https://doi.org/10.1016/s0039-6109(16)38630-3.
13. Rayan GM. Nonoperative treatment of Dupuytren's disease. J Hand Surg. 2008;33(7):1208–10. https://doi.org/10.1016/j.jhsa.2008.05.027.
14. Van Den Berge BA, Werker PMN, Broekstra DC. Limited progression of subclinical Dupuytren's disease: results from a prospective cohort study. Bone Joint J. 2021;103-B(4):704–10. https://doi.org/10.1302/0301-620X.103B4.BJJ-2020-1364.R1.
15. Ketchum LD, Donahue TK. The injection of nodules of Dupuytren's disease with triamcinolone acetonide. J Hand Surg. 2000;25(6):1157–62. https://doi.org/10.1053/jhsu.2000.18493.
16. Yin CY, Yu HHM, Wang JP, Huang YC, Huang TF, Chang MC. Long-term follow-up of Dupuytren disease after injection of triamcinolone acetonide in Chinese patients in Taiwan. J Hand Surg Eur Vol. 2017;42(7):678–82. https://doi.org/10.1177/1753193417690961.
17. van Rijssen AL, Werker PMN. Percutaneous needle fasciotomy in dupuytren's disease. J Hand Surg. 2006;31(5):498–501. https://doi.org/10.1016/j.jhsb.2006.03.174.
18. van Rijssen AL, Ter Linden H, Werker PMN. Five-year results of a randomized clinical trial on treatment in Dupuytren's disease: percutaneous needle fasciotomy versus limited fasciectomy. Plast Reconstr Surg. 2012;129(2):469–77. https://doi.org/10.1097/PRS.0b013e31823aea95.
19. Hurst LC, Badalamente MA, Hentz VR, et al. Injectable collagenase clostridium histolyticum for Dupuytren's contracture. N Engl J Med. 2009;361(10):968–79. https://doi.org/10.1056/NEJMoa0810866.
20. Gilpin D, Coleman S, Hall S, Houston A, Karrasch J, Jones N. Injectable collagenase Clostridium histolyticum: a new nonsurgical treatment for Dupuytren's disease. J Hand Surg. 2010;35(12):2027–2038.e1. https://doi.org/10.1016/j.jhsa.2010.08.007.
21. Peimer CA, Blazar P, Coleman S, Kaplan FTD, Smith T, Lindau T. Dupuytren contracture recurrence following treatment with collagenase clostridium histolyticum (CORDLESS [collagenase option for reduction of Dupuytren long-term evaluation of safety study]): 5-year data. J Hand Surg. 2015;40(8):1597–605. https://doi.org/10.1016/j.jhsa.2015.04.036.
22. Zhang D, Earp BE, Benavent KA, Blazar P. Collagenase treatment of Dupuytren's disease with minimum 5-year follow-up: recurrence, reintervention, and satisfaction. Plast Reconstr Surg. 2020;146(5):1071–9. https://doi.org/10.1097/PRS.0000000000007243.
23. Denkler K. Surgical complications associated with fasciectomy for dupuytren's disease: a 20-year review of the English literature. Eplasty. 2010;10:e15.
24. Crean SM, Gerber RA, Le Graverand MPH, Boyd DM, Cappelleri JC. The efficacy and safety of fasciectomy and fasciotomy for Dupuytren's contracture in European patients: a structured review of published studies. J Hand Surg Eur Vol. 2011;36(5):396–407. https://doi.org/10.1177/1753193410397971.

25. Ruettermann M, Hermann RM, Khatib-Chahidi K, Werker PMN. Dupuytren's disease—etiology and treatment. Dtsch Ärztebl Int. 2021;118(46):781. https://doi.org/10.3238/arztebl.m2021.0325.
26. Rödel F, Fournier C, Wiedemann J, et al. Basics of radiation biology when treating hyperproliferative benign diseases. Front Immunol. 2017;8:519. https://doi.org/10.3389/fimmu.2017.00519.
27. Seegenschmiedt MH, Olschewski T, Guntrum F. Radiotherapy optimization in early-stage Dupuytren's contracture: first results of a randomized clinical study. Int J Radiat Oncol Biol Phys. 2001;49(3):785–98. https://doi.org/10.1016/s0360-3016(00)00745-8.
28. Meredith R, Carlisle J, Dover L, López-Araujo J, Benhabib S, Brezovich I. Dosimetric comparison of radiation methods for palmar fibrosis. J Clin Radiat Oncol. 2017;2(1):1–3. https://doi.org/10.14312/2397-8511.2017-1.
29. Finney R. Dupuytren's contracture. Br J Radiol. 1955;28(335):610–4. https://doi.org/10.1259/0007-1285-28-335-610.
30. Wasserburger K. Therapy of Dupuytren's contracture. Strahlentherapie. 1956;100(4):546–60.
31. Royal College of Radiologists. Recommendations for using radiotherapy for benign disease in the UK. Published online March 2023. https://www.rcr.ac.uk/our-services/all-our-publications/clinical-oncology-publications/recommendations-for-using-radiotherapy-for-benign-disease-in-the-uk/.
32. Keilholz L, Seegenschmiedt MH, Sauer R. Radiotherapy for prevention of disease progression in early-stage Dupuytren's contracture: initial and long-term results. Int J Radiat Oncol Biol Phys. 1996;36(4):891–7. https://doi.org/10.1016/s0360-3016(96)00421-x.
33. Adamietz B, Keilholz L, Grünert J, Sauer R. Radiotherapy of early stage Dupuytren disease. Long-term results after a median follow-up period of 10 years. Strahlenther Onkol. 2001;177(11):604–10. https://doi.org/10.1007/pl00002371.
34. Zirbs M, Anzeneder T, Bruckbauer H, et al. Radiotherapy with soft X-rays in Dupuytren's disease—successful, well-tolerated and satisfying. J Eur Acad Dermatol Venereol. 2015;29(5):904–11. https://doi.org/10.1111/jdv.12711.
35. Schuster J, Saraiya S, Tennyson N, Nedelka M, Mukhopadhyay N, Weiss E. Patient-reported outcomes after electron radiation treatment for early-stage palmar and plantar fibromatosis. Pract Radiat Oncol. 2015;5(6):e651–8. https://doi.org/10.1016/j.prro.2015.06.010.
36. Latusek T, Miszczyk L, Gierlach G, Zając P. An effectiveness evaluation of the palmar fascia irradiation of patients suffering from Dupuytren's disease. Nowotw J Oncol. 2017;67(3):162–7. https://doi.org/10.5603/NJO.2017.0027.
37. Seegenschmiedt MH, Keilholz L, Wielpütz M, Schubert C, Fehlauer F. Long-term outcome of radiotherapy for early stage Dupuytren's disease: a phase III clinical study. In: Eaton C, Seegenschmiedt MH, Bayat A, Gabbiani G, Werker P, Wach W, editors. Dupuytren's disease and related hyperproliferative disorders. Springer: Berlin; 2012. p. 349–71. https://doi.org/10.1007/978-3-642-22697-7_44.
38. Shaffer R, Seegenschmiedt H. Treatment of Dupuytren's disease with post-interventional radiotherapy. Int J Radiat Oncol Biol Phys. 2022;114(3):e423. https://doi.org/10.1016/j.ijrobp.2022.07.1620.
39. Genesis Care Cancer Care Research Pty Ltd. Dupuytren's disease evaluation of preventative or adjuvant radiation therapy; 2023.
40. Burgess T, Wegener E, McClelland B, et al. Adverse events after adjuvant radiation therapy for Dupuytren's disease in the DEPART randomized trial. J Hand Surg Eur Vol. 2025;50(7):891–7. https://doi.org/10.1177/17531934251321393.
41. Ball C, Izadi D, Verjee LS, Chan J, Nanchahal J. Systematic review of non-surgical treatments for early dupuytren's disease. BMC Musculoskelet Disord. 2016;17(1):345. https://doi.org/10.1186/s12891-016-1200-y.
42. Jutkowitz E, Rieke K, Caputo EL, et al. Radiation therapy for benign conditions: a systematic review. Washington, DC: Department of Veterans Affairs (US); 2024.

43. National Institute for Health and Care Excellence. Radiation therapy for early Dupuytren's disease (Interventional Procedure Guidance No. IPG573). Published online 2016. https://www.nice.org.uk/guidance/ipg573.
44. Dupuytren's International Society. Estimate of the risk of cancer caused by radiation therapy of Dupuytren's disease. Dupuytren's International Society, 2019. Published online 2019. www.dupuytren-online.info/downloads_English_website/Risk_of_cancer_with_radiotherapy_of_Dupuytren_Disease.pdf. Accessed 22 Oct 2025.
45. Eng TY, Abugideiri M, Chen TW, et al. Radiation therapy for benign disease. Hematol Oncol Clin North Am. 2020;34(1):205–27. https://doi.org/10.1016/j.hoc.2019.09.005.

Low-Dose Radiotherapy in the Management of Plantar Fasciitis: Mechanisms and Clinical Outcomes

22

Sankalp Singh

22.1 Introduction

22.1.1 Definition and Prevalence

Plantar fasciitis (PF) is a chronic pain syndrome that constitutes 11–15% of all painful foot conditions requiring medical attention [1, 2]. It is the most ubiquitous cause of heel pain in the world and is also referred to as 'calcaneal spur', 'painful heel spur syndrome', and 'jogger's heel'. The nomenclature calcaneal or heel spur was first used by the German doctor Plettner (Ref), who described the exostotic bone formation at the insertion of the plantar fascia at the calcaneal tuberosity in his radiological study from 1900. However, we know now that the presence of a bony spur is not pathognomic for a diagnosis of PF, as nearly 50% of patients lack this radiological finding, while nearly one-third of people with heel spurs are asymptomatic [3].

It is estimated that the global prevalence of this condition is between 4% and 7% with about 10% of the world's population affected by this debilitating disorder during the course of their lifetimes. Unlike other degenerative musculoskeletal disorders, PF can also afflict the younger population in their second and third decades with a peak incidence occurring between 40 and 60 years [4, 5]. The condition is reported to be more common among women than men and also in obese individuals with a Body Mass Index >25 kg/m^2. It is known to occur in both sedentary and highly active individuals, though long-distance running is a risk factor. The incidence in runners has been reported to be between 10% and 22% [1, 2].

Though there is a lack of reliable population-based data on this condition in India, a radiographical study on calcaneal spurs found an incidence of 59% among Indian patients with heel pain, a condition often associated with PF [6]. Recent report also indicated an overall PF prevalence of around 30% in certain Indian

S. Singh (✉)
Department of Radiation Oncology, Army Hospital (Research & Referral), Delhi, India

K. Sood Sharma (ed.), *Radiation Therapy for Benign Disorders*,
https://doi.org/10.1007/978-981-95-6635-8_22

populations with professions associated with prolonged standing and walking, with a higher burden among females and middle-aged adults [7].

The significant pain and functional incapacitation due to PF adversely affects patients' quality of life and activities of daily life including their professional work. This along with repeated visits to medical professionals and prolonged medications and treatment can also lead to significant psychological issues for patients and a considerable burden on a country's healthcare system [4, 8].

22.2 Anatomy and Pathophysiology (Including Risk Factors)

The plantar fascia or aponeurosis is composed of three thick, fibrous bands of connective tissue that arise from the medial portion of the calcaneus, travel along the plantar aspect of the foot, dividing into five segments that extend along each digit and are inserted into the metatarsal heads and the proximal phalanges [9] (Fig. 22.1). The fascia is stretched like a bowstring and forms the base of the longitudinal arch of the foot and plays a crucial part in the biomechanics of the foot. It stores potential energy in the stretched bowstring when the arch is compressed and then releases it as kinetic energy helping to propel the foot forward and giving the body a literal 'spring in the step'. It also acts as a shock absorber every time the foot lands. This dynamic action of the fascia gives both stability and efficiency to our bipedal locomotion.

Plantar fasciitis is multifactorial in etiology. Table 22.1 lists various risk factors associated with this condition. Historically considered an acute inflammatory condition (hence the *-itis* suffix), it is now known to be more of a degenerative disorder

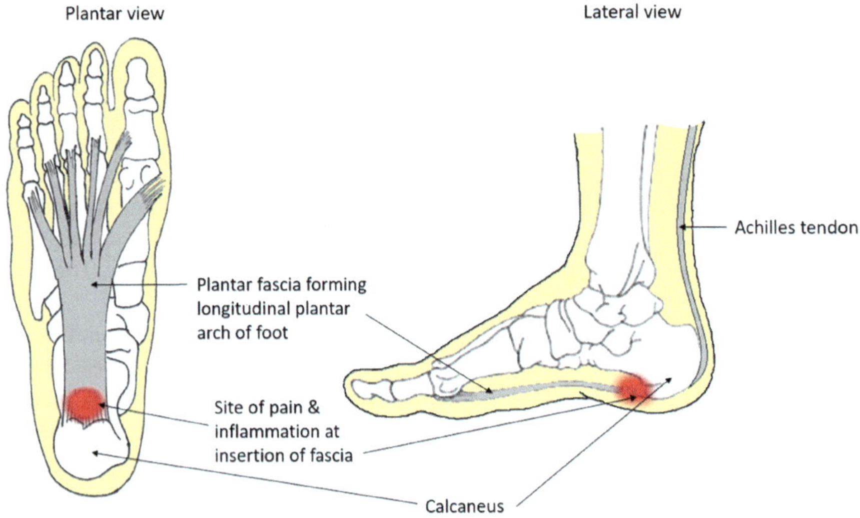

Fig. 22.1 Anatomy of the plantar fascia (aponeurosis) with site of initial pain in plantar fasciitis. (Illustrator—Dr Shashank B. Karvekar)

Table 22.1 Risk factors for development of plantar fasciitis

Obesity (BMI > 27)	Foot deformities
Increasing age	Decreased ankle flexion
Sedentary lifestyle	Ill-fitting or tight shoes
Work-related weight bearing	Flat feet
Long periods of occupational standing	Tightness of Achilles tendon
Long distance running	Shortening of calf muscles

Adapted and modified from: Owens [18]

of the plantar fascia at its insertion into the medial tuberosity of the calcaneus along with the surrounding heel fat pad.

Continuous and inappropriate stress on the fascia because of abnormal stretching due to prolonged standing, long-distance running, mechanical overload due to obesity or work-related weight bearing, shortened calf muscles, and other biomechanical abnormalities of the foot lead to repeated and multiple microtraumas. These microtraumas or microtears initiate a chronic degenerative process in the fascia leading to pain. Healing of these microtraumas through fibrosis causes a decrease in elasticity of the fascia which contributes to the functional incapacitation along with the severe pain [2, 10]. Neovascularization during the healing process, along with fibroblastic activity and chronic mechanical stress, contributes to calcium deposition and the formation of the exostotic calcaneal spur commonly associated with PF.

22.3 Common Symptoms and Diagnosis

The most characteristic symptom of PF is the presence of a sharp pain in the heel early in the morning when the patient takes their first few steps. This hallmark was described as early as 1860 by Zacharie [1]. The pain is usually present in the inferior and medial aspect of the heel but may radiate to involve the entire plantar aspect of the foot. Some sufferers describe the pain as dull aching, burning, or throbbing. It is often severe in the morning and initially gets better after walking for a few hours but can worsen again with increasing activity throughout the day. It can also exacerbate after a period of inactivity, prolonged sitting, or standing [2, 9, 11]. In about a third of cases, bilateral heels are involved. The tensioning of the plantar fascia may also cause restriction of dorsiflexion in severe cases. The severity of the pain is usually enough to cause functional inadequacy and gait disturbance. The symptoms often contribute to negatively impact the quality of life of patients [2, 4, 9].

Diagnosis of PF is typically made clinically. The characteristic symptoms as described above should raise a suspicion which can be confirmed on physical examination. External feature of inflammation, neurological, or vascular deficit are characteristically absent. Palpation would exhibit pain and tenderness at the insertion of the plantar fascia on medial tubercle of calcaneus. Passive dorsiflexion of the foot or toes would also elicit the heel pain. The Windlass test is used to confirm PF in severe cases and involves reproducing the heel pain by passive dorsiflexion of the metatarsophalangeal joint of the big toe while keeping the rest of the foot stabilized [1, 2, 9, 11, 12].

If the diagnosis is established on clinical examination, imaging is ordinarily unnecessary. However, it may be utilized in cases with history or examination suggesting other differential diagnosis or in case of refractory pain despite conservative treatment for a fair amount of time. Differential diagnoses to be considered include traumatic injuries, stress fractures, or retrocalcaneal bursitis.

Conventional lateral radiograph of the foot can reveal the characteristic 'calcaneal heel spur' in around 50% of the affected cases (Fig. 22.2). However, neither are most patients with radiologically diagnosed heel spurs symptomatic, nor is the size or shape of the spur associated with severity or duration of pain or degree of functional limitation. Radiographs may incidentally detect other bony lesions causing the heel pain [2, 3, 11, 13].

Ultrasonography of the affected heel may reveal edema of the aponeurosis as areas of reduced echogenicity during the acute phase. In the chronic stage, thickening or swelling of the plantar fascia (to greater than 4 mm) as well as calcifications in the soft tissue or spurs may be detected. Ultrasonography maybe of greater diagnostic value than x-rays because of the easy visualization of soft-tissue changes and lack of radiation exposure [1, 3, 9].

MRI is rarely used in the routine management of PF but can be of clinical value in chronic cases with persistent pain or when there is a need to differentiate between soft tissue and bony pathologies. Typical MRI findings include

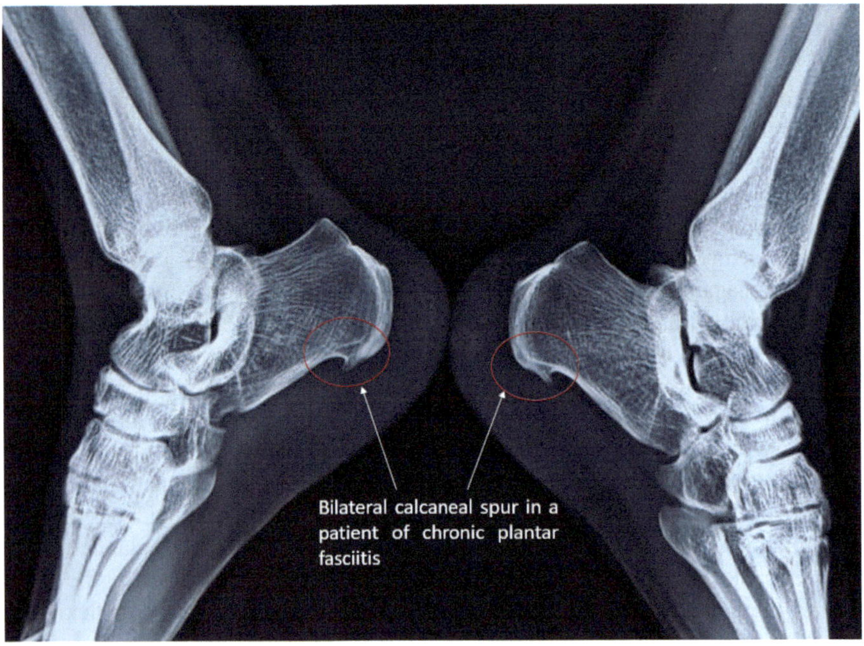

Fig. 22.2 Lateral radiograph of bilateral heels in a 29-year-old male patient, soldier by profession suffering from bilateral plantar fasciitis for 3 years. Bony spurs are clearly evident in both calcaneums arising at the site of insertion of the plantar aponeurosis. (Image courtesy—Dr Sankalp Singh)

thickening of the plantar fascia, with increased signal intensity T2 sequences an intermediate or low signal on T1. Post-contrast enhancement may be seen reflecting inflammation. Fat-suppressed STIR sequences can also detect edema in adjacent soft tissues or bone marrow edema at the calcaneal attachment. MRI is also useful for identifying other associated pathologies such as plantar fascia tears or ruptures and stress fractures of the calcaneus. While MRI provides detailed imaging, it is usually reserved for atypical or refractory cases given its cost and limited impact on initial management [1, 2, 9].

Nuclear scintigraphy is rarely used for PF diagnosis and is limited to atypical cases where findings from other imagings are inconclusive. Use of 99m-Tc-methylene diphosphate (Tc -99m-MDP)-based bone scintigraphy can show pathological uptake at the insertion of the plantar aponeurosis even when no bony changes are visible on radiographs [1, 14, 15].

Routine laboratory bloodwork is non-specific in PF. It is only indicated to rule out differential diagnoses of seronegative spondyloarthropathies in cases of bilateral involvement [1, 16].

22.4 Treatment Approaches

A variety of different effective treatment options are available for PF. The primary goal of all treatment modalities is alleviation of patient's pain. These treatment modalities maybe broadly categorized into conservative, minimally invasive, and surgical (Table 22.2). Though relief or resolution is not absolutely guaranteed with any one modality, most patients respond to therapy with around 82% reported to be relieved by conservative methods at completion of around 12 months of therapy [9, 17].

Table 22.2 Treatment modalities used in the management of plantar fasciitis

Conservative	Minimally invasive	Surgical
Oral analgesics Orthotic concepts Splints Adjustable shoes Silicone insoles Heel pads Physical therapy Weight loss Stretching exercises Resting & reducing physical workload	Extracorporeal Shockwave Therapy (ESWT) Local Injection Corticosteroids +/− anaesthetic Platelet Rich Plasma Botulinum toxin Amniotic fluid Scanning Laser therapy Radiotherapy	Open Endoscopic

22.4.1 Rest and Activity Modification

Since the etiological factors for PF are identified to be mechanical stress of repetitive microtrauma, reduction or removal of this stress can reduce the associated inflammation and pain. Simple solutions like decreasing standing time and non-impact exercises (some examples are swimming and cycling) can reduce the pressure on the affected area. Weight loss in patients with high BMI can similarly decrease the mechanical overloading and relieve pain. This is usually the first and simplest intervention advised to patients during the acute phase of PF. Accurate and appropriate patient education can play a substantial role curbing and controlling this condition at an early stage with minimal physical intervention [9].

Typically, 2 weeks of activity modification to provide rest to the inflamed fascia is prescribed rather than complete bedrest. There is little to no evidence of any advantage of longer rest. Immobilization to rest the foot and take weight off it may be advised in cases of severe pain. A short leg walking boot with controlled ankle motion is used for this purpose but again, not beyond 2 weeks [9, 11, 18].

22.4.2 Physical Therapy and Stretching Exercises

Stretching of the plantar fascia, the ankle joint, the Achilles tendon, and the calf muscles are recommended to relieve pain and increase mobility of plantar fascia. From a bio-mechanical point of view, stretching reduces the continuous tension at the insertion of the fascia. Plantar fascia-specific stretching exercises are proven to be more beneficial than general stretching. Positive outcomes in the form of freedom from pain has been reported from 56% to 92% patients in various studies with results often being durable over several months. Other techniques like taping, application of ice or heat are also used, sometimes by the patient themselves with varying degrees of pain relief [19–22]. Manual physical therapy in the form joint mobilization and soft tissue mobilization with deep tissue massage or trigger-point myofascial release are commonly prescribed and recommended by physical therapy guidelines for treatment of PF. While there is strong evidence in favour of the effectivity of soft tissue mobilization, the evidence in favour of joint mobilization is less robust [9, 23–26].

22.4.3 Orthotics and Supportive Footwear

Shoes, shoe inserts, or foot orthosis that provide appropriate support can relieve pain from PF, provide comfort, and improve functionality though there may be no resolution of the pathology itself. Supportive shoes, orthotics, and inserts like silicone insoles are designed to provide support to the medial part of the plantar arch, relieving the tension in it. Simple, prefabricated silicone heel pads provide a soft support against impact to the painful part of the heel or calcaneum [2, 27–30].

Night splints are designed to provide prolonged stretching while keeping the ankle in dorsiflexion. These can be uncomfortable to wear and are often recommended to be used for 1–3 months. However, there is little evidence for their advantage over other simpler orthotics [1, 9, 30, 31].

22.4.4 Oral Drug Therapy

Along with physical therapy and orthopaedic insoles, drugs like non-steroidal anti-inflammatory drugs (NSAIDs) and acetaminophen are often the first line of therapeutic approach [10]. Being easy and convenient to access and administer, they are relatively popular and in one study from the United States, 70% of patients of PF admitted to using over the counter analgesics [32]. By relieving pain and acute inflammation, drugs can allow patients to be more compliant towards other modalities like physical therapy and exercises. They can be effective for short-term management of PF especially during the early acute phases; however, their continued use may have limited role in terms of recovery [1]. One study reported that addition of NASIDs to stretching and use of insoles added very little advantage over a placebo [33]. Long-term use may also increase risk of gastrointestinal bleed and renal damage. Use of opioids is generally avoided due to their abuse potential but oral steroids given for short periods have shown benefit in reducing pain and disability, particularly in severe cases [34].

22.4.5 Local Injections

Injection of local anaesthetics and steroids into painful musculoskeletal sites has been in use since the 1900s and the 1940s respectively [35, 36]. Injection of local steroids in particular is extensively practised for management of PF and is highly effective in reducing inflammation and provides durable and potent pain relief. The site of injection is usually the point of maximum pain [1]. Steroid injections are often combined with a local anaesthetic to reduce the discomfort of the procedure and provide rapid pain relief while steroids provide the more prolonged analgesic effect [37]. However, there is no evidence that use of local steroids has any effect on the disease process or generation and transmission of pain in PF. The major adverse effect is that repeated steroid injections are associated with a considerable risk of atrophy of plantar fat pad and plantar fascia rupture [36, 38, 39]. Therefore it is recommended to limit the injections to not more than one every 6 months [11, 40, 41].

Other drugs used in local injections for PF with significant degree of success include platelet-rich plasma (PRP) and botulinum toxin [2, 42–44]. There is variable evidence to show whether PRP or corticosteroid injections are better in the short-term (3 months); however, at longer periods of follow-up, there appears to be no difference between the two in terms of outcome [45–47].

22.4.6 Extracorporeal Shockwave Therapy (ESWT)

ESWT employs an electromagnetic mechanism that generates shockwaves by utilizing a magnetic field within a fluid medium. These shockwaves are precisely focussed at the source of pain and are administered in microsecond pressure bursts via a handheld probe [9, 48].

The exact mechanism of ESWT remains unknown but is postulated to work through stimulating expression of angiogenesis-related growth factors that induce neovascularization thereby improving blood supply which enhances cell proliferation, tissue regeneration, and collagen synthesis for repair of musculoskeletal tissues. It is also suggested that ESWT maybe simultaneously destroying unmyelinated nerve fibres and interrupting pain transmission [49–51]. The delivery techniques of ESWT used by different practitioners can have significant variation in terms of the energy used (low, medium or high), number of treatment sessions and the volume treated (only painful area or entire plantar fascia) [52, 53].

The advantages of ESWT are that it is non-invasive, convenient, and cost-effective with no major side-effects though the treatment delivery can be painful and can cause bruising and swelling [54, 55]. In terms of results, ESWT has been shown to be an effective modality in various studies with reduction in pain and improvement in function seen in 65–91% patients [56–58]. The results are generally more long-lasting than those of local steroid injections which tend to reduce after approximately 6 months [59, 60].

22.4.7 Laser Therapy

Low-level laser therapy (LLLT) has emerged as a prominent non-invasive intervention for PF, functioning via photobiomodulation, anti-inflammatory, and regenerative mechanisms. LLLT significantly reduces pain and disability both immediately after therapy and in the short-to-medium term, with meta-analyses showing a clinically meaningful analgesic effect compared to placebo or sham therapy. Its benefits are enhanced further when used as an adjunct to conventional treatments such as stretching and exercise, producing greater pain relief, and functional improvement than exercise alone. Several clinical trials and reviews indicate that LLLT is similar in efficacy to established interventions like extracorporeal shock wave therapy (ESWT), therapeutic ultrasound, and local corticosteroid injections but offers the advantage of minimal adverse effects and good long-term tolerability. When directly compared, both LLLT and corticosteroid injection produce comparable improvements in pain and foot function over 3 months, though LLLT appears superior in reducing local heel tenderness at this time point and avoids the risks of tissue rupture associated with steroids [61–63].

Further, head-to-head randomized controlled trials comparing high-intensity laser therapy (HILT) and LLLT in PF and other musculoskeletal conditions show no consistent overall superiority of one over the other for pain reduction or functional outcomes. One systematic review noted that LLLT might be better for grip strength in other chronic pain syndromes, while HILT can enhance certain tissue or sonographic parameters, but in PF, both modalities are safe, effective, and well-tolerated, producing significant gains in pain, disability, and quality of life. The clinical relevance of LLLT's effects appears to be dependent on proper dosing parameters, as per international recommendations, though long-term outcomes need deeper evaluation. Overall, LLLT stands as a valuable option, equivalent or even preferable to several standard therapies for PF, especially when considering its favourable safety profile and non-invasive nature, making it attractive for wide adoption, including in resource-limited settings [61, 64].

22.4.8 Surgical Treatment

Surgical treatment is usually reserved for treatment of PF only after all conservative or minimally invasive treatments have been attempted unsuccessfully for 6–12 months [2]. As in up to 95% of cases, conservative treatment alone will relieve the patient of symptoms; surgery is offered to a selected few [11, 65, 66].

The primary surgical procedure is an open or endoscopic plantar fasciotomy or 'release' of the plantar aponeurosis. The extent of the fasciotomy varies between partial to complete with some radical procedures involving removal of the bony calcaneal spur as well. The treatment is effective as it relieves the tension directly in the area of the pain and studies have reported success rates of the surgeries in the range of 75–96% with the endoscopically treated patients able to recover faster than those treated with open surgery. Another surgical option for patients with shortened calf muscles is the indirect release of tension by transverse notching of the gastrocnemius muscle fascia [67–70].

However, surgery does not always ensure a successful outcome, and even with good success rates, the overall satisfaction rates of patients are variable and range between 48% and 95% [70, 71]. Possible complications that may occur after surgery include nerve injury, plantar fascia rupture, or flattening of the longitudinal arch [2]. Patients should be adequately informed about the potential complications as well as the possibility of negative outcome before being taken up for surgical treatment.

22.5 Radiotherapy as a Treatment Option

22.5.1 Historical Perspective

The effectivity of low dose radiotherapy (LDRT) in treatment of painful musculoskeletal was first described as early as 1898 [72, 73]. Radiotherapy (RT) has been used for the treatment of various painful musculoskeletal inflammatory disorders since the first half of the twentieth century, and the earliest documented use specifically for PF was in 1924 [74].

However, fear of late effects, especially radiation-induced carcinogenesis and lack of high-level clinical evidence has prevented it from becoming a popular or first-choice modality in most of the world. With improvement of radiotherapy delivery and dosimetry techniques and equipment, as well as better a radiobiological understanding of the anti-inflammatory mechanisms, interest in use of LDRT in treatment of benign diseases has been rekindled recently. Nevertheless, it remains extensively popular for treatment of benign, painful musculoskeletal or degenerative osteoarthritic conditions in some Eastern European countries, especially Germany. In Germany, up to 30% of the daily workload of most radiotherapy centres consists of benign radiotherapy [10, 12, 75–77].

22.5.2 Mechanism of Action in Plantar Fasciitis

The proposed mechanism of action of low-dose radiotherapy (LDRT) in PF is multifactorial. LDRT, delivered in doses ranging from 0.5 to 1.5 Gy per fraction, has been demonstrated in both in vitro and in vivo experimental models to suppress key cellular processes involved in the inflammatory cascade.

LDRT inhibits the activity of inflammatory cells such as macrophages, monocytes, and polymorphonuclear leukocytes by inducing apoptosis. It suppresses the production of pro-inflammatory cytokines including Tumour Necrosis Factor-alpha (TNF-α), Interleukin-1 alpha and beta (IL-1α, IL-1β), and Interleukin-6 (IL-6), while simultaneously promoting the expression of anti-inflammatory cytokines such as Transforming Growth Factor-beta 1 (TGF-β1) and Interleukin-10 (IL-10).

Additionally, LDRT reduces levels of reactive oxygen species (ROS), nitric oxide (NO), and decreases the expression of adhesion molecules, contributing to its overall anti-inflammatory effect. It impairs endothelial cell function by decreasing inducible nitric oxide synthase (iNOS) production and inducing endothelial apoptosis. Furthermore, LDRT reduces leukocyte-endothelial interactions by downregulating adhesion molecules such as L-selectin and E-selectin on endothelial cells, thereby diminishing leukocyte recruitment to sites of inflammation [4, 77–82].

22.5.3 Indications for Radiotherapy in Plantar Fasciitis

Considering general radiation protection guidelines, radiotherapy for treatment of PF is not used as a first-line therapy at present. It is usually indicated in cases where non-radiotherapeutic approaches have not succeeded, and the duration of pain symptoms has been longer than 6 months to rule out any self-limiting conditions. It is generally recommended for patients above the age of 40 years; however, younger age is not an absolute contradiction and treatment with radiotherapy can be offered after careful consideration of risk-benefit ratio [12, 80, 83].

Patients who do not get complete relief after one complete course of LDRT may be offered a second treatment course after a period of 6–12 weeks.

22.5.4 Radiotherapy Techniques and Protocols

22.5.4.1 Radiotherapy Modalities

Over last few decades, substantial volume of clinical evidence has been generated proving the effectivity of radiotherapy in reducing symptoms of PF. These successful results can be achieved using a variety of radiotherapy equipment such as orthovoltage X-ray therapy unit or megavoltage linear accelerators using 4–6 MV photons and telecobalt machines [1, 12, 79, 80, 84, 85]. Both 2-D and 3-D planning has been used effectively for delivery of radiation treatment in PF.

22.5.4.2 Dose Fractionation Schemes

Over the last few decades, there have been a wide variety of fractionation schemes used effectively in treatment of PF with total doses ranging from 3 to 12 Gy and dose per fractions ranging from 0.1 to 1 Gy per fraction.

It was initially observed and recommended by von Pannewitz that the most effective anti-inflammatory effects of radiotherapy for acute inflammatory conditions could be achieved at doses of ≤0.5 Gy per fraction. However, as most patients of PF are only referred for radiotherapy after other treatment options have been attempted, a more chronic inflammatory process is present which appears to better respond to doses of 0.6–1.0 Gy [1, 86].

It has also been observed via in vitro experiments that the anti-inflammatory effect of LDRT is maximum at around 48 h after receiving radiation and reduces subsequently to became negligible after 72 h [81]. This suggests that ideally a gap of 48–72 h should be present between two fractions of LDRT and fits well with the current protocols of 2 fractions per week.

Seegenschmiedt in a retrospective study of orthovoltage treatment (200–250 kV at 20 mA) from 1984 to 1994 compared 3 schedules of 12 Gy in 12 fractions of 1 Gy, 3 Gy in 10 fractions of 0.3 Gy and 5 Gy in 10 fractions of 0.5 Gy. There did not appear to be any statistically significant difference in the three schedules in the rates of complete pain relief; however, the 3 Gy in 10 fractions group had statistically significant higher incomplete or insufficient pain relief and higher rates of delayed responses and recurrences [87].

Niewald et al. in a prospective multicentre randomized control study from 2012 reported that a schedule of 6 Gy in 6 fractions of 1 Gy was more effective and had a longer lasting effect than a schedule of 0.6 Gy in 6 fractions of 0.6 Gy. To rule out the effect of total dose on the results another RCT by the same group compared a schedule of 6 Gy in 6 fractions of 1 Gy delivered twice weekly with 6 Gy in 12 fractions of 0.5 Gy delivered thrice weekly. No difference between the two schedules was found in terms of reduction in patient reported pain or quality of life scores [88].

A prospective randomized control study by Heyd et al. reported that there was no difference in the subjective pain reduction between patients treated by 6 Gy in 6 fractions of 1 Gy or those treated by 3 Gy in 6 fractions of 0.5 Gy. RT was delivered twice weekly in both schedules. Results of this study suggested that while RT is effective in reducing symptoms of PF, the effectiveness may not be proportional to the total dose [89]. Another RCT comparing 6 Gy in 6 fractions of 1 Gy over

3 weeks to 6 Gy in 12 fractions of 0.5 Gy over 4 weeks did not show any difference in symptom relief or quality of life and was closed prematurely [90].

Dose response analysis by Miszczyk et al. of a retrospective patient cohort of PF treated with radiotherapy also did not show any dose-response relation. The total doses and fraction sizes used in the study varied between 1 and 45 Gy and 1 and 3 Gy, respectively. The study also concluded that optimal fraction sizes plateau at 1.5 Gy per fraction while total doses plateau at 9 Gy. Higher doses or fraction sizes did not improve outcome [91].

The present recommended dose schedule is 3–6 Gy of total dose delivered in 6 fractions of 0.5–1 Gy per fraction over 3 weeks with 2 fractions delivered in a week [12, 83]. Going by the principles of radiation protection, the smallest effective fraction size and total dose should be ideally utilized.

However, other schedules like 4 Gy in 8 fractions of 0.5 Gy each [92], 5 Gy in 7 fractions of increasing fraction size (0.25 Gy × 02 + 0.5 Gy × 01 + 1 Gy × 04) [93], larger fraction sizes such as 8 Gy in a single fraction or 8 Gy in 2 fractions of 4 Gy have also been used with effective results reported by several smaller studies [8, 84, 94].

22.5.4.3 Treatment Planning and Delivery

In Germany, while orthovoltage X-ray therapy machines (150–300 kV) were more commonly used for treatment of benign diseases traditionally, over the last 2 decades, linear accelerators using 4–6 MeV photons have become more commonly employed in this role [95].

The treatment position commonly used is 'feet first' with the patient on the treatment couch and with feet towards the gantry of the LINAC. The patient may be placed in supine, lateral decubitus on the side of the involved heel or prone position. The leg to be treated is stretched while the contralateral leg is angled or bent. When using x-rays or orthovoltage equipment, the ipsilateral knee is bent and the foot is placed on the treatment table.

Different types of beam placement can be used for actual treatment delivery. A single anterior-posterior (AP) beam in supine position or a direct plantar beam in prone position centred on anterior part of the calcaneal bone are commonly used for x-ray therapy. The dose reference point is kept at a constant tissue depth (usually 0.5–2 cm) [3, 4, 8, 12].

When using megavoltage machines, a telecobalt or linear accelerator with 4–6 MeV photons may be used. Isocentric lateral parallel opposing portals (90° and 270° in supine position) or parallel opposing fields (0° and 180° in decubitus position) can be employed. The dose prescription is placed at the isocentre which can be at the midpoint of the heel or the centre of the calcaneus [3, 12]. A safety margin of 1–2 cm should also be added. A single AP or plantar beam may also be used on the megavoltage machine but with a 1 cm bolus attached to the edge of the heel to avoid local underdosage [96].

22.5.4.4 Target Volume Delineation

In general, treatment volumes of benign disorders are smaller than those used for cancer treatment. The DEGRO guidelines recommend that for painful enthesiopathies like PF, the target volume should encompass the pain point, the complete involved insertion area of the plantar aponeurosis along with the nearby bony (partial or complete calcaneus) and muscular tissue. A safety margin of 1–2 cm should also be added [3, 12, 80]. Figure 22.3 shows a 3-D treatment plan for a patient with bilateral, chronic, recalcitrant PF.

There is wide variation in the treatment volumes used with some including the entire calcaneus, the plantar aponeurosis plus a 5 mm isotropic margin [78]. The German patterns of care study of radiotherapy for treatment of PF revealed that there was a wide variety of treatment fields between different practitioners without significant changes in outcome [95].

Herman et al. in a retrospective study reported that radiation field size did not have an impact on the treatment outcome of PF [97]. The authors recommended that smaller field sizes encompassing only the painful area with 2-cm margins extending into the neighbouring areas (calcaneus, fascia, fat pad) should be preferred as they were equally effective compared to traditionally larger treatment fields. See Fig. 22.4.

22.5.4.5 Radiation Safety Considerations

There is widespread apprehension globally for the use of radiotherapy for the treatment of benign diseases primarily due to the potential risk of radiation carcinogenesis. However, it should be borne in mind that the evidence supporting this risk comes from data based on the early days of radiotherapy with now obsolete planning techniques and treatments, historical equipment, and limited dosimetry.

Radiation-induced cancers typically emerge after a considerable latency period, making them less prevalent among older patients with shorter life expectancies. The risk of fatal cancer for a 25-year-old is estimated to be nine times greater than for a 75-year-old. Consequently, for younger patients, particularly those under 40, it is crucial to strike a balance between potential risks and benefits [77, 98].

The lifetime probability of developing a radiation induced skin cancer for an average dose of 3 Gy delivered to a surface area of 100 cm^2 (0.006%) is less than the lifetime risk of spontaneous skin cancer (0.2%). The risk of developing sarcoma post-radiotherapy is well-documented but occurs at a very low rate of 0.05% and is rarely reported at doses under 10 Gy [99]. Overall, the risk of developing radiation-induced cancer amongst elderly patients treated with low-dose RT delivered to small volumes of non-oncogenic tissues (heel, joints, tendons, muscle, etc) is minimal [76]. Surenkok et al. calculated the increased carcinogenesis risk factor in 20 patients of PF treated with RT and followed up for between 5 and 29 years, to be 1.3% above the baseline. The evaluation was made based on tissue weighting factors as described by the International Commission on Radiological Protection Publication 60 [100].

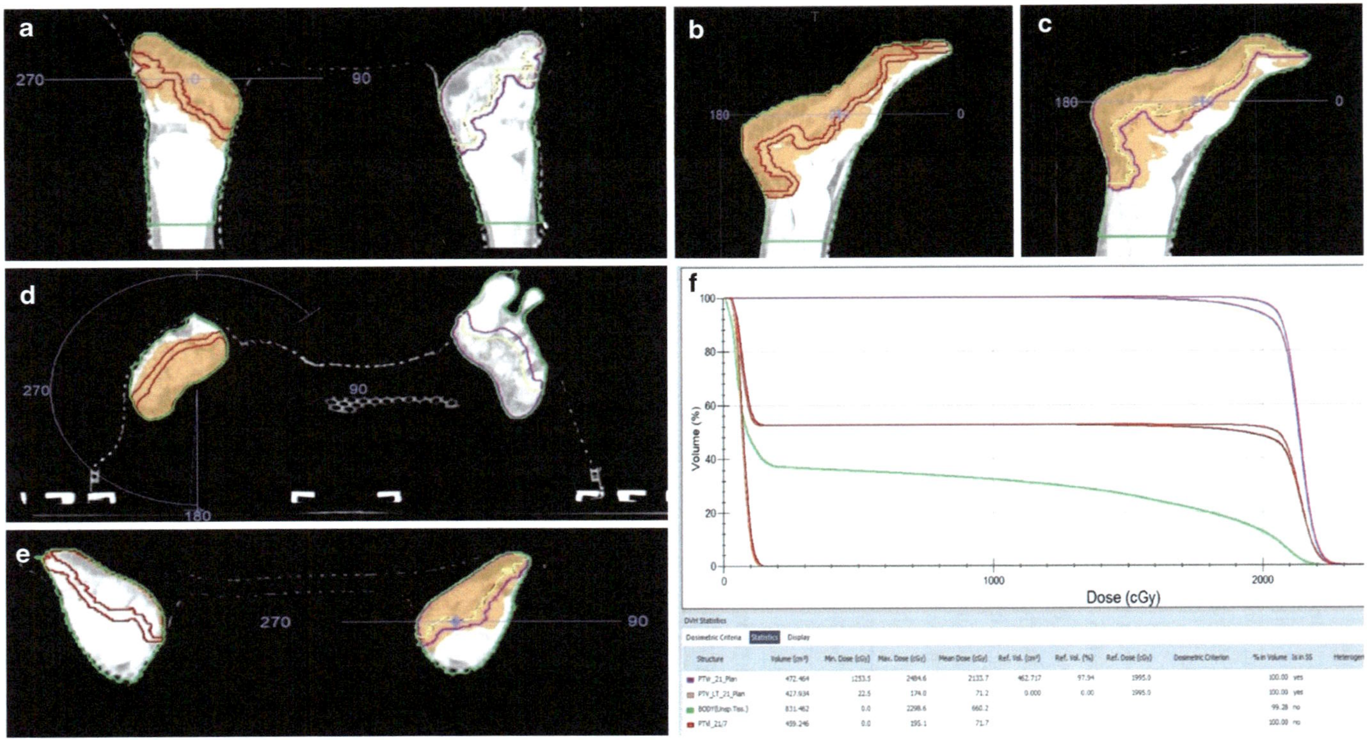

Fig. 22.3 3D treatment planning images of a patient with chronic bilateral plantar fasciitis. Panels A to E show target volume delineation and isodose distribution of bilateral plantar aponeurosis and panel F shows the Dose Volume Histogram of bilateral target volumes. (Images courtesy—Dr. Kanika Sood Sharma)

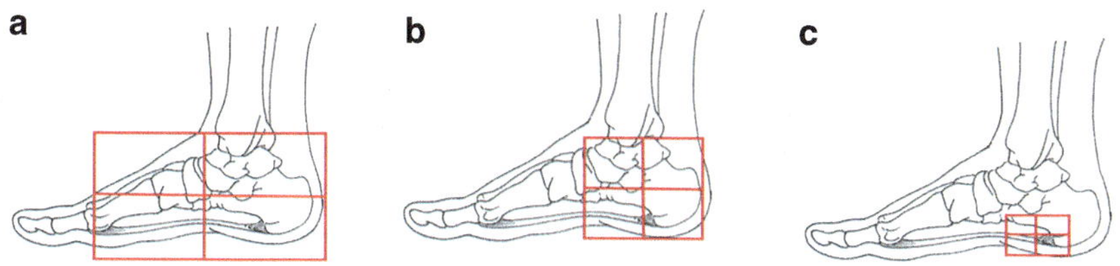

Fig. 22.4 Field sizes in LDRT for plantar fasciitis. (**a**) Traditional field definition including the entire dorsal and middle foot. (**b**) Commonly used field definition covering the entire calcaneus, including insertion of the plantar fascia and the Achilles tendon. (**c**) Small field definition encompassing only the painful area with 2 cm margins with extension into surrounding bone, fat, and fascia. (Illustrator—Dr Shashank B. Karvekar)

Nevertheless, the basic principles of ALARA (As Low As Reasonably Acceptable) in radiotherapy must be applied while planning treatment position and field placements. This includes the use of the smallest necessary field and the lowest effective dose, use of the multiple portals for covering the target volume, orientation of the radiation beam so that the entry and exit beams point away from the patient's body and use of shielding for radiosensitive organs like gonads. Radiation shields like lead aprons may be utilized when appropriate (when using orthovoltage equipment).

22.6 Clinical Evidence for Radiotherapy in Plantar Fasciitis

A large body of evidence on the study of role of radiotherapy in PF is available; however, the majority of studies are either retrospective or have limited sample sizes. The majority of the patients in the study are above the age of 50 years and suffer from refractory PF that has not responded to other therapies. As the goal of treatment is symptom relief, most studies analyse response to treatment immediately after RT and during follow-up commonly using the visual analogue scale (VAS), Calcaneodynia score, and the von Pannewitz scale (VPS) [77].

22.6.1 Prospective Clinical Studies

Schneider et al. treated 62 patients in a prospective study using an RT dose schedule of 5 Gy in 7 fractions. Significant pain relief (≥80% reduction in VAS) was seen in 25%, 60%, and 54% of the treated patients at 6 weeks, 28 months, and 40 months of follow-up demonstrating the effective and long-term results of RT in reducing pain due to PF without any side-effects. Older patients, avoidance of heel stress during treatment and shorter duration of symptoms were associated with better results [93].

Heyd et al. compared a dose of 6 Gy in 6 fractions of 1 Gy over 2 weeks with one of 3 Gy in 6 fractions of 0.5 Gy over the same period. A total of 130 patients were randomized to the high-dose and the low-dose group. At 6-months of follow-up, RT resulted in highly significant reduction of symptoms in both groups. Statistical analysis revealed no significant difference in response to RT between the two groups [89].

Niewald et al. in a multicentre RCT of 66 patients reported that a dose of 6 Gy in 6 fractions of 1 Gy was superior to a dose of 0.6 Gy in 6 fractions of 0.1 Gy in terms of pain relief at 3 months and in terms of retreatment requirement at 48 weeks [88]. In a follow-up RCT of 127 patients by the same authors, no significant difference in reduction in mean pain scores was found between a schedule of 6 Gy in 6 fractions of 1 Gy and one of 6 Gy in 12 fractions of 0.5 Gy with favourable pain relief with both schedules [90]. Both studies used the VAS, Calcaneodynia score, and the SF12 health survey for response assessment. These studies displayed that the superior anti-inflammatory effect of smaller fraction sizes (0.5 Gy) compared to fraction sizes of 1 Gy and above, that is seen in laboratory experiments could not be replicated in a clinical setting.

Similarly, no significant differences were found in immediate, short-term, and long-term pain response between 2 arms of 6 Gy in 6 fractions of 1 Gy and 3 Gy in 6 fractions of 0.5 Gy by Ott et al. in a prospective comparative study of 457 patients followed up for a median period of 32 months [101].

In a comparative RCT, Canyilmaz et al. reported that patients receiving LDRT had statistically significantly better pain relief (66%) than those receiving local steroid +/− anaesthetic injection (28%) [102]. In an RCT from India, 40 sportspersons with chronic, recalcitrant PF were randomized to either LDRT or PRP treatment. There was significant improvement in pain and functional scoring and plantar fascia thickness on ultrasound in both groups at 6 months with no statistically significant difference, suggesting both modalities are equally effective [103]. Chauhan et al. in a prospective single-arm study also from India reported overall pain-relief rates of 96% at 12 months of follow-up among the patients of PF treated with RT with no observed adverse effects [104].

In a single-centre prospective evaluation of RT for PF, epicondylitis and finger osteoarthritis, Rogers et al. reported that patients with PF had statistically significant pain reduction at both rest and during activity. Patients also had significantly faster walking times with a trend towards improved QoL [92]. Table 22.3 summarizes all prospective studies of last two decades.

22.6.2 Retrospective Follow-Up Studies

Seegenschmiedt did not find any significant differences in the rates of complete pain relief between 3 treatment schedules (12 Gy in 12 fractions of 1 Gy; 3 Gy in 10 fractions of 0.3 Gy; and 5 Gy in 10 fractions of 0.5 Gy) in a retrospective study of 141 patients and 170 heels treated over a decade. However, the rates of insufficient pain relief, delayed responses, and recurrences were statistically higher with the lower dose regimen of 3 Gy in 10 fractions making the higher dose regimens preferable [87].

Table 22.3 Summarized data of prospective studies of last two decades on use of RT in treatment of plantar fasciitis

Author Year Country	Type of study	*n*	Avg age (years)	Total dose/ Total fractions (Dose per fraction)	Avg follow-up (months)	Response rates	Adverse effects
Schneider 2004 [93] *Germany*	62	54	5 Gy/7 fx (0.25–1 Gy)	25%	40	Pain relief: 90%	NR
Heyd 2007 [89] *Germany*	RCT	130	59.5	3 Gy/12 fx (0.25 Gy) {50%} 6 Gy in 6 fx (1 Gy) {50%}	6	Pain relief: 88% No difference in response to RT between the 2 arms	NR
Niewald 2012 [88] *Germany*	RCT	62	56	0.6 Gy/6 fx (0.1 Gy) {53%} 6 Gy/6 fx (1 Gy) {47%}	12	Pain relief: 47% (0.6 Gy) 83% (6 Gy)	NR
Ott 2014 [101] *Germany*	RCT	457	55	3 Gy/6 fx (0.5 Gy) {52%} 6 Gy/6 fx (1 Gy) {48%}	32	Pain relief: 98% No difference in long-term response to RT between the 2 arms	NR

(continued)

Table 22.3 (continued)

Author Year Country	Type of study	*n*	Avg age (years)	Total dose/Total fractions (Dose per fraction)	Avg follow-up (months)	Response rates	Adverse effects
Niewald 2015 [90] *Germany*	RCT	117	57	6 Gy/6 fx (1 Gy) {50.4%} 6 Gy/12 fx (0.5 Gy) {49.6%}	3	Pain relief: 66% No difference in pain reduction in 2 arms	No acute side effects
Canyilmaz 2015 [102] *Turkey*	RCT	188	53	RT 6 Gy/6 fx (1 Gy) {66%}. Inj CE + AN {34%}.	12.5	Pain relief: 66% (RT) 28% (Inj)	NR
Gogna 2016 [103] *India*	RCT	40	50–55	RT 6 Gy/6 fx (1 Gy) {50%}. PRP. {50%}	6	Pain relief: 100% No difference in response rates between the 2 groups	No adverse effects observed in either arm
Chauhan 2017 [104] *India*	Prospective single-arm	36	40	6 Gy/6 fx (1 Gy)	12	Pain relief: 96%	No adverse effects observed
Rogers 2020 [92] *Switzerland*	Prospective single-arm	54	52	4 Gy/8 fx (0.5 Gy)	12	Pain relief: 80%	No adverse effects

In a retrospective, patterns-of-care study published from Germany in 2001 data on radiotherapy treatment of PF from 136 institutes and clinical evaluation of 7947 patients, it was reported that both megavoltage as well as orthovoltage radiotherapy were highly effective in pain reduction. Pain reduction was reported in 70% of all patients at 3 months and 65% patients had persistent pain relief with no reported acute or chronic side effects. The authors also reported that 19% patients were offered a second course of RT due to inadequate pain relief or early recurrence of pain [105].

Another retrospective cohort of 327 patients who received 623 irradiation treatments was reported on by Miszczyk et al. 97% of treatments were delivered by orthovoltage machines, and the most common fraction size used was 1.5 Gy (85%). The study reported complete pain relief in 48% and partial relief in 38% of patients in the immediate post-treatment period. At long-term follow-up (mean—74 months) 75% were pain free at rest and 68% were pain free while walking [91].

Similar results were also reported by Muecke et al. in a single-institute study of 117 patients. 84% had reduction of pain in the immediate post-treatment period with 23% becoming pain-free. At 20 months after RT, 90% had pain relief with 75% being pain-free. They also reported that early RT (within 6 months of symptoms) had better outcomes in terms of pain control. In a subsequent multi-centre study of 502 patients, the authors reported an overall 8-year event-free probability of 60.9% after treatment of PF with RT. They also reported that only single course of RT, use of megavoltage photons, and age ≥58 years were significant prognostic factors for pain relief [79, 106].

Several studies have reported that patients who do not benefit or benefit only partially from a first course of radiotherapy can be offered a second course of same dose and fraction size 6–12 weeks after completion of the first course of RT. Hajtmanova et al. reported in a study from Slovakia of 273 patients treated with a dose schedule of 4 Gy in 4 fractions of 1 Gy each with 2–3 fractions per week. Pain relief was experienced by 55.7% patients with one course of RT and 74.5% patients who received a second identical course of RT. The authors also reported that greater benefit of treatment was seen in patients who had been symptomatic for less than 6 months and those who were less than 50 years of age [107].

Schwarz et al. in a small study from Australia reported a 100% pain response for patients of PF treated with a single fraction of 8 Gy by conventional technique, suggesting single fraction radiobiology may be adequate to provide symptom relief in PF [94]. Herman et al. reported in a retrospective study of 250 patients that 70% of the study patients had either complete or partial response to radiotherapy. Age >53 years, duration of symptoms <12 months from start of RT and size of heel spur ≤6.5 mm (or complete absence of the heel spur) increased the possibility of clinical response to RT. Size of the RT treatment field, however, did not have any influence on treatment outcome [97].

Sixty-two patients with painful plantar heel spur were treated by RT using a telecobalt machine by Koca et al. to a dose of 8 Gy in 2 fractions of 4 Gy. At 28 months of follow-up, 58% patients reported complete pain relief and 21% reported partial pain relief. The authors suggested that the simplicity, low-cost, and lack of adverse effects of RT should make it a preferred treatment for painful heel spurs [85]. Uysal reported results of 450 patients treated using a telecobalt machine with a dose schedule of 8 Gy in 2 fractions. RT produced statistically significant pain relief in the study sample with only 2.2% patients requiring a second course of RT due to refractory pain. No radiotherapy related toxicity was reported [84].

Badakshi et al., in a retrospective study of 200 patients of chronic, painful, and refractory PF treated with orthovoltage x-rays to a dose of 3 Gy in 6 fractions over 2 weeks, reported pain relief in 61.4% patients, reduction in mobility restriction in 64.9%, and improved quality of life in 60.8% patients at a mean follow-up of 54 months. The median age of the study population was 70 years, and none of the patients were younger than 65 years [4]. Kedzierawski et al. from Poland in a small study of 47 patients reported complete response from pain in 96% cases with no RT-related side effects. The study also reported re-irradiation in 8% patients [78].

In a retrospective single centre study of 45-years from Turkey, Beyzaodeoglu reported on the treatment of 4904 patients of PF. All patients were treated to a dose of 8 gy in 2 fractions by using a telecobalt machine and 2D treatment planning and delivery. Treatment response was assessed between 3 and 5 weeks after radiation, and 73% patients reported complete relief from pain, 24.2% reported partial relief while 2.8% reported no response [8].

Rudat et al., in a single-centre study of 666 patients and 864 heels, reported that early aggravation of pain after RT (within 3 months) predicts poorer outcomes, but re-radiation benefits a significant proportion (40%) of non-responders and should be offered. They also reported on long-term outcomes that the probability of insufficient pain control (<75% pain control) at 10 years after LDRT was 45.9% with a mean time to insufficient pain control after LDRT was 74 months. No toxicity was reported [108].

Simoes et al., in a recent retrospective review of 12 patients with painful calcaneal spur from Portugal, reported complete pain relief in 100% of patients. The RT dose used was 15 Gy in three fractions of 5 Gy each, though a few other treatment schedules were also used. No RT-related toxicity was encountered [109]. Djiepmo et al. reported RT to be a highly effective treatment modality for PF with no side effects and long duration of response. At a follow-up period of greater than 3 years, 73% were pain-free. The duration of symptoms before start of RT was reported to be a significant prognostic factor [110]. Aynaci et al., in a retrospective study from Turkey, compared patients of PF treated with either RT, local steroid injection or ESWT. At 12 months of follow-up, RT produced more superior pain relief and function improvement compared to other modalities. RT was also associated with longer event-free intervals and less need for further treatment. No RT-related toxicities were reported [111]. Table 22.4 summarizes major retrospective studies of last two decades.

Table 22.4 Summarized data of retrospective studies of last two decades on use of RT in treatment of plantar fasciitis

Author, Year & Country	*n*	Avg age (years)	Total dose/ Total fractions (Dose per fraction)	Second RT course	Average follow-up (months)	Response rates	Adverse effects
Seegenschmiedt 1996 [87] *Germany*	141	55	12 Gy/12 fx (1 Gy) 3 Gy/10 fx (0.3 Gy) 5 Gy/10 fx (0.5 Gy).	NR	36	Complete pain relief: 67–72%	NR
Muecke 2003 [79] *Germany*	117	58	5 Gy/10 fx (0.5 Gy)	11%	20	Pain relief: 90%	None observed
Schwarz 2004 [94] *Australia*	7	66	8 Gy/1 fx (8 Gy)	14%	16	Pain relief: 71%	None observed
Micke 2004 [105] *Germany*	7947	56	2.5–18.75 Gy (0.3–1.5 Gy)	19%	28	Pain relief: 70%	None observed
Miszczyk 2007 [91] *Poland*	327	52	1–45 Gy (1–3 Gy)	29.36%	74	Pain relief: 86%	None observed
Muecke 2007 [106] *Germany*	502	58	OV: 6 Gy/6 fx (1 Gy). MV: 5 Gy/5–10 fx (0.5–1 Gy)	17.5%	26	Pain-free probability at 8 years: 61%	NR
Hajtmanova 2010 [107] *Slovakia*	323	56	4 Gy/4 fx (1 Gy)	44%	3	Pain relief: 74.5%	NR
Hermann 2013 [97] *Germany*	250	53	3–6 Gy/6 fx (0.5–1 Gy)	0%	11	Pain relief: 70%	NR
Koca 2014 [85] *Turkey*	62	57	8 Gy/2 fx (4 Gy)	0%	28	Pain relief: 79%	NR
Badakhshi 2014 [4] *Germany*	171	70	3 Gy/6 Fx (0.5 Gy)	17%	54	Pain relief: 69%	NR

(continued)

Table 22.4 (continued)

Author, Year & Country	*n*	Avg age (years)	Total dose/ Total fractions (Dose per fraction)	Second RT course	Average follow-up (months)	Response rates	Adverse effects
Uysal 2014 [84] *Turkey*	450	52	8 Gy/2 fx (4 Gy)	2%	12	Pain relief: 98%	NR
Kedizierawski 2017 [78] *Poland*	47	61	6 Gy/6 fx (1 Gy)	8%		Pain relief: 100%	None observed
Beyzadeoglu 2019 [8] *Turkey*	4904	51	8 Gy/2 fx (4 Gy)	0%	3–5 weeks	Pain relief: 97%	None observed
Rudat 2021 [108] *Germany*	666	57	3–6 Gy/6 fx (0.5–1 Gy)	28%	16	Pain relief: 68%	Initial pain aggravation in few patients
Aynaci 2021 [111] *Turkey*	205	50–55	6 Gy/6 fx (1 Gy) PGSI. ESWT.	28%	14 12 20	Pain relief: 80.6% 72.3% 63%	None in RT 1 local site infection in PGSI Pain/skin reddening in 16% cases of ESWT
Djiepmo 2022 [110] *Germany*	102	52	3–6 Gy/6 fx (0.5–1 Gy)	16%	94	Complete pain relief: 73%	NR
Simoes 2024 [109] *Portugal*	12	61	15 Gy/3 fx (5 Gy)—Most common	8%	3 weeks	Pain relief: 100%	1 patient Reported transient increase in pain

22.6.3 Systematic Reviews and Meta-analyses

A comprehensive systematic review by the U.S. Department of Veterans Affairs (2015) assessed the effectiveness of radiation therapy for various benign conditions, including PF. The review included randomized controlled trials (RCTs), non-randomized comparative studies, and single-group studies. It concluded that most studies report symptom improvement with LDRT in PF and may improve function as well. Though more high-quality data were recommended for some outcomes, there was no indication from the available evidence that RT should not be considered in refractory cases after other therapies fail [112].

The 2015 DEGRO (Deutsche Gesellschaft für Radioonkologie, or 'German Society for Radiation Oncology') guidelines recommend LDRT as an effective, evidence-based treatment for chronic PF that has not responded to standard conservative therapies. The advised regimen is 3–6 Gy total, given in single fractions of 0.5–1.0 Gy, two to three times per week, with a level of evidence of 1b and grade of recommendation of A. Radiotherapy is generally advised only for patients over 40 years old and with symptoms persisting longer than 3 months, after considering the risks and benefits [12].

The March 2023 Royal College of Radiologists (UK) recommendations for using radiotherapy in benign diseases are supported by high-level evidence. As per these recommendations, RT is considered a safe and effective option for chronic, refractory PF that has lasted more than 6 months and failed conservative treatments. The standard dose suggested is 3–6 Gy in six fractions (0.5–1 Gy per fraction) over 3 weeks [83].

Table 22.3 summarizes the important prospective studies from the last two decades on the use of RT in management of PF, while Table 22.4 summarizes the major retrospective studies from the same period. Table 22.5 summarizes the interpretations that can be drawn and applied in practice about the use of RT in treatment of PF based on the available clinical evidence.

Overall, LDRT is demonstrated to be an effective and durable treatment for chronic PF refractory to conservative therapy, with multiple studies supporting its use in terms of pain control, functional improvement, and long-term symptom relief. Importantly, LDRT for PF is consistently shown to have an excellent safety and low toxicity profile with no significant adverse effects or late complications across large cohorts and long follow-up periods.

Table 22.5 Interpretations and applications about the use of RT in plantar fasciitis management based on available clinical evidence

Efficacy and outcomes	
Pain reduction rates	Significant pain relief (≥80% VAS reduction) was reported in 25–96% of patients depending on the study and follow-up duration. Immediate post-treatment partial or complete pain relief ranged from 48% to 84%. Long-term pain relief at 12–40 months ranged from 60% to 75% in most large cohorts. Randomized controlled trials (RCTs) showed no significant differences in pain relief between dose schedules from 3 to 8 Gy total dose in different fractionations
Functional improvement	Objective improvements in function (walking speed, grip strength) were reported alongside pain relief. Studies specifically measuring gait showed statistically significant faster walking times after LDRT. Radiotherapy was associated with better quality of life scores and reduced mobility restrictions versus steroid injections in comparative studies.
Time to symptom relief	Early pain relief observed as soon as at the end of RT or within 6 weeks after treatment, with continuing improvement up to 6–12 months. Some patients who have an insufficient or partial response after RT or have recurrent pain after the first course of RT can have an improved and longer-lasting response with a second course of RT. therefore, a second course of RT is recommended for such patients.
Durability of treatment response	Persistent pain relief in 65–75% of patients at long-term follow-up (≥12 months, some up to 74 months average). 8-year event-free probability reported at 60.9% in a large multi-Centre series Re-irradiation in 10–19% of patients led to additional pain relief in a significant proportion.
Factors affecting treatment response	Though not seen universally in all studies, older age appears to be associated with a better treatment result with RT. Early initiation of radiotherapy (<6 months symptom duration) is a consistent favourable prognostic factor in several studies. Prevention of stress to heel during radiation treatment is associated with better clinical response to RT. Treatment with megavoltage (MV) beams has been reported to be a significant prognostic factor for pain relief compared to kV or orthovoltage. This is possibly because of the more homogenous dose distribution with MV radiation.

(continued)

Table 22.5 (continued)

Safety and toxicity	
No significant acute or chronic radiation-related toxicity was reported in multiple studies, encompassing thousands of patients treated over decades. Transient local pain flare-ups during or shortly after radiotherapy were occasionally observed but resolved spontaneously without intervention. No cases of secondary malignancies or serious adverse effects related to radiation were reported in any study. Minor skin reactions such as redness were rarely reported and were transient in nature. Re-irradiation up to two or three courses was well tolerated without additional toxicity.	
Comparison with other treatment modalities	
RT vs ESWT	Pain control rates and functional outcome rates were significantly better for patients receiving RT than those receiving ESWT. Time to second treatment was longer in the RT group, indicating durability of response. Though both treatments were safe, higher proportion of patients receiving ESWT experienced transient acute effects.
RT vs local steroid injection	RT achieved significantly better pain relief and control compared to the steroid injection group. RT provided longer event-free intervals, delaying or reducing the need for repeat treatments. Functional scores were superior for patients receiving RT. steroid injections carried minimal risks like injection site infections; RT had no reported toxicities.
RT vs platelet rich plasma (PRP)	Current evidence indicates RT and PRP are equally effective therapeutic options for chronic PF, with similar improvements in pain and function at follow-up.

22.7 Patient Selection and Treatment Decision-Making

All patients must be counselled about the potential of RT-induced late effects and carcinogenesis, however low, and informed consent should be obtained. Despite the nearly negligible risk of such adverse effects with LDRT, it is suggested to reserve RT for patients of PF older than 40 years and those whose symptoms are refractory and recalcitrant to other conservative treatment modalities. Treatment of younger patients can be considered after a thorough consideration and discussion with the patient on the potential risk and benefit of treatment with RT. There is substantial suggestion from literature that outcomes with radiotherapy are better if treatment is initiated within 6 months of treatment onset rather than later [75, 79].

There is significant variation in choosing LDRT as a treatment for PF as per geographical region of residence. In Germany and Eastern Europe, LDRT is a widely recommended and preferred treatment modality; it is rarely prescribed in North America and Western Europe despite the presence of guidelines from the UK's Royal College of Radiologists and Germany's DEGRO [12, 83, 95, 113].

In the context of cost-effectiveness, though radiotherapy involves expensive infrastructure, equipment, and manpower resources, it can provide a substantial economic benefit by reducing pain and improving functional capacity of a large section of the population inflicted by this highly prevalent problem. LDRT typically involves a limited number of sessions, simplistic treatment planning with relatively low resource use compared to prolonged pharmacological treatments or surgical interventions. Its non-invasive nature reduces hospital stay, complications, and rehabilitation costs. Given the limited access to specialized orthopaedic and rehabilitative care in resource-constrained settings, RT can be a financially viable and efficient alternative that improves patient outcomes and reduces the economic burden on healthcare systems in low-to-middle-income countries like India [110].

22.8 Future Directions and Research

It has earlier been mentioned that single fractions and smaller fields can be equally effective in reducing the symptoms of PF [94, 97]. It is thus natural to expect attempts to make LDRT more conformal and focussed. Stereotactic radiotherapy (SRS) would be an ideal modality to cover the small target volumes of PF though the doses that need to be delivered are significantly smaller. An ongoing prospective trial that aims to demonstrate a clinical benefit of LDRT is investigating MRI-based techniques for treatment guidance [114]. Another randomized controlled trial is comparing single-fraction versus fractionated LDRT in PF to assess for its non-inferiority [115].

Being non-invasive, LDRT can easily be combined with other treatment modalities like oral analgesics, physical therapy, exercise, ESWT, LLLT, and injections of steroid or PRP. Future research should focus on the effectivity and safety of such combination therapies as combining LDRT with these modalities can target multiple pain pathways and healing mechanisms, potentially leading to faster recovery and improved long-term outcomes.

22.9 Conclusion

Radiotherapy has established itself as a valuable, evidence-based option for the management of chronic, refractory PF, especially when conventional therapies fail to provide adequate relief. The significant reduction in pain, improvement in function, and long-term safety demonstrated in numerous prospective and retrospective studies support its selective use in appropriate patient populations. Careful patient selection and individualized risk-benefit assessment remain essential, given the very low—but not zero—risk of late radiation effects. With advancements in radiotherapy techniques, optimized protocols, and expanding clinical experience, this modality should play an increasing role in the multidisciplinary treatment of this common benign musculoskeletal disorder.

References

1. Micke O, Ernst-Stecken A, Mucke R, Seegenschmiedt MH. Calcaneodynia: plantar and dorsal heel spur/heel spur syndrome. In: Seegenschmiedt MH, Makoski H, Trott K, Brady L, editors. Radiotherapy for non-malignant disorders. Springer Berlin Heidelberg. p. 295–315.
2. Buchanan BK, Sina RE, Kushner D. Plantar fasciitis. In: StatPearls [Internet]. Treasure Island (FL): StatPearls Publishing; 2025 [cited 2025 Sept 13]. Available from: http://www.ncbi.nlm.nih.gov/books/NBK431073/.
3. Holtmann H, Niewald M, Prokein B, Graeber S, Ruebe C. Randomized multicenter follow-up trial on the effect of radiotherapy for plantar fasciitis (painful heels spur) depending on dose and fractionation – a study protocol. Radiat Oncol [Internet]. 2015 Dec [cited 2025 Sept 13];10(1):23. Available from: https://ro-journal.biomedcentral.com/articles/10.1186/s13014-015-0327-6.
4. Badakhshi H, Buadch V. Low dose radiotherapy for plantar fasciitis. Treatment outcome of 171 patients. Foot [Internet]. 2014 Dec [cited 2025 Sept 13];24(4):172–5. Available from: https://linkinghub.elsevier.com/retrieve/pii/S0958259214000698.
5. Riddle DL, Pulisic M, Pidcoe P, Johnson RE. Risk factors for plantar fasciitis: a matched case-control study. J Bone Joint Surg Am Vol [Internet]. 2003 May [cited 2025 Sept 15];85(5):872–7. Available from: http://journals.lww.com/00004623-200305000-00015.
6. Lourdes RK, Ram GG. Incidence of calcaneal spur in Indian population with heel pain. Int J Res Orthop [Internet]. 2016 Sept 3 [cited 2025 Oct 10];2(3):173. Available from: http://www.ijoro.org/index.php/ijoro/article/view/90.
7. Malik U, Fatima A, Ahmad E, Taqi SZ, Tahir I, Rehman A. Prevalence of plantar Fasciitis pain and its association with quality of work among sales promotion persons at supermarkets: prevalence of plantar Fasciitis and work quality. J Health Rehabil Res [Internet] 2024 Sept 29 [cited 2025 Oct 10];4(3):1–4. Available from: https://jhrlmc.com/index.php/home/article/view/1543.
8. Beyzadeoğlu M, Sağer Ö, Dinçoğlan F, Demiral S, Uysal B, Gamsız H, et al. Evaluation of the radiotherapeutic management of refractory painful heel spur and plantar fasciitis: a single center experience of 45 years. Gulhane Med J [Internet]. 2020 Mar 13 [cited 2025 Sept 13];62(1):8–13. Available from: https://gulhanemedj.org/articles/doi/gulhane.galenos.2019.730.
9. Hasegawa M, Urits I, Orhurhu V, Orhurhu MS, Brinkman J, Giacomazzi S, et al. Current concepts of minimally invasive treatment options for plantar Fasciitis: a comprehensive review. Curr Pain Headache Rep [Internet] 2020 Sept [cited 2025 Sept 13];24(9):55. Available from: https://link.springer.com/10.1007/s11916-020-00883-7.
10. Alépée B, Kaux JF, Colin G, Piret P. Place de la radiothérapie dans le traitement de la fasciite plantaire. Rev Med Liège. 2021;76(12):855-861. Accessed February 13, 2026. https://hdl.handle.net/2268/266834.
11. Gutteck N, Schilde S, Delank KS. Pain on the plantar surface of the foot. Dtsch Arztebl Int [Internet]. 2019 Feb 8 [cited 2025 Sept 13]; Available from: https://www.aerzteblatt.de/10.3238/arztebl.2019.0083.
12. German Cooperative Group on Radiotherapy for Benign Diseases (GCG-BD), Ott OJ, Niewald M, Weitmann HD, Jacob I, Adamietz IA, et al. DEGRO guidelines for the radiotherapy of non-malignant disorders: Part II: Painful degenerative skeletal disorders. Strahlenther Onkol [Internet]. 2015 Jan [cited 2025 Sept 13];191(1):1–6. Available from: http://link.springer.com/10.1007/s00066-014-0757-3.
13. Rubin G, Witten M. Plantar calcaneal spurs. Am J Orthop. 1963;5:38–41.
14. Intenzo CM, Wapner KL, Park CH, Kim SM. Evaluation of plantar fasciitis by three-phase bone scintigraphy. Clin Nucl Med. 1991;16(5):325–8.
15. Williams PL, Smibert JG, Cox R, Mitchell R, Klenerman L. Imaging study of the painful heel syndrome. Foot Ankle. 1987;7(6):345–9.

16. Bergmann JN. History and mechanical control of heel spur pain. Clin Podiatr Med Surg. 1990;7(2):243–59.
17. Teyhen DS, Robertson J. Plantar fasciitis: will physical therapy help my foot pain? J Orthop Sports Phys Ther. 2017;47(2):56.
18. Owens JM. Diagnosis and management of plantar fasciitis in primary care. J Nurse Pract [Internet]. 2017 May [cited 2025 Sept 25];13(5):354–9. Available from: https://linkinghub.elsevier.com/retrieve/pii/S1555415516308297.
19. Rano JA, Fallat LM, Savoy-Moore RT. Correlation of heel pain with body mass index and other characteristics of heel pain. J Foot Ankle Surg. 2001;40(6):351–6.
20. Engkananuwat P, Kanlayanaphotporn R, Purepong N. Effectiveness of the simultaneous stretching of the Achilles tendon and plantar fascia in individuals with plantar fasciitis. Foot Ankle Int. 2018;39(1):75–82.
21. Covey CJ, Mulder MD. Plantar fasciitis: how best to treat? J Fam Pract. 2013;62(9):466–71.
22. Digiovanni BF, Nawoczenski DA, Malay DP, Graci PA, Williams TT, Wilding GE, et al. Plantar fascia-specific stretching exercise improves outcomes in patients with chronic plantar fasciitis. A prospective clinical trial with two-year follow-up. J Bone Joint Surg Am. 2006;88(8):1775–81.
23. Celik D, Kuş G, Sırma SÖ. Joint mobilization and stretching exercise vs steroid injection in the treatment of plantar Fasciitis: a randomized controlled study. Foot Ankle Int. 2016;37(2):150–6.
24. Pollack Y, Shashua A, Kalichman L. Manual therapy for plantar heel pain. Foot. 2018;34:11–6.
25. Grieve R, Palmer S. Physiotherapy for plantar fasciitis: a UK-wide survey of current practice. Physiotherapy. 2017;103(2):193–200.
26. Renan-Ordine R, Alburquerque-Sendín F, de Souza DPR, Cleland JA, Fernández-de-Las-Peñas C. Effectiveness of myofascial trigger point manual therapy combined with a self-stretching protocol for the management of plantar heel pain: a randomized controlled trial. J Orthop Sports Phys Ther. 2011;41(2):43–50.
27. Johnson RE, Haas K, Lindow K, Shields R. Plantar fasciitis: what is the diagnosis and treatment? Orthop Nurs. 2014;33(4):198–204. quiz 205–6.
28. Lee SY, McKeon P, Hertel J. Does the use of orthoses improve self-reported pain and function measures in patients with plantar fasciitis? A meta-analysis. Phys Ther Sport. 2009;10(1):12–8.
29. Martin RL, Davenport TE, Reischl SF, McPoil TG, Matheson JW, Wukich DK, et al. Heel pain-plantar fasciitis: revision 2014. J Orthop Sports Phys Ther. 2014;44(11):A1–33.
30. Wapner KL, Sharkey PF. The use of night splints for treatment of recalcitrant plantar fasciitis. Foot Ankle. 1991;12(3):135–7.
31. Powell M, Post WR, Keener J, Wearden S. Effective treatment of chronic plantar fasciitis with dorsiflexion night splints: a crossover prospective randomized outcome study. Foot Ankle Int. 1998;19(1):10–8.
32. Nahin RL. Prevalence and pharmaceutical treatment of plantar fasciitis in United States adults. J Pain. 2018;19(8):885–96.
33. Donley BG, Moore T, Sferra J, Gozdanovic J, Smith R. The efficacy of oral nonsteroidal anti-inflammatory medication (NSAID) in the treatment of plantar fasciitis: a randomized, prospective, placebo-controlled study. Foot Ankle Int. 2007;28(1):20–3.
34. Goff JD, Crawford R. Diagnosis and treatment of plantar fasciitis. Am Fam Physician. 2011;84(6):676–82.
35. Hench PS, Kendall EC, Slocumb CH, Polley HF. The effect of a hormone of the adrenal cortex (17-hydroxy-11-dehydrocorticosterone: compound E) and of pituitary adrenocortical hormone in arthritis: preliminary report. Ann Rheum Dis. 1949;8(2):97–104.
36. Shanthanna H, Busse JW, Thabane L, Paul J, Couban R, Choudhary H, et al. Local anesthetic injections with or without steroid for chronic non-cancer pain: a protocol for a systematic review and meta-analysis of randomized controlled trials. Syst Rev. 2016;5:18.

37. Wong SHS, Wong CSM, Li TTL. Steroids in regional analgesia. Expert Opin Pharmacother. 2010;11(17):2839–48.
38. Sellman JR. Plantar fascia rupture associated with corticosteroid injection. Foot Ankle Int. 1994;15(7):376–81.
39. Tsai WC, Hsu CC, Chen CPC, Chen MJL, Yu TY, Chen YJ. Plantar fasciitis treated with local steroid injection: comparison between sonographic and palpation guidance. J Clin Ultrasound. 2006;34(1):12–6.
40. Kim C, Cashdollar MR, Mendicino RW, Catanzariti AR, Fuge L. Incidence of plantar fascia ruptures following corticosteroid injection. Foot Ankle Spec. 2010;3(6):335–7.
41. David JA, Sankarapandian V, Christopher PR, Chatterjee A, Macaden AS. Injected corticosteroids for treating plantar heel pain in adults. Cochrane Database Syst Rev. 2017;6(6):CD009348.
42. Majidi L, Saeb F, Alaei B, Khateri S, Ezzati Amini E, Nikoo MR. Comparison of the effectiveness of local corticosteroid injection and extracorporeal shockwave therapy in patients with pes anserine bursitis: an open-label randomized clinical trial. Med J Islam Repub Iran. 2023;37:10.
43. Karakılıç GD, Aras M, Büyük F, Bakırcı EŞ. Prolotherapy versus phonophoresis and corticosteroid injections for the treatment of plantar fasciitis: a randomized, double-blind clinical trial. J Foot Ankle Surg. 2023;62(6):922–7.
44. Sneed D, Wong C. Platelet-rich plasma injections as a treatment for Achilles tendinopathy and plantar fasciitis in athletes. PM R. 2023;15(11):1493–506.
45. Shetty SH, Dhond A, Arora M, Deore S. Platelet-rich plasma has better long-term results than corticosteroids or placebo for chronic plantar Fasciitis: randomized control trial. J Foot Ankle Surg. 2019;58(1):42–6.
46. Uğurlar M, Sönmez MM, Uğurlar ÖY, Adıyeke L, Yıldırım H, Eren OT. Effectiveness of four different treatment modalities in the treatment of chronic plantar fasciitis during a 36-month follow-up period: a randomized controlled trial. J Foot Ankle Surg. 2018;57(5):913–8.
47. Singh P, Madanipour S, Bhamra JS, Gill I. A systematic review and meta-analysis of platelet-rich plasma versus corticosteroid injections for plantar fasciopathy. Int Orthop. 2017;41(6):1169–81.
48. Theodore GH, Buch M, Amendola A, Bachmann C, Fleming LL, Zingas C. Extracorporeal shock wave therapy for the treatment of plantar fasciitis. Foot Ankle Int. 2004;25(5):290–7.
49. Hsu RWW, Hsu WH, Tai CL, Lee KF. Effect of shock-wave therapy on patellar tendinopathy in a rabbit model. J Orthop Res. 2004;22(1):221–7.
50. Wang CJ. An overview of shock wave therapy in musculoskeletal disorders. Chang Gung Med J. 2003;26(4):220–32.
51. Ogden JA, Alvarez RG, Levitt R, Marlow M. Shock wave therapy (Orthotripsy) in musculoskeletal disorders. Clin Orthop. 2001;387:22–40.
52. Wang YC, Chen SJ, Huang PJ, Huang HT, Cheng YM, Shih CL. Efficacy of different energy levels used in focused and radial extracorporeal shockwave therapy in the treatment of plantar fasciitis: a meta-analysis of randomized placebo-controlled trials. J Clin Med. 2019;8(9):1497.
53. Scheuer R, Friedrich M, Hahne J, Holzapfel J, Machacek P, Ogon M, et al. Approaches to optimize focused extracorporeal shockwave therapy (ESWT) based on an observational study of 363 feet with recalcitrant plantar fasciitis. Int J Surg. 2016;27:1–7.
54. Roerdink RL, Dietvorst M, van der Zwaard B, van der Worp H, Zwerver J. Complications of extracorporeal shockwave therapy in plantar fasciitis: systematic review. Int J Surg. 2017;46:133–45.
55. Rompe JD, Küllmer K, Riehle HM, Herbsthofer B, Eckardt A, Bürger R, et al. Effectiveness of low-energy extracorporal shock waves for chronic plantar fasciitis. Foot Ankle Surg [Internet] 1996 [cited 2025 Sept 25];2(4):215–21. Available from: https://linkinghub.elsevier.com/retrieve/pii/S126877319680004X.
56. Wang CJ. Extracorporeal shockwave therapy in musculoskeletal disorders. J Orthop Surg. 2012;7:11.

57. Kudo P, Dainty K, Clarfield M, Coughlin L, Lavoie P, Lebrun C. Randomized, placebo-controlled, double-blind clinical trial evaluating the treatment of plantar fasciitis with an extracoporeal shockwave therapy (ESWT) device: a North American confirmatory study. J Orthop Res. 2006;24(2):115–23.
58. Lou J, Wang S, Liu S, Xing G. Effectiveness of extracorporeal shock wave therapy without local anesthesia in patients with recalcitrant plantar Fasciitis: a meta-analysis of randomized controlled trials. Am J Phys Med Rehabil. 2017;96(8):529–34.
59. Sun K, Zhou H, Jiang W. Extracorporeal shock wave therapy versus other therapeutic methods for chronic plantar fasciitis. Foot Ankle Surg. 2020;26(1):33–8.
60. Hocaoglu S, Vurdem UE, Cebicci MA, Sutbeyaz ST, Guldeste Z, Yunsuroglu SG. Comparative effectiveness of radial extracorporeal shockwave therapy and ultrasound-guided local corticosteroid injection treatment for plantar fasciitis. J Am Podiatr Med Assoc. 2017;107(3):192–9.
61. Naterstad IF, Joensen J, Bjordal JM, Couppé C, Lopes-Martins RAB, Stausholm MB. Efficacy of low-level laser therapy in patients with lower extremity tendinopathy or plantar fasciitis: systematic review and meta-analysis of randomised controlled trials. BMJ Open [Internet] 2022 Sept [cited 2025 Oct 10];12(9):e059479. Available from: https://bmjopen.bmj.com/lookup/doi/10.1136/bmjopen-2021-059479.
62. Zare Bidoki M, Vafaeei Nasab MR, Khatibi Aghda A. Comparison of high-intensity laser therapy with extracorporeal shock wave therapy in the treatment of patients with plantar fasciitis: a double-blind randomized clinical trial. Iran J Med Sci [Internet]. 2024 Mar [cited 2025 Oct 10];49(3). Available from: https://doi.org/10.30476/ijms.2023.98042.2991.
63. Yetişir A, Kozanoğlu E, Kelle B. Comparison of effects of low level laser therapy and local corticosteroid injection in the treatment of plantar fasciitis. Turk J Phys Med Rehabil [Internet]. 2023 Mar 1 [cited 2025 Oct 10];1(1):8–14. Available from: https://www.ftrdergisi.com/uploads/pdf/pdf_4422.pdf.
64. Saleh MS, Shahien M, Mortada H, Elaraby A, Hammad YS, Hamed M, et al. High-intensity versus low-level laser in musculoskeletal disorders. Lasers Med Sci [Internet]. 2024 July 11 [cited 2025 Oct 10];39(1):179. Available from: https://link.springer.com/10.1007/s10103-024-04111-1.
65. Kinley S, Frascone S, Calderone D, Wertheimer SJ, Squire MA, Wiseman FA. Endoscopic plantar fasciotomy versus traditional heel spur surgery: a prospective study. J Foot Ankle Surg. 1993;32(6):595–603.
66. Quaschnick MS. The diagnosis and management of plantar fasciitis. Nurse Pract. 1996;21(4):50–4. 60–3, quiz 64–5.
67. Tomczak RL, Haverstock BD. A retrospective comparison of endoscopic plantar fasciotomy to open plantar fasciotomy with heel spur resection for chronic plantar fasciitis/heel spur syndrome. J Foot Ankle Surg. 1995;34(3):305–11.
68. Morton TN, Zimmerman JP, Lee M, Schaber JD. A review of 105 consecutive uniport endoscopic plantar fascial release procedures for the treatment of chronic plantar fasciitis. J Foot Ankle Surg. 2013;52(1):48–52.
69. Fishco WD, Goecker RM, Schwartz RI. The instep plantar fasciotomy for chronic plantar fasciitis. A retrospective review. J Am Podiatr Med Assoc. 2000;90(2):66–9.
70. Davies MS, Weiss GA, Saxby TS. Plantar fasciitis: how successful is surgical intervention? Foot Ankle Int. 1999;20(12):803–7.
71. Abbassian A, Kohls-Gatzoulis J, Solan MC. Proximal medial gastrocnemius release in the treatment of recalcitrant plantar fasciitis. Foot Ankle Int. 2012;33(1):14–9.
72. Sokoloff N. Röntgenstrahlen gegen Gelenkrheumatismus. Fortschr Geb Rontgenstr Nuklearmed. 1898;1:209–13.
73. Stenbek O. On the treatment of rheumatism of chronic arthritis with X-rays. Läk Fören Förh. 1898;1:117.
74. Brenner DJ. Exploring two two-edged swords. Radiat Res. 2012;178(1):7–16.
75. Seegenschmiedt MH, Micke O, Muecke R, German Cooperative Group on Radiotherapy for Non-malignant Diseases (GCG-BD). Radiotherapy for non-malignant disorders: state of the art and update of the evidence-based practice guidelines. Br J Radiol. 2015;88(1051):20150080.

76. G-Colin_2024_French.
77. Álvarez B, Montero Á, Aramburu F, Calvo E, Ángel De La Casa M, Valero J, et al. Radiotherapy for ostheoarticular degenerative disorders: when nothing else works. Osteoarthr Cartil Open [Internet]. 2020 Jan [cited 2025 Sept 13];1(3–4):100016. Available from: https://linkinghub.elsevier.com/retrieve/pii/S2665913119300196.
78. Kędzierawski P, Stando R, Macek P. Retrospective evaluation of the effectiveness of radiotherapy in patients with plantar fascitis (heel spurs). Rep Pract Oncol Radiother [Internet]. 2017 May [cited 2025 Sept 13];22(3):209–11. Available from: https://linkinghub.elsevier.com/retrieve/pii/S1507136716301729.
79. Mücke R, Schönekaes K, Micke O, Seegenschmiedt MH, Berning D, Heyder R. Low-dose radiotherapy for painful heel spur: retrospective study of 117 patients. Strahlenther Onkol [Internet]. 2003 Nov [cited 2025 Sept 13];179(11):774–8. Available from: http://link.springer.com/10.1007/s00066-003-1126-9.
80. German Cooperative Group on Radiotherapy for Benign Diseases (GCG-BD), Reinartz G, Eich HT, Pohl F. DEGRO practical guidelines for the radiotherapy of non-malignant disorders – Part IV: Symptomatic functional disorders. Strahlenther Onkol [Internet]. 2015 Apr [cited 2025 Sept 26];191(4):295–302. Available from: http://link.springer.com/10.1007/s00066-014-0789-8.
81. Arenas M, Sabater S, Hernández V, Rovirosa A, Lara PC, Biete A, et al. Anti-inflammatory effects of low-dose radiotherapy: Indications, dose, and radiobiological mechanisms involved. Strahlenther Onkol [Internet]. 2012 Nov [cited 2025 Sept 26];188(11):975–81. Available from: http://link.springer.com/10.1007/s00066-012-0170-8.
82. Rödel F, Frey B, Manda K, Hildebrandt G, Hehlgans S, Keilholz L, et al. Immunomodulatory properties and molecular effects in inflammatory diseases of low-dose X-irradiation. Front Oncol [Internet]. 2012 [cited 2025 Sept 26];2. Available from: http://journal.frontiersin.org/article/10.3389/fonc.2012.00120/abstract.
83. rcr-publications_recommendations-for-using-radiotherapy-for-benign-disease-in-the-uk_march-2023.
84. Uysal B, Beyzadeoglu M, Sager O, Demıral S, Gamsız H, Dıncoglan F, et al. Role of radiotherapy in the management of heel spur. Eur J Orthop Surg Traumatol [Internet] 2015 Feb [cited 2025 Sept 26];25(2):387–9. Available from: http://link.springer.com/10.1007/s00590-014-1482-4.
85. Koca T, Aydın A, Sezen D, Başaran H, Karaca S. Painful plantar heel spur treatment with co-60 teletherapy: factors influencing treatment outcome. Springerplus [Internet] 2014 Dec [cited 2025 Sept 26];3(1):21. Available from: https://springerplus.springeropen.com/articles/10.1186/2193-1801-3-21.
86. Lindner H, Freislederer R. Long term results of radiotherapy of degenerative joint diseases (author's transl). Strahlentherapie. 1982;158(4):217–23.
87. Seegenschmiedt MH, Keilholz L, Katalinic A, Stecken A, Sauer R. Heel spur: radiation therapy for refractory pain--results with three treatment concepts. Radiology [Internet]. 1996 July [cited 2025 Sept 13];200(1):271–6. Available from: http://pubs.rsna.org/doi/10.1148/radiology.200.1.8657925.
88. Niewald M, Seegenschmiedt MH, Micke O, Graeber S, Muecke R, Schaefer V, et al. Randomized, multicenter trial on the effect of radiation therapy on plantar fasciitis (painful heel spur) comparing a standard dose with a very low dose: mature results after 12 months' follow-up. Int J Radiat Oncol [Internet]. 2012 Nov [cited 2025 Sept 26];84(4):e455–62. Available from: https://linkinghub.elsevier.com/retrieve/pii/S0360301612008486.
89. Heyd R, Tselis N, Ackermann H, Röddiger SJ, Zamboglou N. Radiation therapy for painful heel spurs: results of a prospective randomized study. Strahlenther Onkol [Internet]. 2007 Jan [cited 2025 Sept 13];183(1):3–9. Available from: http://link.springer.com/10.1007/s00066-007-1589-1.
90. Niewald M, Holtmann H, Prokein B, Hautmann MG, Rösler HP, Graeber S, et al. Randomized multicenter follow-up trial on the effect of radiotherapy on painful heel spur (plantar fasciitis) comparing two fractionation schedules with uniform total dose: first results after three

months' follow-up. Radiat Oncol [Internet]. 2015 Dec [cited 2025 Sept 13];10(1):174. Available from: http://www.ro-journal.com/content/10/1/174.

91. Miszczyk L, Jochymek B, Wozniak G. Retrospective evaluation of radiotherapy in plantar fasciitis. Br J Radiol [Internet]. 2007 Oct [cited 2025 Sept 13];80(958):829–34. Available from: https://academic.oup.com/bjr/article/80/958/829-834/7443832.
92. Rogers S, Eberle B, Vogt DR, Meier E, Moser L, Gomez Ordoñez S, et al. Prospective evaluation of changes in pain levels, quality of life and functionality after low dose radiotherapy for epicondylitis, plantar fasciitis, and finger osteoarthritis. Front Med [Internet]. 2020 May 19 [cited 2025 Sept 13];7:195. Available from: https://www.frontiersin.org/article/10.3389/fmed.2020.00195/full.
93. Schneider O, Stückle CA, Bosch E, Gott C, Adamietz IA. Effectiveness and prognostic factors of radiotherapy for painful plantar heel spurs. Strahlenther Onkol [Internet]. 2004 Aug [cited 2025 Sept 13];180(8):502–9. Available from: http://link.springer.com/10.1007/s00066-004-1204-7.
94. Schwarz F, Christie DR, Irving M. Are single fractions of radiotherapy suitable for plantar fasciitis? Australas Radiol [Internet]. 2004 June [cited 2025 Sept 13];48(2):162–9. Available from: https://onlinelibrary.wiley.com/doi/10.1111/j.1440-1673.2004.01292.x.
95. Micke O, Seegenschmiedt MH, German Cooperative Group on Radiotherapy for Benign Diseases. Radiotherapy in painful heel spurs (plantar fasciitis)--results of a national patterns of care study. Int J Radiat Oncol Biol Phys. 2004;58(3):828–43.
96. Hermann RM, Bruns F, Nitsche M. Low-dose radiotherapy of painful heel spur/plantar fasciitis as an example of treatment effects in benign diseases. In: Onal C, editor. Radiotherapy [Internet]. InTech; 2017 [cited 2025 Oct 10]. Available from: http://www.intechopen.com/books/radiotherapy/low-dose-radiotherapy-of-painful-heel-spur-plantar-fasciitis-as-an-example-of-treatment-effects-in-b.
97. Hermann RM, Meyer A, Becker A, Schneider M, Reible M, Carl UM, et al. Effect of field size and length of plantar spur on treatment outcome in radiation therapy of plantar fasciitis: the bigger the better? Int J Radiat Oncol [Internet]. 2013 Dec [cited 2025 Sept 13];87(5):1122–8. Available from: https://linkinghub.elsevier.com/retrieve/pii/S0360301613030770.
98. Mazonakis M, Damilakis J. Cancer risk after radiotherapy for benign diseases. Phys Med [Internet]. 2017 Oct [cited 2025 Sept 27];42:285–91. Available from: https://linkinghub.elsevier.com/retrieve/pii/S1120179717300157.
99. McKeown SR, Hatfield P, Prestwich RJ, Shaffer RE, Taylor RE. Radiotherapy for benign disease; assessing the risk of radiation-induced cancer following exposure to intermediate dose radiation. Br J Radiol [Internet]. 2015 Dec [cited 2025 Sept 27];88(1056):20150405. Available from: https://academic.oup.com/bjr/article/7445374.
100. Surenkok S, Dirican B, Beyzadeoglu M, Oysul K. Heel spur radiotherapy and radiation carcinogenesis risk estimation. Radiat Med. 2006;24(8):573–6.
101. Ott OJ, Jeremias C, Gaipl US, Frey B, Schmidt M, Fietkau R. Radiotherapy for benign calcaneodynia: long-term results of the Erlangen Dose Optimization (EDO) trial. Strahlenther Onkol. 2014;190(7):671–5.
102. Canyilmaz E, Canyilmaz F, Aynaci O, Colak F, Serdar L, Uslu GH, et al. Prospective randomized comparison of the effectiveness of radiation therapy and local steroid injection for the treatment of plantar Fasciitis. Int J Radiat Oncol [Internet] 2015 July [cited 2025 Sept 13];92(3):659–66. Available from: https://linkinghub.elsevier.com/retrieve/pii/S0360301615001716.
103. Gogna P, Gaba S, Mukhopadhyay R, Gupta R, Rohilla R, Yadav L. Plantar fasciitis: a randomized comparative study of platelet rich plasma and low dose radiation in sportspersons. The Foot [Internet]. 2016 Aug [cited 2025 Sept 13];28:16–9. Available from: https://linkinghub.elsevier.com/retrieve/pii/S0958259216300438.
104. Chauhan AK, Verma Y, Sangwan SS, Kumar D, Kaur P. Efficacy of external beam radiotherapy for the management of refractory plantar fasciitis: a prospective study. Int J Curr Res. 2017;9:51230–6.

105. Micke O, Seegenschmiedt MH. Radiotherapy in painful heel spurs (plantar fasciitis)—results of a national patterns of care study. Int J Radiat Oncol [Internet]. 2004 Mar [cited 2025 Oct 5];58(3):828–43. Available from: https://linkinghub.elsevier.com/retrieve/pii/S0360301603016201.
106. Muecke R, Micke O, Reichl B, Heyder R, Prott FJ, Seegenschmiedt MH, et al. Demographic, clinical and treatment related predictors for event-free probability following low-dose radiotherapy for painful heel spurs—a retrospective multicenter study of 502 patients. Acta Oncol. 2007;46(2):239–46.
107. Hajtmanová E, Kinclová I, Kostková L, Hajtman A, Péc M. Low-dose radiotherapy in the treatment of plantar fasciitis. Klin Onkol. 2010;23(2):104–10.
108. Rudat V, Tontcheva N, Kutz G, Orovwighose TO, Gebhardt E. Long-term effect and prognostic factors of a low-dose radiotherapy of painful plantar calcaneal spurs: a retrospective unicenter study. Strahlenther Onkol [Internet]. 2021 Oct [cited 2025 Sept 13];197(10):876–84. Available from: https://link.springer.com/10.1007/s00066-020-01741-6.
109. Simões S, Ramos S, Carvalho F, Costa MA, Fardilha C, Costa P. The role of radiotherapy in relieving pain caused by calcaneal spur. Int J Radiol Radiat Ther [Internet]. 2024 Apr 19 [cited 2025 Sept 13];11(2):30–1. Available from: https://medcraveonline.com/IJRRT/the-role-of-radiotherapy-in-relieving-pain-caused-by-calcaneal-spur.html.
110. Djiepmo F, Tamaskovics B, Bölke E, Peiper M, Haussmann J, Neuwahl J, et al. Low-dose radiation treatment for painful plantar enthesophyte: a highly effective therapy with little side effects. Eur J Med Res [Internet]. 2022 Dec [cited 2025 Oct 7];27(1):28. Available from: https://eurjmedres.biomedcentral.com/articles/10.1186/s40001-022-00642-x.
111. Aynacı Ö. Comparison of effectiveness of radiation therapy, local steroid injection, and extracorporeal shock wave therapy in patients with plantar fasciitis: a multicenter study. Turk J Oncol [Internet] 2021 [cited 2025 Sept 13]; Available from: http://onkder.org/pdf/pdf_TOD_1238.pdf.
112. Jutkowitz E, Rieke K, Caputo EL, Yan SX, Rudolph J, Mai HJ, et al. Radiation therapy for benign conditions: a systematic review. Washington, DC: Department of Veterans Affairs (US); 2024.
113. Yıldırım HC, Dinçbaş FÖ, Demircan V, Beyzadeoğlu M, Tekçe E, Yazıcı G, et al. Radiotherapy for benign diseases in Turkey: a patterns of care survey of the Turkish Society for Radiation Oncology (TROD 05-002). Strahlenther Onkol. 2024;200(2):143–50.
114. University of Erlangen-Nürnberg Medical School. Establishment and evaluation of standardized clinical, biological and imaging parameters to assess the response of ldrt in heel spur with plantar fasciitis [Internet]. clinicaltrials.gov; 2025 May [cited 2025 Oct 10]. Report No.: NCT06969820. Available from: https://clinicaltrials.gov/study/NCT06969820.
115. Masaryk Memorial Cancer Institute. Optimization of fractionation schedules of heel spur radiotherapy: monocentric prospective. Randomized Open-label Trial [Internet]. clinicaltrials.gov; 2023 Oct [cited 2025 Oct 10]. Report No.: NCT06104410. Available from: https://clinicaltrials.gov/study/NCT06104410.

Keoid

23

Ashok Kumar

23.1 Introduction

Keloid is a type of scar that forms beyond the boundaries of the original wound, and often it is raised, thick, soft to firm, shiny and may or may not be itchy. This is a benign condition which results in disfiguration and can cause discomfort. It is a type of hyperplastic scar that is due to collagen overgrowth responding to any kind of injury including burns. It can be asymptomatic but may also sometimes cause major discomfort like intractable pruritus, disfigurement, pain, and allodynia and may lead to a psychological distress. Risk factors for keloids can range from dark skin pigmentation, African/Asian ethnic background, family history, genetic predisposition (Ch 2q23 and 7p11), anatomic wound sites, infections, burns, repeated surgeries, and chronic wounds.

23.2 Brief History

Smith's papyrus (2500–3000 BC) first described this condition, and the term c'heloide was coined by Alibert in 1806 to differentiate it from other malignant conditions since these lesions were seen as expanding crab-claw-like formations. In 1790, it was described as 'Dartres de graisse' due to its 'greasy eruptions', in a book by Noël Retz.

A. Kumar (✉)
Department of Radiation Oncology, Holy Family Hospital, Okhla, Delhi, India

K. Sood Sharma (ed.), *Radiation Therapy for Benign Disorders*,
https://doi.org/10.1007/978-981-95-6635-8_23

23.3 Epidemiology

The studies on demographic distribution of keloids are not contributory to make a definitive assumption; however, keloids are affected by geographic and ethnic distribution. As per the available literature, incidence rates vary from 0.09% in England to 16 % in Zaire [1, 2]; however, the basis of these assumptions is not clear in the studies performed. However, in Kenya, the keloid prevalence is 8.5% among people with normally pigmented skins [3] in contrast to Japan, where it is around 0.1% [4]. Thus, it is safe to say that average incidence is around 10 % in Africa, up to 0.1 % in Asian population and <0.1 % in other countries. A specific type of keloid ACNE KELOIDALIS NUCHAE (AKN) is very common in blacks than other population, and it can be attributed to the high skin pigmentation with greater susceptibility to keloid formation.

Genetic risk factors play a role in keloid genesis and are associated with certain gene mutations and polymorphisms [5] along with the familial tendency to develop keloids. Rubinstein-Taybi syndrome (RSTS), the Ehlers-Danlos syndrome, the Lowe syndrome, and the novel X-linked syndrome are diseases which are associated with high risk of keloid development. Certain environmental factors which contribute to keloid development include mechanical injury, surgery, and piercing among the few. The most common site includes anterior chest (49 %), scapula (27%), lower jaw/neck (12%), upper arm (5%), dorsal region (3%), lower abdomen (5%), femoral region (2%), knee (0.5%), and upper abdomen (0.5%) [6]. Anatomical sites with skin tension also contribute to various shapes and sizes of keloids; hence, chest wall keloids are typically butterfly in shape, with dumbbell shape on scapular site with ball shaped lesions on earlobes (Figs. 23.1, 23.2, 23.3, 23.4, 23.5, 23.6, 23.7, 23.8, 23.9 and 23.10).

An analysis of data from the United States National Ambulatory Medical Care Survey from 1990 to 2009 that included 85,50,000 visits for keloids showed that when examining the number of visits per 100,000 United States residents according to ethnicity, African Americans and Asian Americans made the highest number of visits for keloids, nearly 2.5 times as high as non-Hispanic White Americans, respectively [7].

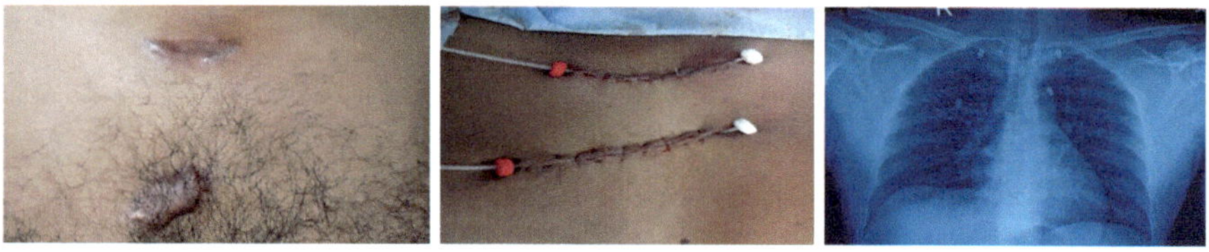

Fig. 23.1 38 years old male, case of polyarthritis with nodules over anterior chest, progressed to keloids. Treated with Injection Kenakort and silicone gel sheet for two years. Now treated with surgical excision and interstitial brachytherapy to a dose of 12 GY over 2 days. (Image Courtesy: Dr. (Brig) Pallabh Chaterjee, Prof & Sr. Consultant, Plastic Surgery)

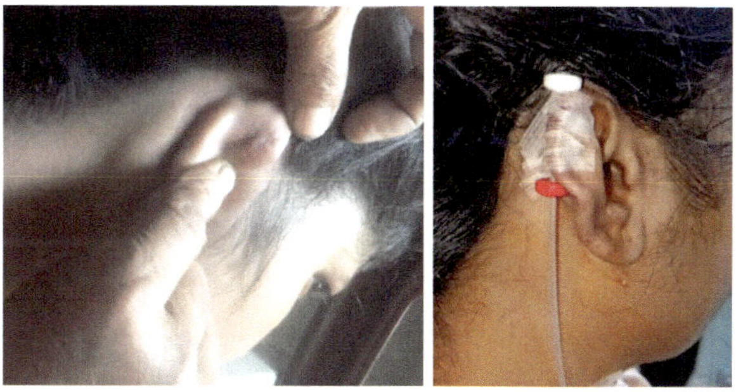

Fig. 23.2 A nodule shaped ear lobe keloid in a young female post ear piercing. Treated with steroid injections for two years and then treated with surgical excision and interstitial brachytherapy. (Image Courtesy: Dr. (Lt Col) Nilima Mishra, MBBS, PGDHHM, PGDMLS)

Fig. 23.3 Keloid development over anterior chest post carcinoma breast surgery (Image Courtesy: Dr. (Wing Commander) Nikhil Thakur, Assistant Professor, Radiation Oncology, Command Hospital, Bengaluru)

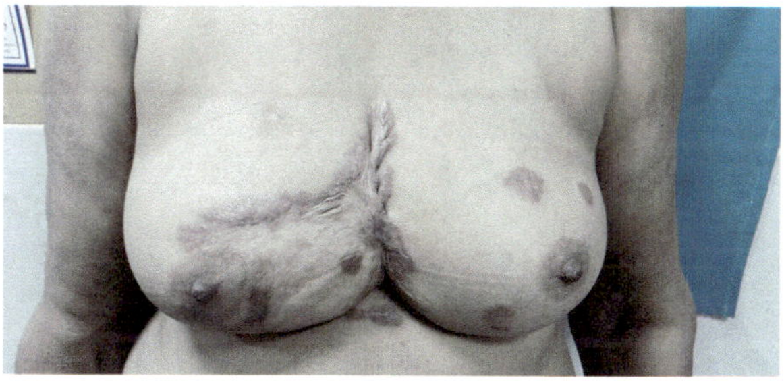

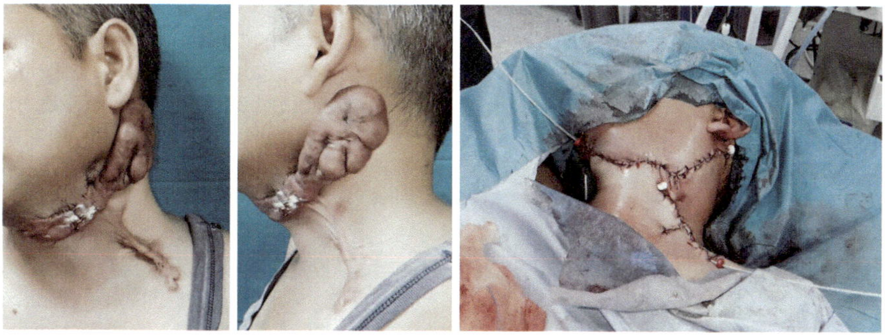

Fig. 23.4 A young patient developed keloids post-surgery for carcinoma oral cavity with neck node dissection. He was managed with steroid injections and silicone gel sheets for over 1 year. Finally, surgery and post-operative interstitial brachytherapy was performed. (Image Courtesy: Dr. (Lt Col) Manish Sandhu, Consultant Radiation Oncology, Command Hospital, Lucknow)

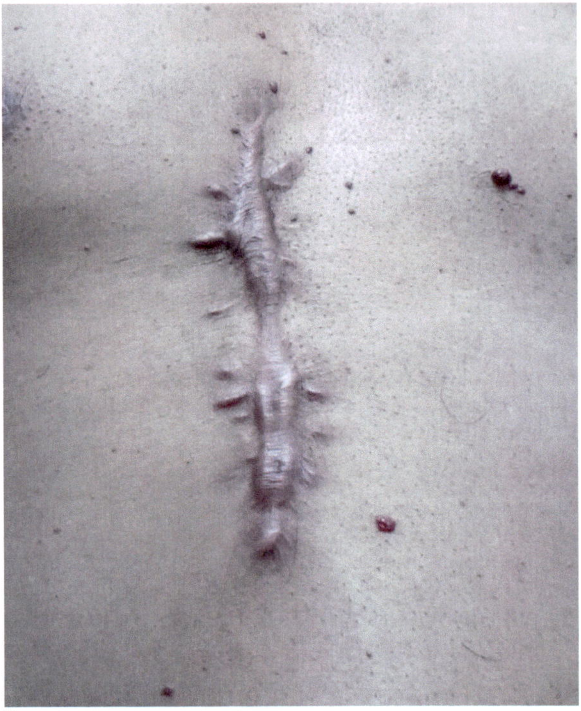

Fig. 23.5 Keloid after a boil over anterior chest and upper abdomen (Image Courtesy: Dr. (Col) Bharat Mishra, Professor, Dept of Plastic Surgery, AFMC, Pune)

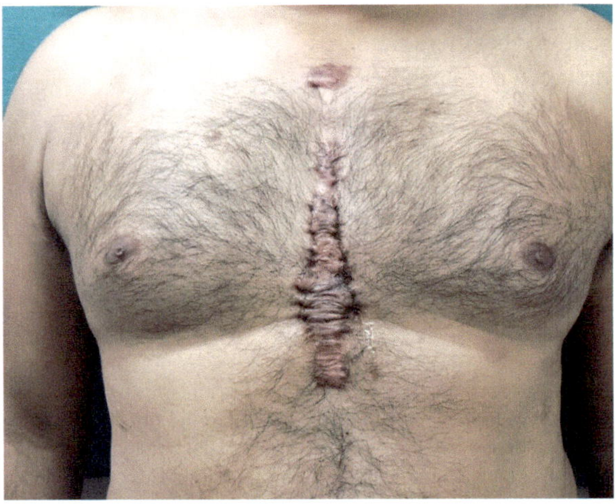

Fig. 23.6 Anterior chest keloid post-surgery for heart condition (Image Courtesy: Dr. (Col) Pranay Pratap, Associate Professor, Dept of Plastic Surgery, AFMC, Pune

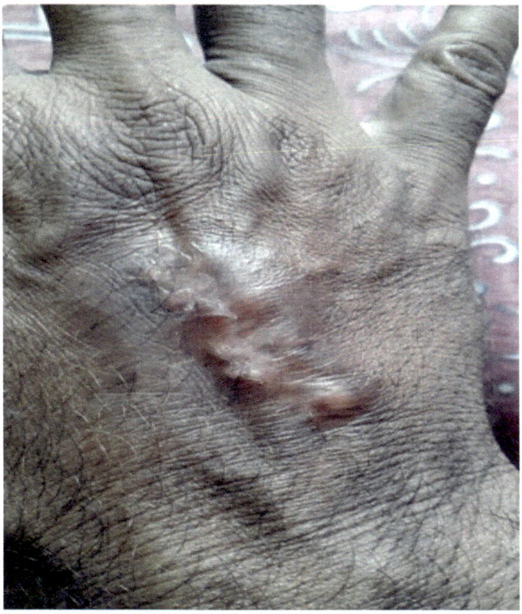

Fig. 23.7 Keloid over dorsal aspect of hand post burn injury (Image Courtesy. (Sqn Ldr) Prabhjeet Singh Bathla, Assistant Professor, Radiation Oncology, Command Hospital, Bengaluru)

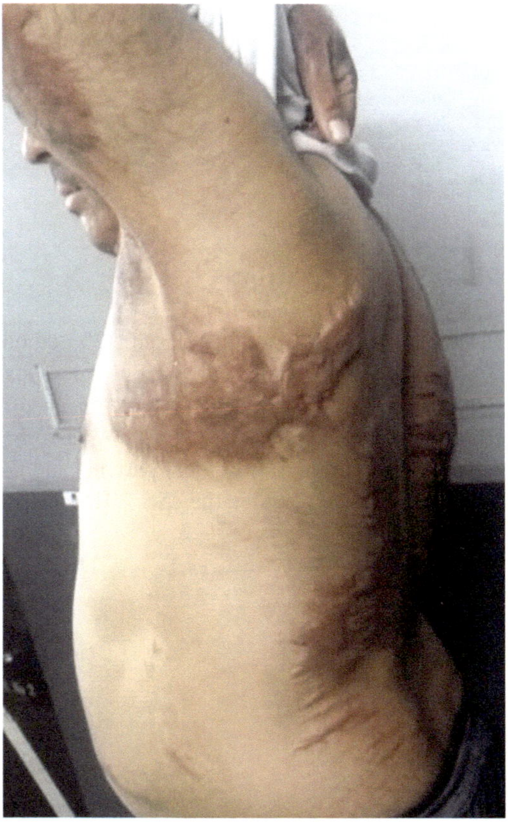

Fig. 23.8 Keloid post-burn injury (Image Courtesy: Dr. (Lt Col.) Mayuri Jain, Consultant, Radiation Oncology, Command Hospital, Lucknow)

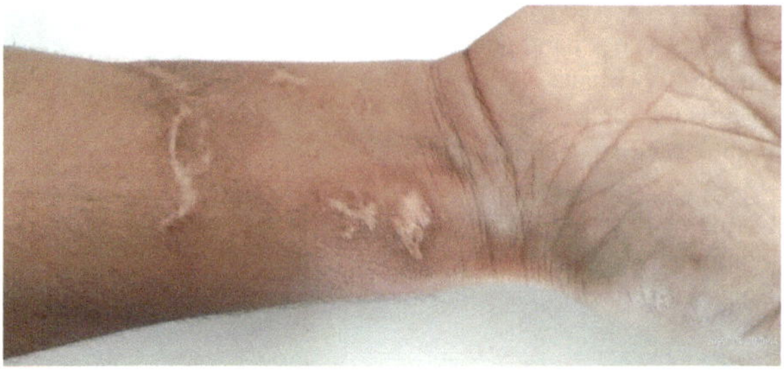

Fig. 23.9 Keloid post suicidal attempt (Image Courtesy: Dr. (Lt Col.) Rekha Vashisth, Consultant, Radiation Oncology, Command Hospital, Pune)

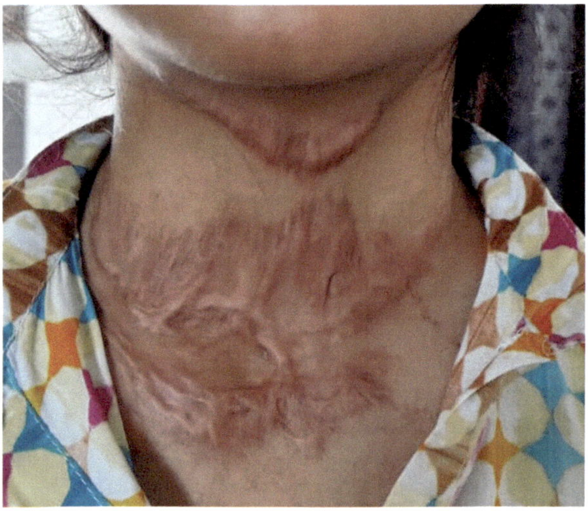

Fig. 23.10 Keloid post burn injury (Image Courtesy: Dr. (Surg Lt Cdr) Bhanu Prakash M, Consultant, Radiation Oncology, INHS Asvini)

23.4 Classification

Scars have been traditionally classified based on their clinical features (Table 23.1). To help unify the clinical definition of keloids and hypertrophic scars, the Japan Scar Workshop (JSW) created a tool for objectively diagnosing keloids and hypertrophic scars. This tool, called the JSW 2015 Scar Scale (JSS 2015), involves scoring the risk factors of individual patients and the lesion characteristics. Studies are needed to assess whether the JSS 2015 can accurately diagnose keloids in other populations.

Table 23.1 Classification and clinical features of hypertrophic scars and keloids [24]

Scar type	Characteristics	Maturation
Mature	Light or flat	
Immature	Red/pruritic/painful/elevated	May mature later or get pigmentated
Linear hypertrophic	Red/raised/pruritic/confined to scar border/matures to rope-like appearance/mature scar that has a wider area	Rapid increase in size within 3-6 months/may regress after a few/matures in 2 years' time
Widespread hypertrophic (burn scar)	Wide/red/raised/pruritic/remains within borders of injury	
Minor keloid	Focally raised/pruritic/ extends beyond scar border/genetic component/typical site—earlobes	May develop after one year of injury/does not regress spontaneously/high recurrence rate
Major keloid	Large/painful/pruritic/extends beyond border/can result from minor trauma	Does not regress spontaneously/keeps on progressing in size

23.5 Pathophysiology

It is characterised by accelerated proliferation of fibroblasts due to the impaired balance between the proliferation and apoptosis. It is also important to note that endothelial dysfunction mediated by propagation of the inflammatory response in the scar tissue is also an important factor leading to development of keloids.

23.6 Etiology and Pathogenesis

Keloids are hyperproliferative disorders which are due to chronic inflammation and the absence of tumour cells or structural atypia suggests that these are hyperplastic disorder which are stimulated by external or internal injury. The injury to reticular layer of dermis is the main inciting c-factor for the development of keloids in predisposed individuals. However, the exact pathogenesis of keloid development is still not understood, but it does involve the dysregulation of the wound healing process. The disruption of the vascular endothelium leading to vascular permeability during the vascular phase of wound healing, resulting in the continued influx of inflammatory cells and factors which results in local inflammation and fibrotic activity, may be the most important causative factor for the development of keloids and hypertrophic scars [8–10].

Also, at the molecular level cytokines and growth factors including TGF B, VEGF, PDGF, IL 6, and IL 8 have been found in these scars; however, the exact mechanism is still to be understood [11–13].

Other mechanisms associated with keloid development include mechanical stretching leading to abnormal scar formations; particular body locations, for example anterior chest, scapula, etc.; and uncommon regions including scalp, anterior leg, and upper eyelid, where there is no scope for mechanical stretches [14]. The shape and size of keloid development also depend upon the direction of stretching forces which suggests that skin tension augments the cutaneous inflammation which generates a leading edge and spreading of the scar. [6, 14, 15]. In the end, it is the inflammatory cytokines, inflammation, vascular permeability, and production of extracellular matrix which is involved in the pathogenesis of keloid development. Other factors contributing are cutaneous infections, genetic factors, age, sex hormones, and hypertension.

Importantly the reticular layer displays inflammation, angiogenesis, and large amounts of hyalinized collagen [16].

23.7 Diagnosis

Keloids are diagnosed on the basis of clinical features and history which gives the nature of injury which led to the development of keloid. Keloids may develop after a long time post any trivial injury also.

23.8 Clinical Features

They present as indurated, elevated, and erythematous with shiny surface with either red in colour in white individuals or violet or black in dark-skinned individuals. Keloids generally develop horizontally beyond the original wound margins with continued growth pattern. The shapes can vary depending upon the location to either linear, butterfly or crab like features, or sometimes they may appear as dumbbell-shaped. It can also present as a nodular shape or cauliflower shape. In comparison to the hypertrophic scars, keloid scar generally continues to grow despite reaching the plateau phase in contrast to the hypertrophic scar which starts regressing after reaching the plateau phase of growth.

Symptomatically keloids are associated with local pain and itching with poor aesthetics. There may sometimes be persisting pain which is uncommon, and it may be due to underlying infection or inflammation.

The most important diagnostic tool to assess the keloid scar is taking a detailed history to know the exact cause; it may arise from a negligible wound which predates many months before the scar formation.

A very simple tool to assess the scar, which can either be a hypertrophic scar or a keloid scar, is the Japan Scar Workshop (JSW) 2015 Scar Scale (JSS 2015) [17, 18]. The scale includes information on 12 variables, including demographics, aetiology, location, clinical features, and subjective symptoms, each of which is assigned a score of 0 to 3. An overall score of 6 to 15 indicates characteristics of a hypertrophic scar vis a vis a score of ≥16 points indicate keloid characteristics. A scores <6 indicates mature scars.

Other conditions which may mimic keloid scar includes benign and malignant cutaneous tumours, chondroid syringoma, dermatofibrosarcoma protuberans, cutaneous squamous cell carcinoma, juvenile xanthogranuloma, psudolymphoma, nodular scleroma, and lobomycosis. [19]

23.9 Management

Management of keloid depends upon the severity of disease and ranges from conservative management to more aggressive medical, surgical, and post-surgical radiotherapeutic management (Table 23.2). The main aim of keloid treatment is to prevent recurrences, improving aesthetics and reducing inflammation.

Keloid management requires a comprehensive and coordinated approach since the recurrence rates are high, inadequate knowledge about its pathogenesis, and any single modality is ineffective in complete cure. Post-operative radiation has now been a standard approach, which includes either external beam radiation with electrons or interstitial brachytherapy.

Multiplication times of fibroblasts is 44 h, and that of keloid tissue is 30 h, and rapidly proliferating cells are more sensitive to radiation; hence radiation should be employed in the management as soon as possible and should start within 24 h of surgery for the best results. [20, 21]

Since recurrences post adjuvant radiation are approximately 20% as compared to surgery alone, wherein the recurrence rates are as high as 50–99%, Mankowski et al. showed that recurrences are lower with using adjuvant radiation [22–25]. Radiation does come with its property of inducing secondary malignancies, esp. in paediatric age group and patients may develop sarcomas, basal cell carcinoma, and thyroid and breast malignancies, though the propensity and incidence rates are very low, and it is an acceptable modality of management across the globe [26–32].

Table 23.2 Available treatment options

Conservative:	Invasive:
1. Injections	1. Surgery
a. Corticosteroids	a. +/– Radiation
b. Fluorouracil	b. +/– injection
c. Bleomycin	2. Radiation therapy
d. Interferon alfa–2b	a. External beam radiation
2. Dressings	b. Brachytherapy
a. Occlusive	1. Low dose rate or high dose rate
b. Silicone sheet	2. Interstitial or surface mould
3. Topical	3. Use of radioisotopes
a. Silicone gel	c. Heavy ion therapy
b. Imiquimod	3. Others
	a. Cryotherapy: Laser/Co2/Argon/Nd:YAG/Er:YAG

Small-to-moderate sized keloids of approximately <20 cm^2 are managed with conservative therapies which includes intralesional corticosteroids injection or intralesional chemotherapeutic agents [19]. Intralesional corticosteroid injections like triamcinolone acetonide 5–10 mg combined with a local anaesthetic [28] are used in combination with tape/plaster for small keloids and are targeted at the keloid border rather than the centre of the keloid initially, and later when the central hard portion softens, then the injection is given in the centre of keloid and is repeated every three to four weeks till the time the keloid scar has flattened. To enhance the effect of intralesional corticosteroids, topical fluorouracil or botulinum toxins can be used [23, 33–35].

Apart from the above smaller keloids can also be managed esp. in children with the use of tape/plasters containing topical corticosteroid like flurandrenolide at the dose of 4 mcg/cm^2. Another agent deprodone propionate plasters can also be used. These tapes should be used for a minimum of three months for complete resolution of smaller lesions [28, 36, 37].

Topical corticosteroid creams along with laser therapy have also shown benefit in the management of smaller keloids [38–40].

Use of intralesional chemotherapy drugs like fluorouracil or bleomycin along with combination of triamcinolone injections have also been found effective in the post-operative management [35, 41–43]. In such cases, the dosages used for fluorouracil is 1.5–5 mg/ml and for bleomycin 1 mg/ml are used in combination with triamcinolone injections at dosages of 2–10 mg/ml. adverse effects include keloid necrosis, ulcerations, pain, crusting, hyperpigmentation, and dermal atrophy.

Apart from the above medical interventions, surgical approach alone entails high risks of recurrences; hence postoperative adjuvant management in the form of radiation therapy, corticosteroid injections or tape/plasters is used. The major issues with surgical excision are cosmetic concerns and recurrences.

In cases of large keloids, the aim of therapy is complete excision of the keloid, reducing the thick areas of keloid and disrupting the tension on the scar with the use of flaps. Since there is very high recurrence rate in cases of large keloids post-surgery, adjuvant radiation with long-term tape fixation of scar is recommended for management [24].

In specific regions like ear lobes, it is removed by wedge excision and primary closure; in auricular region of ear and in cases of digital keloids, core excision is done [19, 28, 44–47].

23.10 Role of Radiation Therapy

Radiation therapy has been used post-operatively either with external beam radiation or by interstitial brachytherapy. The reason behind using adjuvant radiation is to reduce the neovascularisation and suppress the inflammatory mediators around the wound, hence promoting adequate healing [8].

External beam radiation therapy is given either by superficial x-rays or orthovoltage x-rays or electron beam therapy. Electron therapy is a more preferred modality of giving external beam radiation due to its inherent radiobiological properties and depth of penetration [48, 49]. Concerns of long-term toxicity and development of secondary malignancies are always an issue; however, the incidence reported is very low or negligible.

Radiation dose: Radiation doses are carefully designed for areas with a high risk of recurrences, like anterior chest wall, upper back, and shoulders wherein a dose schedule of 18 Gy for three fractions is preferred over three days giving a biologically equivalent dose of approximately 30Gy. In areas with low risk of recurrences, such as ear lobes, the dosages can be modified to either 8 Gy in single fraction or 12–15 Gy in two fractions over two days.

External beam radiation can also be used as a monotherapy; however, the dose given is higher and is generally limited in older patients with large diffuse keloids to alleviate the symptoms of itching and pain.

The recurrence rates even after surgery and post-operative radiation ranges from 9% to 22% based on various literatures and published studies [50–52].

23.11 Radiotherapeutic Techniques:

Since post-operatively fibroblasts and collagen fibres are highly radiosensitive, and radiation induces permanent damage to the fibroblast proliferation and collagen synthesis which in turns blocks the cell cycle and induces apoptosis which then prevents keloid recurrences [24, 28]. Radiation increases the levels of reactive oxygen species, superoxide, hydrogen peroxide, and hydroxyl radicals which at the micromolecular level damages the DNA, inhibits the fibroblast proliferation, and in turn inhibits keloid recurrence.

Post-operatively radiation is either given by external beam or by brachytherapy. External beam radiation is given either by X-rays or electrons [22, 53, 54].

Use of X-rays started in 1961 by De Bearman and Gourgerot [55] and later by Cosman et al. who performed this therapy immediately after surgery with a recurrence rate of 21% and disease control rate up to 88%. In a series by Son et al., delivering 8 Gy in a single fraction had a recurrence rate of only 6 %. There is a very limited data available on use of X rays in the management of keloids; however, it had its place in the management due to its shorter treatment time and requirements of lower dosages. It had its own adverse effects in terms of damage to the surrounding normal tissues and greater penetration, a lack of strict radiotherapy protocols, and common consensus. Despite the above, x-ray therapy can be used safely and effectively.

With the advent of technology and improvement in radiation devices, X-rays have now been largely replaced by electron beam therapy due to its property of depth dose of up to 5 cm only, decreased toxicity to surrounding normal structures and deeper tissues; however, the recurrence pattern is almost similar to the X-rays. The energy used in electron therapy is 4–6 MeV. In a study by Ogawa et al. [56] the local recurrence rate was 5–20 % for various sites, including earlobes, chest, and other areas. In another study by Wang et al. [57] with total electron dose of 12 Gy in various sites, the local recurrence rate was only 8%. Usually, the dose schedule used in electron therapy is 18 Gy in three fractions with less commonly used schedule of 18 Gy in a single fraction to 15 GY in 2 fractions [58].

Brachytherapy has been in vogue since 1960s, and either interstitial or surface placement near the target site provides more focused treatment along with preventing toxicity to surrounding normal tissues [59]. By placing the brachytherapy catheters in the surgical scar bed with depth dose distribution limited to 5 mm – 1 cm region all around, it provides the most conformal type of radiation delivery, thus avoiding dosages to the underlying normal structures. High dose rate (HDR) brachytherapy is most commonly used. Previously low dose rate (LDR) brachytherapy over 24–72 h had been used with equal efficacy and outcomes; however, it was inconvenient to the patient in terms of long treatment times and poor patient compliance as compared to the HDR BT which is preformed within 24 h of surgery with shorter treatment times. As per the available literature, surgery combined with HDR BT has resulted in better patient outcomes with reduced recurrence rates [60]. In patients who failed surgery and adjuvant external beam radiation, redoing surgery followed by HDRBT had a local control rate of over 88% [61]. In a study by Garg et al which compared failed postoperative external beam radiation in keloids, HDR -BT had a local control rate of 88% [61]. In another study with HDR-BT doses of 6 Gy in three fractions resulted in a local control rate of up to 94% [62]. HDR-BT has been used extensively in uneven keloids with better symptom relief and less costly [63].

Another modality of treatment is surface mould brachytherapy using P32, Sr 90, or Y90 with recurrence rates up to 20% and with the benefit of being non-invasive, having lower side effects and can be modelled as per the shape of the lesion [64, 65].

With the advancement of technology, the use of heavy ion therapy has resulted in a cure rate approaching approximately 95% with minimal to no complications; however, the reported studies are very limited. In a study by Chen et al., 16 patients were enrolled in the study and were given 16 Gy at 2 GY per fraction regime, and follow-up to three years resulted in a cure rate of 95% [66]. The unique features of heavy ion therapy may in future be a foremost treatment modality for keloids and many other benign conditions.

23.11.1 Safety and Adverse Risk Profile

There may be early and late adverse effects of radiation either in the form of external beam therapy or brachytherapy and includes early complications of erythema, desquamation, and hyperpigmentation. Late complications which may appear after many weeks includes permanent hyperpigmentation, capillary dilatation, subcutaneous fibrosis, and chronic ulcerations which may be related to the dose delivered [26, 67].

Application of local aloe vera gels or glycerol post-treatment has been found to be effective in promoting and improving skin rejuvenation process.

Another complication of post-operative adjuvant radiation is the risk of developing secondary malignancies. In a study by Ogawa et al., five cases of secondary tumour were found in patients treated for keloid; however, the relationship between development of secondary malignancy and keloid was not well understood [28]. There have been many studies which have proved that the risk of secondary malignancy and keloid has very minimal to no association [26, 65, 68–70].

A close clinical follow-up is warranted for these patients. If any signs of recurrence (e.g., scar induration) are noted, the simple tape should immediately be replaced with steroid tape/plaster and, if necessary, intralesional injections of triamcinolone or chemotherapeutic agents.

Preventing a scar formation is a very important aspect of keloid management and it includes promoting rapid wound healing since a healing time of more than three weeks is an important factor for keloid development, management of burn wounds , preventing improper surgical incisions like linear incisions should not run in the direction of skin tension, using horizontal incisions for abdominal surgeries rather the vertical incisions, using z platies where linear incisions are unavoidable, use of local flaps to reduce potential tension, use of non-absorbable sutures in subcutaneous plane and most importantly patient education regarding importance of avoiding stretching and to prevent any kind of inflammation infection, avoiding hot baths post-surgery and to avoid body piercing for patients who are prone to keloid development.

23.12 Conclusion

In conclusion, postoperative radiotherapy is an effective method in prevention of keloid recurrence than other treatment modalities like surgery alone or other non-invasive methods. Also, in improvement of aesthetics, post-operative radiotherapy has proven to be an effective management in minimising the gross disfigurements. Furthermore, adjuvant EBRT and brachytherapy have shown equal and effective control rates. However, despite the similar recurrence rates of external and brachytherapy, brachytherapy is gradually increasing in clinical use due to the convenience and lower cost of treatment, leading to high patient compliance. Heavy ion radiotherapy is a new application in keloid. There are very few literature reports on its efficacy and safety, but based on the only literature available, it has a low recurrence rate and complication rate. As per the available literature, adjuvant therapy should be started soon after surgical excision in order to maximise the control rate and recurrences.

References

1. Kelly AP. Keloids. Dermatol Clin. 1988;6(3):413–24.
2. Louw L. Keloids in rural Black South Africans. Part 1: general overview and essential fatty acid hypotheses for keloid formation and prevention. Prostaglandins Leukot Essent Fatty Acids. 2000;63(5):237–45.

3. Kiprono SK, Chaula BM, Masenga JE, Muchunu JW, Mavura DR, Moehrle M. Epidemiology of keloids in normally pigmented Africans and African people with albinism: population-based cross-sectional survey. Br J Dermatol. 2015;173(3):852–4.
4. Ogawa R. Importance of epidemiologic investigation on keloids. Scar Management. 2009;3:62–4.
5. Shih B, Bayat A. Genetics of keloid scarring. Arch Dermatol Res. 2010;302(5):319–39.
6. Ogawa R, Okai K, Tokumura F, Mori K, Ohmori Y, Huang C, Hyakusoku H, Akaishi S. The relationship between skin stretching/contraction and pathologic scarring: the important role of mechanical forces in keloid generation. Wound Repair Regen. 2012;20(2):149–57.
7. Davis SA, Feldman SR, McMichael AJ. Management of keloids in the United States, 1990–2009: an analysis of the National Ambulatory Medical Care Survey. Dermatol Surg. 2013;39:988.
8. Ogawa R, Akaishi S. Endothelial dysfunction may play a key role in keloid and hypertrophic scar pathogenesis—Keloids and hypertrophic scars may be vascular disorders. Med Hypotheses. 2016;96:51.
9. Demir T, Takada H, Furuya K, et al. Role of skin stretch on local vascular permeability in murine and cell culture models. Plast Reconstr Surg Glob Open. 2022;10:e4084.
10. Huang C, Liu L, You Z, et al. Endothelial dysfunction and mechanobiology in pathological cutaneous scarring: lessons learned from soft tissue fibrosis. Br J Dermatol. 2017;177:1248.
11. Huang C, Ogawa R. The vascular involvement in soft tissue fibrosis-lessons learned from pathological scarring. Int J Mol Sci. 2020;21
12. Jagadeesan J, Bayat A. Transforming growth factor beta (TGFbeta) and keloid disease. Int J Surg. 2007;5:278.
13. Berman B, Maderal A, Raphael B. Keloids and hypertrophic scars: pathophysiology, classification, and treatment. Dermatol Surg. 2017;43(Suppl 1):S3.
14. Huang C, Ogawa R. Fibroproliferative disorders and their mechanobiology. Connect Tissue Res. 2012;53:187.
15. Ogawa R. Mechanobiology of scarring. Wound Repair Regen. 2011;19(Suppl 1):s2.
16. Ogawa R. Keloid and hypertrophic scars are the result of chronic inflammation in the reticular dermis. Int J Mol Sci. 2017;18.
17. Japan Scar Workshop Scar Scale 2015 (Classification and Evaluation of Keloids and Hypertrophic Scars). http://www.scar-keloid.com/pdf/JSW_scar_scale_2015_EN.pdf. Accessed on 1 Apr 2022.
18. Ogawa R, Akita S, Akaishi S, et al. Diagnosis and treatment of keloids and hypertrophic scars-japan scar workshop consensus document 2018. Burns Trauma. 2019;7:39.
19. Ogawa R, Akaishi S, Hyakusoku H. Differential and exclusive diagnosis of diseases that resemble keloids and hypertrophic scars. Ann Plast Surg. 2009;62:660.
20. Bautista Hernandez Y, Villavicencio Queijero MA, Quezada Bautista AA, Vazquez TA. Surface brachytherapy in the treatment of keloid scars in Mexico. Rep Pract Oncol Radiother. 2020;25:133–8. https://doi.org/10.1016/j.rpor.2019.11.002.
21. Xu J, Yang E, Yu N-Z, Long X. Radiation therapy in keloids treatment: history, strategy, effectiveness, and complication. Chin Med J. 2017;130:1715–21. https://doi.org/10.4103/0366-6999.209896.
22. Jones ME, Ganzer CA, Bennett D, Finizio A. Surgical excision of keloids followed by in-office superficial radiation therapy: prospective study examining clinical outcomes. Plast Reconstr Surg Glob Open. 2019;7:e2212. https://doi.org/10.1097/GOX.0000000000002212.
23. Jfri A, Rajeh N, Karkashan EA. Case of multiple spontaneous keloid scars. Case Rep Dermatol. 2015;7:156–60. https://doi.org/10.1159/000437249.
24. Mustoe TA, Cooter RD, Gold MH, Richard Hobbs FD, Ramelet AA, Shakespeare PG, et al. International clinical recommendations on scar management. Plast Reconstr Surg. 2002;110:560–71. https://doi.org/10.1097/00006534-200208000-00031.
25. Mankowski P, Kanevsky J, Tomlinson J, Dyachenko A, Luc M. Optimizing radiotherapy for keloids: a meta-analysis systematic review comparing recurrence rates between dif-

ferent radiation modalities. Ann Plast Surg. 2017;78:403–11. https://doi.org/10.1097/SAP.0000000000000989.
26. Mazonakis M, Damilakis J. Cancer risk after radiotherapy for benign diseases. Phys Med. 2017;42:285–91. https://doi.org/10.1016/j.ejmp.2017.01.014.
27. Rödel F, Fournier C, Wiedemann J, Merz F, Gaipl US, Frey B, et al. Basics of radiation biology when treating hyperproliferative benign diseases. Front Immunol. 2017;8:519. https://doi.org/10.3389/fimmu.2017.00519.
28. Ogawa R, Yoshitatsu S, Yoshida K, Miyashita T. Is radiation therapy for keloids acceptable? The risk of radiation-induced carcinogenesis. Plast Reconstr Surg. 2009;124:1196–201. https://doi.org/10.1097/PRS.0b013e3181b5a3ae.
29. Recalcati S, Caccialanza M, Piccinno R. Postoperative radiotherapy of auricular keloids: a 26-year experience. J Dermatol Treat. 2011;22:38–42. https://doi.org/10.3109/09546630903460278.
30. McKeown SR, Hatfield P, Prestwich RJ, Shaffer RE, Taylor RE. Radiotherapy for benign disease; assessing the risk of radiation-induced cancer following exposure to intermediate dose radiation. Br J Radiol. 2015;88:20150405. https://doi.org/10.1259/bjr.20150405.
31. Leer JWH, van Houtte P, Davelaar J. Indications and treatment schedules for irradiation of benign diseases: a survey. Radiother Oncol. 1998;48:249–57. https://doi.org/10.1016/S0167-8140(98)00051-6.
32. Gold MH, Berman B, Clementoni MT, Gauglitz GG, Nahai F, Murcia C. Updated international clinical recommendations on scar management: part 1– evaluating the evidence. Dermatol Surg. 2014;40:817–24. https://doi.org/10.1111/dsu.0000000000000049.
33. Trisliana Perdanasari A, Torresetti M, Grassetti L, et al. Intralesional injection treatment of hypertrophic scars and keloids: a systematic review regarding outcomes. Burns Trauma. 2015;3:14.
34. Ren Y, Zhou X, Wei Z, et al. Efficacy and safety of triamcinolone acetonide alone and in combination with 5-fluorouracil for treating hypertrophic scars and keloids: a systematic review and meta-analysis. Int Wound J. 2017;14:480.
35. Morelli Coppola M, Salzillo R, Segreto F, Persichetti P. Triamcinolone acetonide intralesional injection for the treatment of keloid scars: patient selection and perspectives. Clin Cosmet Investig Dermatol. 2018;11:387.
36. Ogawa R. The most current algorithms for the treatment and prevention of hypertrophic scars and keloids: a 2020 update of the algorithms published 10 years ago. Plast Reconstr Surg. 2022;149:79e.
37. Ogawa R, Akashi S. Effectiveness of corticosteroid tape/plaster for keloids and hypertrophic scars—comparative study of fludroxycortide and deprodone tape/plasters. Scar Manag. 2016;10:55.
38. Cavalié M, Sillard L, Montaudié H, et al. Treatment of keloids with laser-assisted topical steroid delivery: a retrospective study of 23 cases. Dermatol Ther. 2015;28:74.
39. Marsden CW. Fluocinolone acetonide 0.2 per cent cream—a co-operative clinical trial. Br J Dermatol. 1968; 80:614.
40. Kraeva E, Ho D, Jagdeo J. Successful treatment of keloid with fractionated carbon dioxide (CO_2) laser and laser-assisted drug delivery of triamcinolone acetonide ointment in an african-american man. J Drugs Dermatol. 2017;16:925.
41. Sun P, Lu X, Zhang H, Hu Z. The efficacy of drug injection in the treatment of pathological scar: a network meta-analysis. Aesthetic Plast Surg. 2021;45:791.
42. Bijlard E, Steltenpool S, Niessen FB. Intralesional 5-fluorouracil in keloid treatment: a systematic review. Acta Derm Venereol. 2015;95:778.
43. Jiang ZY, Liao XC, Liu MZ, et al. Efficacy and safety of intralesional triamcinolone versus combination of triamcinolone with 5-fluorouracil in the treatment of keloids and hypertrophic scars: a systematic review and meta-analysis. Aesthetic Plast Surg. 2020;44:1859.
44. Ogawa R, Huang C, Akaishi S, et al. Analysis of surgical treatments for earlobe keloids: analysis of 174 lesions in 145 patients. Plast Reconstr Surg. 2013;132:818e.

45. Al Aradi IK, Alawadhi SA, Alkhawaja FA, Alaradi I. Earlobe keloids: a pilot study of the efficacy of keloidectomy with core fillet flap and adjuvant intralesional corticosteroids. Dermatol Surg. 2013;39:1514.
46. Ogawa R, Akaishi S, Dohi T, et al. Analysis of the surgical treatments of 63 keloids on the cartilaginous part of the auricle: effectiveness of the core excision method. Plast Reconstr Surg. 2015;135:868.
47. Kaku C, Matsunaga N, Kuribayashi S, Ogawa R. Toe keloids treated with core excision, postoperative radiotherapy, and steroid plaster. Plast Reconstr Surg Glob Open. 2020;8:e3085.
48. Enhamre A, Hammar H. Treatment of keloids with excision and postoperative X-ray irradiation. Dermatologica. 1983;167:90.
49. Akita S, Akino K, Yakabe A, et al. Combined surgical excision and radiation therapy for keloid treatment. J Craniofac Surg. 2007;18:1164.
50. Ogawa R, Tosa M, Dohi T, et al. Surgical excision and postoperative radiotherapy for keloids. Scars Burn Heal. 2019;5:2059513119891113.
51. Mankowski P, Kanevsky J, Tomlinson J, et al. Optimizing radiotherapy for keloids: a meta-analysis systematic review comparing recurrence rates between different radiation modalities. Ann Plast Surg. 2017;78:403.
52. Berman B, Nestor MS, Gold MH, et al. A retrospective registry study evaluating the long-term efficacy and safety of superficial radiation therapy following excision of keloid scars. J Clin Aesthet Dermatol. 2020;13:12.
53. Ogawa R. The most current algorithms for the treatment and prevention of hypertrophic scars and keloids. Plast Reconstr Surg. 2010;125:557–68. https://doi.org/10.1097/PRS.0b013e3181c82dd5.
54. Miles OJ, Zhou J, Paleri S, Fua T, Ramakrishnan A. Chest keloids: effect of surgical excision and adjuvant radiotherapy on recurrence, a systematic review and meta-analysis. ANZ J Surg. 2021;91:1104–9. https://doi.org/10.1111/ans.16561.
55. Bearman RD. Cheloides des maqueuses. Ann Dermatol Syphilol. 1906;7:151.
56. Ogawa R, Miyashita T, Hyakusoku H, Akaishi S, Kuribayashi S, Tateno A. Postoperative radiation protocol for keloids and hypertrophic scars: statistical analysis of 370 sites followed for over 18 months. Ann Plast Surg. 2007;59:688–91. https://doi.org/10.1097/SAP.0b013e3180423b32.
57. Wang Y, Ma J, Zhang Z, Shen H. Combined surgical excision and electron external beam radiation improves the treatment of keloids: a descriptive study. Dermatol Ther. 2020;33:e13494. https://doi.org/10.1111/dth.13494.
58. Papanikolaou N. Handbook of radiotherapy physics: theory and practice. Med Phys. 2008;35:4281. https://doi.org/10.1118/1.2969650.
59. Alam M, Nanda S, Mittal BB, Kim NA, Yoo S. The use of brachytherapy in the treatment of nonmelanoma skin cancer: a review. J Am Acad Dermatol. 2011;65:377–88. https://doi.org/10.1016/j.jaad.2010.03.027.
60. Guix B, Henrìquez I, Andrés A, Finestres F, Tello JI, Martìnez A. Treatment of keloids by high-dose-rate brachytherapy: a seven-year study. Int J Radiat Oncol. 2001;50:167–72. https://doi.org/10.1016/S0360-3016(00)01563-7.
61. Garg MK, Weiss P, Sharma AK, Gorla GR, Jaggernauth W, Yaparpalvi R, et al. Adjuvant high dose rate brachytherapy (Ir-192) in the management of keloids which have recurred after surgical excision and external radiation. Radiother Oncol. 2004;73:233–6. https://doi.org/10.1016/j.radonc.2004.04.010.
62. Jiang P, Baumann R, Dunst J, Geenen M, Siebert F-A, Niehoff P, et al. Perioperative interstitial high-dose-rate brachytherapy for the treatment of recurrent keloids: feasibility and early results. Int J Radiat Oncol. 2016;94:532–6. https://doi.org/10.1016/j.ijrobp.2015.11.008.
63. De Cicco L, Vischioni B, Vavassori A, Gherardi F, Jereczek-Fossa BA, Lazzari R, et al. Postoperative management of keloids: low-dose-rate and high-dose-rate brachytherapy. Brachytherapy. 2014;13:508–13. https://doi.org/10.1016/j.brachy.2014.01.005.

64. Liao Y, Dorafshar AH, Bernard D, Kim T, Camden NB, Wang D. High-dose rate interstitial brachytherapy vs external beam radiation for the treatment of complex keloids. Med Dosim. 2022;47:158–60. https://doi.org/10.1016/j.meddos.2022.01.003.
65. Wagner W, Alfrink M, Micke O, Schäfer U, Schüller P, Willich N. Results of Prophylactic irradiation in patients with resected keloids: a retrospective analysis. Acta Oncol. 2000;39:217–20. https://doi.org/10.1080/028418600430806.
66. Chen Y, Feng D, Wang X, Xue J, Chen X. Postoperative carbon ion radiotherapy for keloids: a preliminary report of 16 cases and review of the literature. Wounds. 2014;26:264–72.
67. Bijlard E, Verduijn GM, Harmeling JX, Dehnad H, Niessen FB, Meijer OWM, et al. Optimal high-dose-rate brachytherapy fractionation scheme after keloid excision: a retrospective multicenter comparison of recurrence rates and complications. Int J Radiat Oncol. 2018;100:679–86. https://doi.org/10.1016/j.ijrobp.2017.10.044.
68. Sakamoto T, Oya N, Shibuya K, Nagata Y, Hiraoka M. Dose-response relationship and dose optimization in radiotherapy of postoperative keloids. Radiother Oncol J Eur Soc Ther Radiol Oncol. 2009;91:271–6.
69. Xu J, Yang E, Yu NZ, Long X. Radiation therapy in keloids treatment: history, strategy, effectiveness, and complication. Chin Med J. 2017;130:1715–21.
70. Van Leeuwen MC, Stokmans SC, Bulstra AE, Meijer OW, Heymans MW, Ket JC, Ritt MJ, van Leeuwen PA, Niessen FB. Surgical excision with adjuvant irradiation for treatment of keloid scars: a systematic review. Plastic and reconstructive surgery. Glob. Open. 2015;3:e440.

Langerhans Cell Histiocytosis

24

Aditi Tanwar, Pankaj Gupta, and Mimansha Patel

24.1 Background

Langerhans cell histiocytosis (LCH) is a rare, clonal, inflammatory neoplastic disease characterized by the abnormal accumulation and proliferation of immature myeloid dendritic cells that exhibit immunophenotypic markers similar to epidermal Langerhans cells [1]. These pathological cells are CD1a+, S100+, and Langerin (CD207) + and possess distinctive Birbeck granules visible under electron microscopy [5]. LCH presents with a wide clinical spectrum, ranging from isolated, self-limiting unifocal lesions to devastating multisystem organ involvement with life-threatening consequences [2]. The enigmatic nature of LCH lies in its ability to mimic both reactive inflammatory disorders and aggressive malignancies, making diagnosis and management particularly challenging.

LCH primarily affects children, with peak incidence occurring between 1 and 4 years of age [2]. However, adult cases, often with distinct pulmonary manifestations, are increasingly recognized [6]. Advances in molecular genetics have revolutionized the understanding of its pathophysiology, especially with the identification of BRAFV600E and other MAPK pathway mutations [3, 10], firmly establishing LCH as a clonal myeloid neoplasm. The introduction of targeted therapies has marked a paradigm shift in treatment strategies, especially for refractory and high-risk cases [4, 8].

A. Tanwar (✉)
Department of Radiation Oncology, Dharamshila Narayana Superspeciality Hospital, New Delhi, India

P. Gupta
Department of Pathology, Amaltas Institute of Medical Sciences, Dewas, Madhya Pradesh, India

M. Patel
Department of Oral Pathology, Triveni Dental College, Bodri, Bilaspur, Chhattisgarh, India

K. Sood Sharma (ed.), *Radiation Therapy for Benign Disorders*,
https://doi.org/10.1007/978-981-95-6635-8_24

24.1.1 Epidemiology

LCH remains a rare disorder with variable incidence across different populations and age groups. In pediatric populations, the incidence is estimated at 4–8.9 per million children under the age of 15 annually, with a peak between ages 1 and 4 years [1, 2]. Adult-onset LCH is less common, with an incidence of approximately 0.07 per million adults annually [2]. However, increased recognition and refined diagnostic criteria have led to improved case identification in adults, particularly among smokers with pulmonary involvement [6].

A slight male predominance is observed across most studies (M:F ratio of 1.2–2:1), although some subtypes like cutaneous or endocrine LCH may exhibit a more balanced gender distribution [2]. Population-based studies from the UK and France have highlighted differences in incidence based on socioeconomic status and ethnicity. Hispanic ethnicity and lower socioeconomic conditions have been associated with higher incidence and poorer outcomes, potentially reflecting delayed access to healthcare, environmental exposures, or genetic predisposition [2, 7].

Interestingly, familial cases and associations with other malignancies or immune disorders have been documented, raising questions about underlying genetic susceptibilities [3]. Ongoing genomic surveillance may offer insights into the risk stratification of vulnerable populations [10].

24.1.2 Historical Background

The nomenclature and classification of langerhans cell histiocytosis have undergone several transformations over the past century, reflecting the evolving understanding of the disease [6].

The earliest reports of the condition date back to 1868, when Paul Langerhans first described the eponymous epidermal dendritic cells [5]. However, it wasn't until the early twentieth century that distinct clinical syndromes involving abnormal histiocytes were formally recognized:

Letterer–Siwe Disease (1924): Described as an acute disseminated form of histiocytosis predominantly affecting infants and young children. It was associated with systemic symptoms, hepatosplenomegaly, lymphadenopathy, cytopenias, and often rapid progression leading to death [2].

Hand–Schüller–Christian Disease (1928): Identified by its classic triad of lytic bone lesions, exophthalmos, and central diabetes insipidus. This form was considered more chronic and often affected children aged 2–6 years [2].

Eosinophilic Granuloma (1940): Represented the benign, localized osseous manifestation of LCH seen in older children and young adults, often presenting as isolated bone lesions with a good prognosis [2].

In 1953, pathologist Louis Lichtenstein proposed the term "Histiocytosis X" to encompass these three overlapping syndromes, as their cellular origin was unclear.

This term remained in usage for several decades until ultrastructural studies and immunophenotyping in the 1970s and 1980s revealed the characteristic Birbeck granules and surface markers CD1a and Langerin, confirming the Langerhans cell lineage of the pathological histiocytes [5].

As immunologic and genetic insights into the disease deepened, the Histiocyte Society in 1987 formally adopted the term "Langerhans Cell Histiocytosis," [6], emphasizing the clonal nature of the abnormal cells and providing a unified framework for diagnosis, staging, and treatment. Subsequently, large multicenter studies such as the LCH I, II, and III trials and the establishment of the Euro Histio Network contributed significantly to the standardization of management protocols [6].

The early twenty-first century witnessed a revolutionary leap in the molecular understanding of LCH with the discovery of *BRAFV600E* mutations in more than half of LCH cases [3, 10], aligning the disease more closely with other neoplastic disorders. Subsequent identification of *MAP 2 K1* and other kinase pathway mutations solidified the reclassification of LCH as a neoplastic condition with inflammatory features.

Today, LCH is classified by the World Health Organization (WHO) under *clonal hematopoietic disorders*, reflecting its molecular and clinical behavior. This evolution from an ill-defined inflammatory disorder to a genetically characterized myeloid neoplasm underscores the importance of ongoing research and multidisciplinary collaboration in understanding and managing LCH [3, 10].

24.1.3 Rationale for Role of Radiation in LCH

There is an interplay of various mechanisms at the molecular level that suggest the use of radiation in benign diseases. Role of radiation in managing benign diseases is multifaceted, involving:

1. Enhanced capillary permeability and tissue perfusion (perfusion theory).
2. Elimination of inflammatory cells and modulation of mediators (fermentative theory).

Under normal conditions, inflammatory responses are regulated by a tightly sequential process that depends on the production of inflammatory mediators, cell adhesion molecules expression, and leukocyte-endothelial cell interaction: rolling, adhesion, and migration to the interstitial space [15].

During the rolling phenomenon, leukocytes are activated through local inflammatory mediators, slowing the blood flow and stimulating immunocompetent cells to migrate to the surrounding tissue, regulated by membrane-bound receptors (selectins), producing cytokines responsible for vasodilatation and vascular permeability (Interleukine-1 (IL-1), Tumor Necrosis Factor-α (TNF-α), Nitric Oxide (NO)). These factors are responsible for edema, erythema, and pain.

When LD-RT is applied (<1 Gy), it inhibits the expression of Inducible Nitric Oxide Synthase (iNOS) and that reduces endothelial cell-leukocyte interactions as well as vasodilatation. Other anti-inflammatory cytokines are produced (IL-10, Transforming Growth Factor-β1 (TGF-β1), increasing apoptosis and diminishing NO production. TGF-β1 is known to be an endogenous important factor in inflammatory regulation.

There is also a decreased expression of adhesion molecules (P-, L-, E- Selectins, Intercellular Adhesion Molecule (ICAM), Vascular Cell Adhesion Molecule (VCAM)), and lower secretion of CCL20 (C-C motif chemokine ligand 20) of neutrophiles, which correlates to a lower adhesion to endothelial cells.

1. Modulation of the autonomic nervous system (neuroregulatory theory).
2. Alterations in tissue composition (electrochemical theory).
3. Inhibition of excessive cell growth (antiproliferative effect at 8-10Gy)-irradiation produces a delay in cell mitotic cycle that prevents cellular growth in the irradiated tissue during a dose-dependent period of time.
4. Immunomodulatory theory—A regulation of lymphocytes antigenic stimulus takes place over 10Gy, suppressing the local autoimmune process [16].

The therapeutic benefits of radiation likely stem from a synergy of these mechanisms, rather than a single dominant effect.

24.2 Etiopathogenesis

The pathogenesis of LCH involves a complex interplay between clonal proliferation of mutated myeloid dendritic cells and dysregulated inflammatory signaling. Initially thought to be a reactive inflammatory disease, it is now established as a clonal neoplasm driven predominantly by somatic mutations in the mitogen-activated protein kinase (MAPK) pathway [3, 6, 7].

(a) Molecular Genetics

BRAFV600E Mutation: Found in 50–60% of LCH cases, this activating mutation leads to constitutive phosphorylation of MEK and ERK, promoting cellular proliferation, survival, and resistance to apoptosis [3, 10].

MAP 2 K1 Mutations: Present in 20–25% of BRAF-negative cases, these mutations also result in ERK activation [9]. (Refer to Fig. 24.1).

Other MAPK Pathway Mutations: NRAS, ARAF, KRAS, and ERBB3 mutations have also been identified in smaller subsets.

Gene Fusions and In-Frame Deletions: Emerging data suggests additional mechanisms like BRAF fusions and deletions may contribute to the pathogenesis [10].

These mutations are often detected in hematopoietic progenitor cells, supporting the concept that LCH arises from early myeloid precursors rather than mature langerhans cells [3, 12]. This explains the systemic dissemination of the disease in multisystem cases.

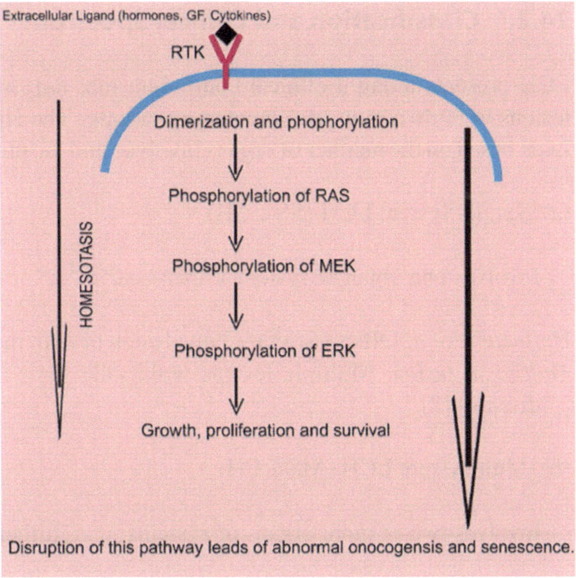

Fig. 24.1 Cascade of events in RTK (Receptor Tyrosine kinase), RAS MEK ERK phosphorylation in normal homeostasis. (Original image by the co-author Dr. Pankaj Gupta)

(b) Immune Dysregulation

LCH lesions are not composed exclusively of neoplastic cells. They also include eosinophils, T lymphocytes, macrophages, and multinucleated giant cells. This suggests a significant inflammatory component. Regulatory T cells (Tregs) are expanded in LCH lesions, and the pathological dendritic cells express immune checkpoint ligands like PD-L1, contributing to local immune evasion and chronic inflammation [7, 13].

(c) Cytokine and Chemokine Profile

LCH cells secrete and respond to a range of pro-inflammatory cytokines including IL-1β, IL-6, TNF-α, and osteopontin. These mediators facilitate the recruitment of immune cells and contribute to granuloma formation, tissue damage, and systemic symptoms [7].

(d) Developmental Timing

The stage at which a MAPK mutation arises in the hematopoietic lineage appears to influence disease severity. Early mutations in hematopoietic stem cells are associated with high-risk multisystem disease and neurodegeneration, whereas later mutations in tissue-restricted progenitors tend to produce localized disease [12].

24.2.1 Classification and Clinical Spectrum

LCH presents along a clinical continuum that ranges from self-limiting unifocal lesions to multisystem life-threatening disease. The Histiocyte Society categorizes LCH based on the number of organs involved and the presence of "risk organs." [2, 6]

(a) Single-System LCH (SS-LCH)

Involves one organ or system, either as a:

Unifocal lesion: Often a solitary bone lesion or skin rash.
Multifocal lesion: Multiple lesions within the same organ (e.g., multifocal bone disease) [2].

(b) Multisystem LCH (MS-LCH)

Involves two or more organs or systems. It is further divided into:

Low-risk MS-LCH: No involvement of risk organs.
High-risk MS-LCH: Involves risk organs—liver, spleen, or bone marrow—which significantly impacts prognosis [3].

(c) Pulmonary LCH (PLCH)

Primarily affects adult smokers. Considered a distinct entity due to its association with tobacco exposure. Presenting features include cough, dyspnea, and nodulocystic lung lesions [6]. Spontaneous regression can occur with smoking cessation [7].

(d) Neurodegenerative LCH (ND-LCH)

A rare and poorly understood manifestation of CNS involvement. Characterized by behavioral changes, ataxia, or cognitive decline. MRI shows cerebellar and basal ganglia abnormalities. Associated strongly with BRAFV600E mutations in circulating myeloid cells [3, 14].

(e) Other Special Forms

Diabetes insipidus from hypothalamic–pituitary axis involvement [2].
Oral-facial granulomatosis in pediatric and adult LCH.

LCH must be evaluated using a structured staging approach involving clinical, radiological, and histological assessment to identify the extent of disease and classify the risk category appropriately [2, 6].

24.2.2 Clinical Presentation

The clinical manifestations of LCH are highly variable and depend on the site and extent of organ involvement. LCH can be asymptomatic or present with life-threatening organ dysfunction. Presentations also vary with age, with children often exhibiting more aggressive systemic disease and adults more commonly presenting with isolated or pulmonary forms.

(a) Skeletal System

Bone lesions are the most common presentation, occurring in up to 80% of cases [2]. These lesions are typically lytic and may be painful, especially in weight-bearing bones such as the femur or pelvis. Craniofacial bones, especially the skull and mandible, are frequently involved [5]. In the jaw, lesions may mimic aggressive periodontitis or periapical pathology.

(b) Skin and Mucous Membranes

Skin involvement occurs in approximately 40–50% of patients and may present as scaly papules, eczematous patches, or seborrhea-like eruptions [2]. Lesions may ulcerate or crust and are often distributed on the scalp, trunk, or intertriginous areas. Mucosal ulcerations of the oral cavity and genitalia can occur.

(c) Endocrine System

Involvement of the hypothalamic–pituitary axis leads to *central diabetes insipidus* (CDI), seen in approximately 20–25% of patients [2]. Symptoms include polyuria and polydipsia. CDI is often irreversible and may precede other manifestations of systemic disease.

(d) Pulmonary System

Pulmonary LCH is primarily observed in adult smokers and may present with nonspecific symptoms like chronic cough, dyspnea, or chest pain [6]. Imaging often reveals bilateral cysts and nodules, and pneumothorax may be a presenting feature.

(e) Hepatosplenic and Hematologic Involvement

Hepatosplenomegaly, cholestasis, jaundice, and cytopenias indicate risk-organ involvement and portend a poorer prognosis [3]. Liver dysfunction can mimic autoimmune hepatitis or primary sclerosing cholangitis.

(f) Central Nervous System

CNS involvement may occur in the form of mass lesions or as *neurodegenerative LCH (ND-LCH),* presenting with ataxia, tremors, behavioral disturbances, and cognitive decline [14]. MRI findings often include T2 hyperintensity in the basal ganglia and cerebellum.

24.2.3 Histopathology and Immunohistochemistry

Histological examination remains the gold standard for diagnosis. LCH lesions are granulomatous and contain Langerhans-like cells admixed with eosinophils, neutrophils, lymphocytes, and multinucleated giant cells [5].

(a) Microscopic Features

Langerhans cells are medium to large with oval or reniform (kidney-shaped) nuclei, longitudinal grooves ("coffee-bean" appearance), and pale eosinophilic cytoplasm [5] (refer to Figs. 24.2 and 24.3).

Lesions often show necrosis, hemorrhage, and fibrosis depending on chronicity [5].

(b) Immunohistochemical Markers

Immunohistochemistry plays a crucial role in confirming diagnosis:

CD1a: Expressed on the surface of pathological langerhans cells, used routinely in diagnostic panels [5].

Langerin (CD207): A definitive marker responsible for the formation of Birbeck granules, highly specific for Langerhans cells [5].

S100 protein: Though less specific, it is consistently expressed in LCH cells and helpful when used in combination with CD1a and Langerin [5].

(c) Electron Microscopy.

Birbeck granules are rod-shaped, tennis racket-like cytoplasmic organelles considered pathognomonic of Langerhans cells. They are rarely used in modern diagnosis due to IHC reliability [5].

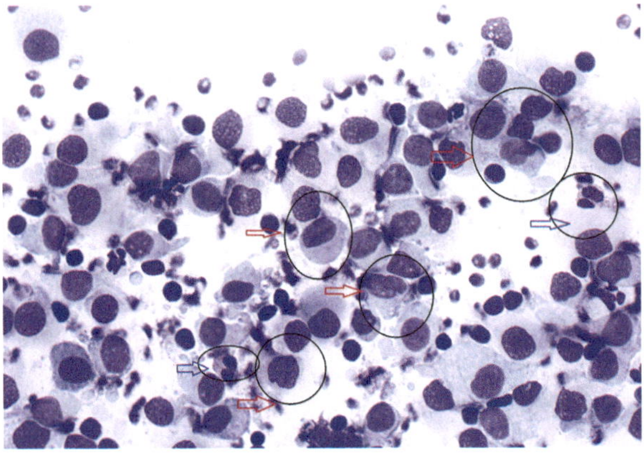

Fig. 24.2 Cytology image showing scattered histiocytes with cleaving and grooving (red arrows) and eosinophils (blue arrows)

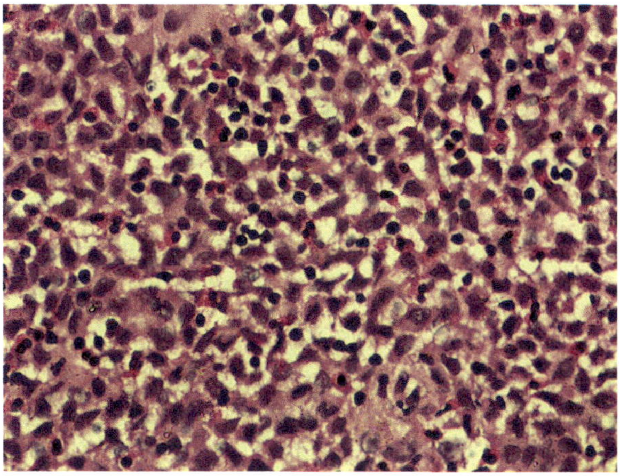

Fig. 24.3 H&E-stained (400x) image showing scattered histiocytes with nuclear grooves and cleaved nuclei, admixed with scattered eosinophils. (Image courtesy Dr.Prerna Arora Nipun Path Lab)

24.2.4 Diagnostic Work-Up

A thorough and standardized diagnostic approach is crucial for accurate classification, risk stratification, and therapy planning [6, 10].

(a) Biopsy

Tissue biopsy is the cornerstone of diagnosis and should be performed on the most accessible and representative lesion. Histopathology and immunohistochemistry (CD1a$^+$, Langerin$^+$, S100$^+$) confirm the diagnosis of LCH [5]. Samples may also be used for genetic mutation analysis.

(b) Molecular Testing

Detection of *BRAFV600E* and *MAP 2 K1* mutations in biopsy tissue or peripheral blood guides prognosis and therapeutic decisions [3, 9].

Circulating cell-free DNA or cfDNA testing is emerging as a tool for detecting minimal residual disease [10, 12].

(c) Imaging

Skeletal survey or whole-body MRI to assess bone lesions.

Chest CT in suspected pulmonary cases.

FDG-PET/CT provides comprehensive disease mapping and response assessment [11].

MRI brain and pituitary if neuroendocrine or CNS symptoms are present [14].

(d) Laboratory Investigations

Complete blood count (CBC), liver function tests, renal profile, coagulation studies.

Endocrine testing: Includes serum electrolytes, urine specific gravity, osmolality, and serum antidiuretic hormone for suspected central diabetes insipidus [2].

Bone marrow biopsy: Indicated in multisystem LCH with cytopenias or risk organ involvement [3].

Together, these evaluations form the foundation for classifying patients into single-system or multisystem LCH, identifying risk organ involvement, and personalizing treatment protocols accordingly [6].

24.2.5 Differential Diagnosis

Due to its diverse clinical presentation and histological appearance, LCH can mimic several malignant and benign disorders. Accurate differentiation is critical for proper management.

Ewing Sarcoma: Often presents as a painful bone mass with systemic symptoms; lacks CD1a and Langerin expression and demonstrates EWSR1 gene rearrangements on molecular testing [5].
Chronic Osteomyelitis: Presents with localized bone pain, fever, and elevated inflammatory markers; typically bacterial in origin with supportive cultures.
Lymphoma/Leukemia: May involve bone marrow or extranodal tissue with systemic B symptoms; immunophenotyping differentiates from LCH [5].
Metastatic Neuroblastoma: Common in young children, often affecting bones; histology and immunohistochemistry (neuroendocrine markers) aid in diagnosis.
Rosai-Dorfman Disease: Characterized by massive lymphadenopathy and histiocytes with emperipolesis; CD1a-negative and S100-positive.
Juvenile Xanthogranuloma: Typically affects skin of infants and young children; histiocytes are CD1a-negative and Langerin-negative.

Histopathology, supported by immunohistochemistry and molecular diagnostics, remains the definitive method for distinguishing LCH from these entities [5, 6].

24.3 Treatment

Management of LCH depends on the disease extent, organ involvement, and presence of risk organ dysfunction. Treatment aims to induce remission, prevent reactivation, and reduce long-term morbidity [3, 6].

(a) Single-System LCH (SS-LCH)
Unifocal Bone Lesions: Observation, surgical curettage, or intralesional corticosteroids, use of radiotherapy. Prognosis is excellent.
Skin-Limited LCH: Topical steroids or nitrogen mustard; radiating the superficial lesions with electron therapy, systemic therapy if resistant.
(b) Multisystem LCH (MS-LCH)

Without Risk Organ Involvement:
First-line: Vinblastine and prednisone for 6–12 months.
Maintenance: 6-mercaptopurine added for relapse prevention.

With Risk Organ Involvement:
Induction therapy: Vinblastine, prednisone, and methotrexate [4, 8].
Salvage regimens: Cladribine, cytarabine, or doxorubicin-based protocols [3].
Patients with poor response at 6 weeks require therapy intensification.

(c) Pulmonary LCH (PLCH)

Smoking cessation is paramount and often leads to disease stabilization or resolution [6].

Progressive disease may be treated with cladribine or cytarabine; lung transplantation is reserved for advanced fibrotic cases.

(d) Neurodegenerative LCH (ND-LCH)

Challenging to treat; limited response to standard chemotherapy.

Investigational therapies include BRAF/MEK inhibitors, immunomodulators, and intrathecal methotrexate in clinical trials [14].

(e) Targeted Therapies

BRAF Inhibitors (e.g., vemurafenib, dabrafenib) demonstrate high response rates in BRAFV600E-positive LCH [4, 8].

MEK Inhibitors (e.g., trametinib, cobimetinib) are effective in MAP 2 K1-mutant or refractory cases [9].

Ongoing trials are evaluating the efficacy of combining BRAF and MEK inhibitors for sustained disease control.

Early identification of risk organ involvement and tailoring therapy based on molecular findings have significantly improved treatment outcomes in LCH. Biopsy Tissue: biopsy is the cornerstone of diagnosis and should be performed on the most accessible and representative lesion. Histopathology and immunohistochemistry ($CD1a^+$, $Langerin^+$, $S100^+$) confirm the diagnosis of LCH [5]. Samples may also be used for genetic mutation analysis.

24.4 Role of Radiation Therapy in LCH

The clinical presentation of LCH varies widely from single system bone lesion to multisystem disease. Hence a variety of treatment options are available ranging from observation to systemic therapy, stem cell trasplant, etc. However, with the advent of molecular detailing of the disease, the treatment approach for langerhans cell histiocytosis (LCH) has evolved significantly, transitioning from: empiricism (based on histologic findings alone) to precision (targeted approaches driven by genetic mutations). This shift enables more effective and personalized treatment strategies for LCH patients. Amid the multiple treatment options available, radiation therapy continues to be a valuable and effective treatment option though its usage has declined owing to a plethora of systemic options available. Moreover, majority of the clinicians are a little skeptical about usage of radiation in children fearing the risk of developmental abnormalities due to damage to endochondral ossification centers and secondary malignancies. There are no randomized trials exploring the role of radiation in LCH; the available information is based on the case series and case reports published worldwide.

24.4.1 Indications of Radiation in LCH

1. Painful bone lesions
2. Risk of pathological fracture
3. Spinal cord compression
4. Extraosseous soft tissue involvement
5. Progressive disease with compressive or painful symptoms
6. Localized lesions not amenable to surgery either due to cosmetic reasons or risk of loss organ function
7. Skin lesions that cannot be surgically excised or relapse after treatment

24.4.2 Techniques of Radiation

The techniques of radiation have evolved over decades from two-dimensional conventional portals to three-dimensional conformal therapy to IMRT (intensity modulated radiotherapy) to IGRT (image guided radiotherapy). During the earlier decades, radiation was used to treat the bone lesions of LCH using two-dimensional conventional portals using cobalt 60 teletherapy. But with the advent of improvement in techniques of radiation, there is an increase in the use of conformal therapy [17]. In view of the proximity to critical structures in intracranial presentation of LCH, the role of stereotaxy has also been explored. Stereotactic radiosurgery (SRS) has increasingly been used to treat CNS pathologies, sometimes replacing surgery. For localized cranial LCH lesions, while surgery is often preferred, SRS is emerging as a viable option, with several reported cases. However, due to the rarity of LCH, more evidence is needed to establish effectiveness of stereotaxy in adult patients [18, 19].

24.4.3 Intensity-Modulated Radiation Therapy (IMRT)

Intensity-modulated radiation therapy (IMRT) delivers precise radiation doses using dynamic multi-leaf collimators (MLCs) that adjust during beam delivery. This technique achieves superior dose conformity, reducing toxicity through:

Inverse planning algorithms, division of targets into subfields, intensity-modulated fields. IMRT can be delivered via: step-and-shoot method (static beam delivery) and dynamic method (continuous MLC movement).

While IMRT offers advanced precision, it also presents challenges, including longer treatment times, increased integral dose and potential risk of secondary malignancies, and intrafraction motion uncertainties, which can be mitigated with Image-Guided Radiation Therapy (IGRT) integration.

24.4.4 Image-Guided Radiation Therapy (IGRT)

Image-guided radiation therapy (IGRT) utilizes advanced imaging technologies to ensure precise tumor targeting. By accounting for patient and tumor movement, IGRT reduces targeting errors. Techniques like cone-beam CT enable real-time adjustments, ensuring safe and effective treatments.

Benefits of IGRT include enhanced precision, reduced normal tissue toxicity, and improved tumor control [20]. While IGRT has limitations, such as increased imaging dose and longer treatment times, its advantages make it a crucial component of modern radiation therapy, particularly in high-precision treatments like SBRT and SRS.

24.4.5 Stereotactic Body Radiotherapy (SBRT)

SBRT is an excellent option for cases requiring re-irradiation or high-dose treatments in fewer sessions. This technique delivers radiation with millimeter-level accuracy, focusing intensely on the tumor. It allows for steep dose gradients, minimizing radiation exposure to adjacent critical structures.

24.4.6 Electron Therapy

Electron beam therapy is used to treat superficial tumors; the skin lesions that are a common presentation in LCH can be effectively treated with electrons. Treatments with this approach are generally single field, with the gantry angle selected such that the incident electron beam is perpendicular to the treatment target to maximize depth of electron penetration [21]. Electron beam energy is selected such that a therapeutic isodose line (often 80% or 90% of the prescribed dose) will adequately cover the deep aspect of the tumor target.

24.4.7 Dose and Fractionation Schedules

Although no specific randomized trials have been conducted to establish the dose of radiation in LCH, with the data extrapolated from the case series and case reports, a low dose of radiation in the range of 10–30 Gy (1.8–3 Gy per fraction) has been found to be beneficial mainly for bone lesions.

Multisystem LCH involving lymph nodes, brain, thyroid, skin, etc. may require higher doses of radiation.

Also, higher dose per fraction (stereotactic radiosurgery) has also been seen beneficial in localized bone lesions with limited intracranial extension.

24.5 Review of Literature

Although there is an absence of any randomized controlled trial evaluating the efficacy of radiation as a part of the treatment schedule for LCH. But a number of case series and case reports have been published indicating the significant role of radiation in palliating the symptoms of single-system disease as well as progressive multisystem disease.

The first successful use of roentgen therapy for the treatment of LCH was described by Sosman in the year 1930. the defects in the skull bone were shown to decrease with the use of X-rays although finally the patient succumbed to his disease [23].

In the year 2001, Schiebe et al. [24] evaluated the role of low doses of radiation in a 75-year-old woman who presented with oral LCH. Within 2 weeks of completion of radiation, there was a rapid regression of mucosal ulcerations and improvement of symptoms. External beam radiotherapy with total doses between 10 and 20 Gy seems to be effective for local control of this disease.

Another attempt for evaluating the role of radiation in the treatment of symptomatic LCH affecting the temporal bone was evaluated by Zoldre et al. [25] in 2009. They reported complete remission of symptoms of sensorineural hearing loss in these patients after the use of low dose of radiation.

In a study in 2010 by Atalar et al. [26], different treatment approaches for the treatment of LCH were analyzed including the role of radiation (RT). RT was used in combination with surgery and chemotherapy and also as a standalone modality and was found to be a useful option in palliative setting in LCH patients.

In a study by Meyer et al. [27], the role of low dose of radiation was evaluated for cranial base lesion which was histopathologically confirmed to be LCH. A dose as low as 9 Gy with 1.8 Gy daily fraction was found to reduce the symptoms as well as remineralization of the affected bone was seen within 6 months of treatment.

In the year 2013, Jan kriz et al. [28] reported the role of radiation in LCH. They reported the results on 80 patients irradiated over a span of 45 years. A median total dose of 15 Gy (range 3–50.4 Gy) was delivered with median single fraction of 2 Gy (range 1.8–3 Gy). Radiation was found to be a very safe and effective treatment option and shows sufficient local control even at low doses.

Laird et al. [29] in the year 2018 studied the effectiveness of radiation as a treatment modality for single system as well as multisystem LCH. Bone, brain, skin, lymphnode, thyroid, and nasopharynx were the sites that were irradiated. Median dose was 11.4 Gy (range, 7.5–50.4 Gy). After a median follow-up of 45 months, there were no local failures in the bone lesions whereas other sites like skin, lymphnodes, and brain showed local failures indicating that bone lesions are well controlled with low doses of radiation, whereas disease in other tissues might require higher doses of radiation or additional treatment modalities.

Ghuijs et al. [30] in the year 2022 analyzed the use of low dose of radiation therapy in a lytic bone lesion refractory to surgical interventions and progressive with significant soft tissue extension to the surrounding musculature. A dose as low as 20 Gy in 10 fractions was significant enough to produce a complete remission of the disease.

24.5.1 Prognosis

The prognosis of LCH varies widely depending on patient age, disease extent, and treatment response [3, 6]:

(a) Favorable Factors
Single-system disease (especially isolated bone) [2].
Rapid response to first-line therapy [2].
Absence of risk organ involvement [3].
(b) Poor Prognostic Indicators

Multisystem disease with liver, spleen, or bone marrow involvement [3].
Presence of BRAFV600E mutation in circulating cells [10].
Delayed response or resistance to initial therapy [4].
Early-onset neurodegenerative manifestations [14].

(c) Survival and Outcomes
SS-LCH: >90% 5-year survival [2].
MS-LCH (no risk organ): 85–90% survival [2].
MS-LCH (risk organ): 65–75% survival with relapse in 30–50% [3].
Long-term sequelae: Endocrine dysfunction, neurocognitive delay, skeletal deformities [2, 14].

The overarching goal is early diagnosis, risk-adapted therapy, and comprehensive follow-up to minimize morbidity and improve quality of life [4, 6].

24.6 Future Directions

Recent advances in understanding and managing Langerhans Cell Histiocytosis have significantly reshaped its clinical outlook. Molecular and immunologic research continues to unravel the pathogenesis, offering novel targets for precision medicine [10, 13].

(a) Molecular Diagnostics

Cell-free DNA (cfDNA) testing now enables non-invasive mutation detection and monitoring of minimal residual disease (MRD) [10, 12].

Circulating BRAFV600E mutation is being studied as a biomarker for disease burden, risk stratification, and relapse prediction.

(b) Targeted Therapy Developments

Vemurafenib and *dabrafenib*, BRAF inhibitors, have demonstrated high response rates in BRAFV600E-mutant LCH, especially in refractory or high-risk patients [4, 9].

MEK inhibitors (e.g., trametinib, cobimetinib) offer treatment alternatives in MAP 2 K1-mutant or BRAF-negative cases.

Combination therapy with BRAF and MEK inhibitors has shown promise in reducing relapse rates and improving progression-free survival.

(c) Advancements in Radiotherapy techniques

Even in the presence of multiple systemic agents available for treatment of LCH, radiation has continued to be an effective option for painful and progressive lesions. The use of stereotaxy for smaller lesions has been found to be beneficial in intracranial and bone lesions in a few case reports. Its potential can be explored in extracranial sites as well. The use of proton therapy has been found to be beneficial in other pediatric tumors. The precise adjustability of proton therapy minimizes radiation-related long-term side effects and reduces the risk of secondary malignancies, ultimately enhancing quality of life of the survivor [22]. Hence its role can be exploited in randomized controlled trials in pediatric LCH as well.

(d) Immunological Insights

Increased expression of *PD-L1* on LCH cells and *PD-1, LAG-3,* and *TIM-3* on exhausted T-cells within lesions suggests a role for *immune checkpoint modulation* [7, 13].

Clinical trials investigating *anti-PD-1 therapy* are underway.

(e) Imaging and Biomarker Advancements

PET/CT is now widely used for staging and treatment monitoring, superior to traditional bone scans [11].

MRI brain with advanced sequences is preferred in evaluating neurodegenerative LCH [14].

Osteopontin levels in CSF have emerged as a potential biomarker for CNS involvement.

(f) Pediatric vs. Adult LCH Paradigms

Adult-onset LCH, especially pulmonary LCH, is now viewed as a distinct clinicopathologic entity.

Genomic studies reveal that adult LCH has higher mutational burden and more complex kinase alterations than pediatric LCH [14].

24.7 Conclusion

Langerhans cell histiocytosis is a clonal myeloid neoplasm with highly variable clinical behavior and systemic impact [1, 2]. Once considered an enigmatic inflammatory disease, LCH is now recognized as a mutation-driven disorder that arises from aberrant activation of the MAPK/ERK pathway [3].

The clinical spectrum ranges from unifocal bone lesions to multisystem disease with risk organ involvement, necessitating a tailored diagnostic and therapeutic approach [2, 6]. Molecular profiling has become essential for identifying actionable mutations such as BRAFV600E and MAP 2K1 [3, 9] and is now guiding the use of targeted therapies like BRAF and MEK inhibitors [4, 8].

Histopathological confirmation through biopsy and immunohistochemistry remains central to diagnosis, while advanced imaging and laboratory investigations inform staging and prognosis [5, 11]. Treatment strategies are stratified based on risk and range from local therapies to intensive chemotherapy and biologics [2, 3]. Despite excellent outcomes in low-risk patients, those with high-risk multisystem disease or neurodegenerative involvement require close surveillance and access to innovative therapies [14].

With ongoing advances in genomics, immunotherapy, and imaging, the role of radiation is also evolving in progressive and painful disease. There are no definite treatment protocols for LCH; the future of LCH management continues to evolve toward precision oncology [3, 7]. Early diagnosis, multidisciplinary care, and long-term follow-up remain the cornerstones of improved outcomes in this rare but impactful disorder.

References

1. Allen CE, Merad M, McClain KL. Langerhans-cell histiocytosis. N Engl J Med. 2018;379(9):856–68.
2. Rodriguez-Galindo C, Allen CE. Langerhans cell histiocytosis. Blood. 2020;135(16):1319–31.
3. Berres ML, Lim KP, Peters T, et al. BRAF-V600E expression in precursor versus differentiated dendritic cells defines clinically distinct LCH risk groups. J Exp Med. 2014;211(4):669–83.
4. Donadieu J, Larabi IA, Tardieu M, et al. Vemurafenib for refractory multisystem Langerhans cell histiocytosis in children: an international observational study. J Clin Oncol. 2019;37(31):2857–65.
5. Picarsic J, Jaffe R. Nosology and pathology of Langerhans cell histiocytosis. Hematol Oncol Clin North Am. 2015;29(5):799–823.
6. Emile JF, Abla O, Fraitag S, et al. Revised classification of histiocytoses and neoplasms of the macrophage-dendritic cell lineages. Blood. 2016;127(22):2672–81.
7. Hogstad B, Berres ML, Chakraborty R, et al. RAF/MEK/ERK pathway suppresses dendritic cell migration and traps dendritic cells in LCH lesions. J Exp Med. 2018;215(1):319–36.
8. Heritier S, Jehanne M, Leverger G, et al. Vemurafenib use in an infant for high-risk Langerhans cell histiocytosis. JAMA Oncol. 2015;1(6):836–8.
9. Chakraborty R, Hampton OA, Shen X, et al. Mutually exclusive recurrent somatic mutations in MAP 2K1 and BRAF support a central role for ERK activation in LCH pathogenesis. Blood. 2014;124(19):3007–15.

10. Badalian-Very G, Vergilio JA, Degar BA, et al. Recurrent BRAF mutations in LCH. Blood. 2010;116(11):1919–23.
11. Ginhoux F, Merad M. Ontogeny and homeostasis of Langerhans cells. Immunol Cell Biol. 2010;88(4):387–92.
12. Durham BH, Roos-Weil D, Baillou C, et al. Functional evidence for derivation of systemic histiocytic neoplasms from hematopoietic stem/progenitor cells. Blood. 2017;130(2):176–80.
13. Senechal B, Elain G, Jeziorski E, et al. Expansion of regulatory T cells in patients with LCH. PLoS Med. 2007;4(8):e253.
14. McClain KL, Picarsic J, Chakraborty R, et al. CNS LCH: common hematopoietic origin for neurodegeneration and mass lesions. Cancer. 2018;124(12):2607–20.
15. Micke O. Heinrich Seegenschmiedt and the German working group on radiotherapy of benign diseases. Consensus guidelines for radiation therapy of benign diseases—a multi-center approach. Int J Radiation Oncology Biol Phys. 2002;52(2):496–513.
16. Royo LT, Redondo GA, Pianetta MÁ, et al. Low-dose radiation therapy for benign pathologies. Rep Pract Oncol Radiother. 2020;25(2):250–4.
17. James Laird BA, Jennifer Ma BA, Karen Chau BA, et al. Outcome after radiation therapy for Langerhans cell Histiocytosis is dependent on site of involvement. Int J Radiat Oncol Biol Phys. 2018;100(3):670–8.
18. Tripathi M, Maskara P, Deora H, et al. Role of stereotactic radiosurgery in intracranial histiocytosis: a systematic review of literature of an emerging modality for localized disease. World Neurosurg. 2021;150:64–70.
19. Park DJ, Marianayagam NJ, Yener U, et al. Stereotactic radiosurgery for localized cranial Langerhans cell Histiocytosis: a single institution experience and review of literature. World Neurosurg. 2023;172:e476–82.
20. De Los Santos J, Popple R, Agazaryan N, Bayouth JE, Bissonnette JP, Bucci MK, Dieterich S, Dong L, Forster KM, Indelicato D, Langen K. Image guided radiation therapy (IGRT) technologies for radiation therapy localization and delivery. Int J Radiation Oncol Biol Phys. 2013;87(1):33–45.
21. Elledge CR, Alcorn SR, et al. 8-treatment planning in palliative radiotherapy. Palliative Radiation Oncology; 2024. p. 65–74.
22. Thomas H, Timmermann B, et al. Paediatric proton therapy. Br J Radiol. 2020;93(1107):20190601.
23. Sosman MC, et al. Xanthomatosis (Schuller-Christian's disease; lipoid histiocytosis). JAMA. 1932;98(2):110–7. https://doi.org/10.1001/jama.1932.02730280018005.
24. Schiebe M, Schroeder HG, Hoffmann W, et al. Irradiation of histiocytosis X confined to the oral mucosa. Strahlenther Onkol. 2001;177(1):48–50.
25. Zlodre JK, Rennie ATM, Ramsden JD, et al. Langerhans' cell histiocytosis of the temporal bone: successful treatment of sensorineural hearing loss with low-dose radiotherapy. J Laryngol Otol. 2009;123(6):676–9.
26. Atalar B, Miller RC, Dincbas FO, et al. Adult langerhans cell histiocytosis of bones: a rare cancer network study. Acta Orthop Belg. 2010;76(5):663–8.
27. Meyer A, Stark M, Karstens JH, et al. Langerhans cell Histiocytosis of the cranial base: is low-dose radiotherapy effective? Case Rep Oncol Med. 2012;2012:789640.
28. Kriz J, Eich HT, Bruns F, et al. Radiotherapy in langerhans cell histiocytosis—a rare indication in a rare disease. Radiat Oncol. 2013;8:233.
29. Laird J, Ma J, Chau K, et al. Outcome after radiation therapy for Langerhans cell histiocytosis is dependent on site of involvement. Int J Radiat Oncol Biol Phys. 2018;100(3):670–8.
30. Ghuijs W, Kemps PG, Capala ME, et al. Aggressive unifocal bone Langerhans cell histiocytosis with soft tissue extension both responsive to radiotherapy: a case report. Radiat Oncol. 2022;17:137. https://doi.org/10.1186/s13014-022-02108-0.

Aneurysmal Bone Cyst

25

Vansh Arora

25.1 Pathogenesis

Historically considered a reactive vascular condition, aneurysmal bone cysts (ABCs) are now recognized to have a neoplastic component in many primary cases, driven by specific genetic alterations. ABCs can be primary, arising de novo, or secondary, occurring within pre-existing lesions such as giant cell tumors, fibrous dysplasia, osteoblastoma, or chondroblastoma. Primary ABCs are frequently associated with a chromosomal translocation, t(16;17)(q22;p13), resulting in overexpression of the ubiquitin-specific protease 6 (USP6) gene. This genetic aberration activates matrix metalloproteinases (MMPs), which degrade the extracellular matrix, promoting bone resorption and cystic cavity formation [1] (Fig. 25.1).

The vascular nature of ABCs significantly contributes to their pathogenesis. Aberrant, dilated vascular channels within the lesion increase venous pressure, leading to hemorrhage and the formation of large, blood-filled cystic spaces lacking true endothelial lining. These spaces are separated by fibrous septa containing fibroblasts, osteoclast-like multinucleated giant cells, and reactive woven bone. These cellular elements drive osteolytic expansion and stimulate further vascular and fibro-osseous proliferation. Vascular endothelial growth factor (VEGF) expression within the lesion enhances angiogenesis, fueling lesion growth [2].

Pathologically, ABCs are characterized by cavernous, blood-filled spaces, fibrous septa rich in giant cells and fibroblasts, and areas of immature bone formation. Radiologically, they present with a characteristic "blow-out" appearance, marked by cortical thinning and expansile ballooning, reflecting their aggressive local behavior [3]. These features collectively contribute to the clinical challenges of managing ABCs, particularly in anatomically sensitive locations such as the spine or pelvis, where surgical intervention may pose significant risks.

V. Arora (✉)
DrNB Medical Oncology Trainee, Dharamshila Narayana Hospital, Delhi, India

K. Sood Sharma (ed.), *Radiation Therapy for Benign Disorders*,
https://doi.org/10.1007/978-981-95-6635-8_25

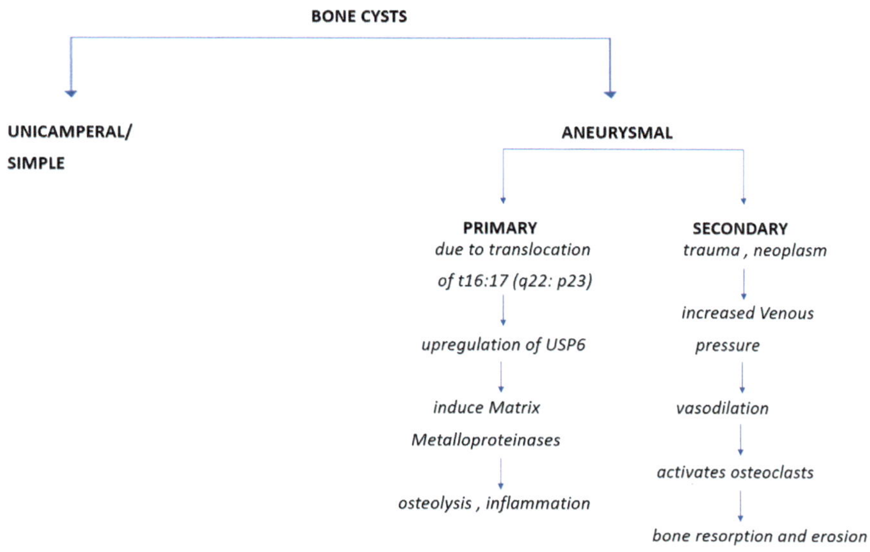

Fig. 25.1 Types of bone cysts and pathogenesis of ABC

25.2 Role of Radiotherapy

While surgical excision and curettage remain the cornerstone treatments for aneurysmal bone cysts (ABCs), complete resection is not always feasible due to anatomical constraints or patient-specific factors. Radiotherapy (RT) has emerged as an effective adjuvant or salvage therapy for inoperable, recurrent, or surgically high-risk ABCs. Although historically approached with caution due to concerns about long-term complications, particularly in younger patients, advancements in imaging, conformal planning, and delivery techniques have significantly enhanced RT's safety and efficacy [4].

RT targets the highly vascular and proliferative components of ABCs, leveraging ionizing radiation to induce DNA damage in mesenchymal and endothelial cells. This triggers apoptosis, reducing stromal proliferation and angiogenesis, which are critical to lesion growth. As the cellular components degenerate, cystic spaces collapse, followed by fibrous and osseous remodeling, leading to lesion stabilization or regression [5]. Low-dose RT, typically ranging from 18–30 Gy, has been shown to induce endothelial apoptosis and fibrosis, halting internal hemorrhage and preventing lesion revascularization, thus achieving long-term control [6].

Indications for RT Include:

Inoperable lesions in complex anatomical sites (e.g., skull base, spine, or sacrum), where surgery risks damage to critical structures.

Recurrent disease following failed surgery or sclerotherapy, particularly when reoperation increases morbidity.

Medically unfit patients unable to tolerate anesthesia or surgery due to comorbidities.

High-morbidity surgical sites, where resection could cause significant functional or cosmetic deficits, such as neurological impairment in spinal ABCs or facial deformities in skull base lesions.

Compared to alternatives like sclerotherapy or embolization, RT offers a non-invasive approach with high local control rates, particularly when delivered using modern techniques [7]. Sclerotherapy, while effective, often requires multiple sessions and has variable outcomes depending on lesion vascularity. Embolization, though useful for vascular lesions, is limited by anatomical accessibility and technical expertise. Surgery, despite its curative potential, carries a 10–30% recurrence risk after curettage [8].

Patient selection is critical. RT is most suitable for older children and adults with residual or recurrent ABCs, or when surgery is contraindicated. In children under five, RT is generally avoided due to risks of growth plate damage and secondary malignancies, unless no viable alternatives exist [9]. Biopsy confirmation is essential to rule out malignant mimics like telangiectatic osteosarcoma or giant cell tumors with secondary aneurysmal changes [10].

Limitations and challenges include the rare but serious risk of radiation-induced sarcoma, though this is minimized with low doses used for benign lesions. Growth disturbances in skeletally immature patients and limited prospective data also pose challenges. Most evidence comes from retrospective series, underscoring the need for larger trials [11].

Modern RT Techniques, such as intensity-modulated radiotherapy (IMRT), image-guided radiotherapy (IGRT), and stereotactic body radiotherapy (SBRT), enhance precision by tailoring radiation to the tumor volume, sparing adjacent structures. These advancements have improved outcomes, with studies reporting long-term control and minimal toxicity in complex ABC cases [12].

25.3 Radiation Technique in ABC Management

External beam radiotherapy (EBRT) is the primary modality, with SBRT and IMRT increasingly used for lesions near critical structures. Immobilization ensures accuracy, using thermoplastic masks for head/neck lesions or vacuum cushions for spinal/pelvic sites. Planning involves CT-based simulation with MRI fusion for precise delineation of cystic components. The gross tumor volume (GTV) encompasses the visible lesion, with a clinical target volume (CTV) adding a 0.5–1 cm margin for microscopic spread, and a planning target volume (PTV) including an additional 0.3–0.5 cm for setup errors. Dose and fractionation typically involve 18–30 Gy in 1.8–2 Gy daily fractions, though hypofractionated regimens (12–16 Gy in 3–4 fractions) are explored for favorable cases [13]. Dose constraints prioritize minimizing exposure to critical structures (e.g., spinal cord $\leq$45 Gy, growth plates $<$15 Gy) to prevent long-term sequelae [14].

25.4 Toxicity Profile and Risk Minimization

Radiotherapy (RT) for aneurysmal bone cysts (ABCs) is generally well-tolerated due to low doses and focused treatment volumes. However, given the young age of many patients and the benign nature of ABCs, minimizing acute and long-term toxicities is paramount to maintain a favorable risk–benefit profile [15].

Acute Toxicities are minimal, typically including:

Mild skin erythema in the irradiated field, which resolves spontaneously.
Fatigue, which is transient and managed with supportive care.

Late toxicities, though rare, are more significant:

Growth arrest or deformity: Irradiation of epiphyseal growth plates in children can cause limb length discrepancies or angular deformities, particularly in those under 10 [16].

Radiation-induced malignancy: While rare with low doses (18–30 Gy), secondary malignancies remain a theoretical risk, with latency periods spanning decades [17].

Fibrosis and osteoradionecrosis: These are uncommon but can cause stiffness or compromised bone integrity, especially in weight-bearing bones [18].

Risk Mitigation Strategies

Advanced Techniques: IMRT, volumetric modulated arc therapy (VMAT), and SBRT ensure precise dose delivery, sparing critical structures like the spinal cord or growth plates [19].

Dose Constraints: Adhering to limits (e.g., spinal cord <45 Gy, growth plates <15 Gy) minimizes long-term risks [20].

Multidisciplinary Planning: Collaboration among radiation oncologists, orthopedic surgeons, and radiologists optimizes treatment safety [21].

Long-Term Monitoring: Regular imaging (MRI/CT) and functional assessments are essential to detect recurrence, growth issues, or late radiation effects early [22].

By leveraging modern techniques and vigilant follow-up, RT can be a safe and effective option for ABC management, particularly in challenging cases.

25.5 Review of Literature and Case Studies

Although surgery remains the primary treatment for aneurysmal bone cysts (ABCs), radiotherapy (RT) is increasingly recognized as an effective option for inoperable, recurrent, or high-risk cases. Evidence from retrospective series and case reports highlights RT's efficacy and safety, particularly in anatomically complex sites like the spine, sacrum, or skull base.

Papagelopoulos et al. (2001) reported a series of spinal ABCs treated with external beam radiotherapy (EBRT) at 30 Gy. All patients achieved complete local control without recurrence, and no long-term radiation-related complications were observed, supporting RT's safety in well-selected cases [23]. Similarly, Boriani et al. (1992) described nine patients with sacral ABCs treated with adjuvant RT after incomplete resection or biopsy. Doses ranged within a conservative therapeutic window, resulting in significant symptomatic relief and lesion stabilization, with no reported radiation-induced complications [24].

Raskin et al. (2013) further corroborated RT's utility in a retrospective review of patients with recurrent or inoperable ABCs. Doses of 24–30 Gy in 1.8–2 Gy fractions achieved excellent local control, with no significant long-term sequelae, positioning RT as a minimally invasive alternative to repeated surgery [25].

A case from our institution illustrates RT's potential. A 16-year-old male with a recurrent cervical spine ABC at C2–C3 presented with neurological symptoms, including upper limb weakness and gait instability, following subtotal resection. Due to surgical risks near the spinal cord, intensity-modulated radiotherapy (IMRT) was administered at 28 Gy in 14 fractions, with MRI fusion for precise targeting. Spinal cord dose constraints were strictly followed. Follow-up imaging at 3 and 6 months showed cystic collapse and osseous remodeling, with complete neurological recovery by 6 months. At 3 years, the patient remained disease-free without radiation-related toxicity or spinal deformity, highlighting IMRT's efficacy in delicate sites.

These studies and cases demonstrate RT's role in achieving durable local control and symptomatic relief in challenging ABCs. Low-dose regimens (24–30 Gy) minimize complications, and modern techniques like IMRT enhance precision. However, long-term surveillance is crucial, particularly in younger patients, to monitor for rare risks like secondary malignancies [26].

25.6 Future Directions

The future of radiotherapy (RT) for aneurysmal bone cysts (ABCs) is promising, driven by technological advancements, molecular insights, and personalized approaches. Innovations such as proton therapy, stereotactic radiotherapy (SRT), molecular targeting, and artificial intelligence (AI)-based planning aim to enhance efficacy, reduce toxicity, and optimize outcomes. Multicentric studies and registries are essential to standardize protocols and solidify RT's role [27].

Proton therapy leverages the Bragg peak to deliver radiation with minimal exit dose, sparing healthy tissues. This is particularly beneficial for pediatric patients with ABCs in sensitive sites like the spine or pelvis, reducing risks of growth disturbances or secondary malignancies [28]. Early studies suggest comparable local control to traditional RT with lower toxicity [29].

Stereotactic radiotherapy (SRT), including stereotactic body radiotherapy (SBRT) and stereotactic radiosurgery (SRS), enables high-dose delivery in fewer fractions with submillimeter precision. This approach is ideal for inoperable or recurrent ABCs, minimizing treatment duration and side effects, though clinical trials are needed for validation [30].

Molecular targeting capitalizes on ABCs' molecular drivers, such as USP6 gene rearrangements and angiogenic pathways. Combining RT with anti-angiogenic agents or USP6 inhibitors could enhance radiosensitivity, allowing lower doses and reduced toxicity [31]. Preclinical studies are exploring these synergies, with potential to transform ABC management [32].

AI-based planning uses predictive analytics to tailor RT to individual patient and tumor characteristics, optimizing dose distribution and minimizing toxicity. AI can also identify patients best suited for RT versus other therapies, streamlining clinical decision-making [33].

Research and standardization: The rarity of ABCs limits large-scale data. Multicentric prospective studies and registries are critical to define RT's efficacy, optimal dosing, and long-term outcomes, paving the way for standardized protocols [34].

These advancements promise precise, effective, and low-toxicity RT for ABCs, but rigorous research is needed to integrate them into clinical practice and improve patient outcomes.

25.7 Conclusion

Aneurysmal bone cysts (ABCs) are benign, locally aggressive lesions with a high recurrence risk, particularly in complex anatomical sites. While surgery is the primary treatment, radiotherapy (RT) offers a vital alternative for inoperable, recurrent, or high-morbidity cases. Modern techniques like proton therapy and stereotactic radiotherapy enable precise, low-dose delivery, achieving effective local control with minimal toxicity, especially in pediatric or spinal cases. These approaches have transformed RT into a safe and viable option, though long-term risks, such as secondary malignancies, necessitate vigilant follow-up. Current evidence, supported by retrospective studies, endorses RT's cautious use in carefully selected patients. Multidisciplinary collaboration among radiation oncologists, orthopedic surgeons, and molecular researchers is essential to optimize treatment plans. Ongoing research, including multicentric studies and registries, will further define RT's role, refine dosing strategies, and establish standardized protocols. By leveraging technological and molecular advancements, RT continues to evolve as a cornerstone in managing challenging ABCs, offering hope for improved outcomes in this rare condition.

References

1. Oliveira AM, Perez-Atayde AR, Inwards CY, et al. USP6 and CDH11 oncogenes identify the neoplastic cell in primary aneurysmal bone cysts and are absent in so-called secondary aneurysmal bone cysts. Am J Pathol. 2004;165(5):1773–80.
2. Leithner A, Windhager R, Lang S, et al. Aneurysmal bone cyst: a population-based epidemiologic study and literature review. Clin Orthop Relat Res. 1999;363:176–9.

3. Rapp TB, Ward JP, Alaia MJ. Aneurysmal bone cyst. J Am Acad Orthop Surg. 2012;20(4):233–41.
4. Feigenberg SJ, Marcus RB Jr, Zlotecki RA, et al. Radiation therapy for benign tumors and tumor-like conditions of bone. Cancer Control. 2001;8(6):509–17.
5. Mendenhall WM, Zlotecki RA, Scarborough MT, et al. Aneurysmal bone cyst: treatment with radiotherapy. Int J Radiat Oncol Biol Phys. 2006;66(3):S128.
6. Bush CH, Adler Z, Drane WE, et al. Percutaneous radionuclide ablation of aneurysmal bone cysts. AJR Am J Roentgenol. 2010;194(5):W479–83.
7. Rossi G, Rimondi E, Bartalena T, et al. Selective arterial embolization of 36 aneurysmal bone cysts of the skeleton with percutaneous sclerotherapy. Skeletal Radiol. 2010;39(2):161–7.
8. Mankin HJ, Hornicek FJ, Ortiz-Cruz E, et al. Aneurysmal bone cyst: a review of 150 patients. J Clin Oncol. 2005;23(27):6756–62.
9. Marcove RC, Sheth DS, Takemoto S, et al. The treatment of aneurysmal bone cyst. Clin Orthop Relat Res. 1995;311:157–63.
10. Sciot R, Dorfman H, Brys P, et al. Cytogenetic-morphologic correlations in aneurysmal bone cyst, giant cell tumor of bone and combined lesions. Mod Pathol. 2000;13(11):1206–10.
11. Gibbs CP Jr, Hefele MC, Peabody TD, et al. Aneurysmal bone cyst of the extremities: factors related to local recurrence after curettage with a high-speed burr. J Bone Joint Surg Am. 1999;81(12):1671–8.
12. Harrop JS, Schmidt MH, Boriani S, et al. Aggressive "benign" primary spine neoplasms: Osteoblastoma, aneurysmal bone cyst, and giant cell tumor. Spine (Phila Pa 1976). 2009;34(22 Suppl):S39–47.
13. Chang CY, Kattapuram SV, Chen TH, et al. Radiographic evaluation and treatment of aneurysmal bone cysts. Radiol Clin North Am. 2011;49(6):1245–58.
14. DeLaney TF, Liebsch NJ, Pedlow FX, et al. Phase II study of high-dose photon/proton radiotherapy in the management of spine sarcomas. Int J Radiat Oncol Biol Phys. 2009;74(3):732–9.
15. Halperin EC, Perez CA, Brady LW. Principles and practice of radiation oncology. 6th ed. Philadelphia: Lippincott Williams & Wilkins; 2013.
16. Esiashvili N, Goodman M, Marcus RB Jr. Changes in incidence and survival of Ewing sarcoma patients over the past 3 decades: Surveillance Epidemiology and End Results data. J Pediatr Hematol Oncol. 2008;30(6):425–30.
17. Tucker MA, D'Angio GJ, Boice JD Jr, et al. Bone sarcomas linked to radiotherapy and chemotherapy in children. N Engl J Med. 1987;317(10):588–93.
18. Paulino AC, Nguyen TX, Mai WY, et al. Dose response and local control of Ewing sarcoma and osteogenic sarcoma with radiotherapy. Int J Radiat Oncol Biol Phys. 2007;69(3):S121.
19. Timmermann B, Schuck A, Niggli F, et al. Spot-scanning proton therapy for malignant soft tissue tumors in childhood: first experiences at the Paul Scherrer Institute. Int J Radiat Oncol Biol Phys. 2007;67(2):497–504.
20. Hall EJ, Giaccia AJ. Radiobiology for the radiologist. 7th ed. Philadelphia: Lippincott Williams & Wilkins; 2012.
21. Boriani S, De Iure F, Campanacci L, et al. Aneurysmal bone cyst of the mobile spine: report on 41 cases. Spine (Phila Pa 1976). 2001;26(1):27–35.
22. Donaldson WF, O'Connor GA, Rodabaugh R, et al. Aneurysmal bone cyst: a review of 26 cases. Orthopedics. 1997;20(8):715–20.
23. Papagelopoulos PJ, Choudhury SN, Frassica FJ, et al. Treatment of aneurysmal bone cysts of the pelvis and sacrum. J Bone Joint Surg Am. 2001;83(11):1674–81.
24. Boriani S, Bandiera S, Biagini R, et al. Aneurysmal bone cyst of the spine: treatment by curettage and bone grafting. Chir Organi Mov. 1992;77(4):365–71.
25. Raskin KA, Schwab JH, Mankin HJ, et al. Aneurysmal bone cyst: long-term outcomes and predictors of recurrence. Clin Orthop Relat Res. 2013;471(6):1895–904.
26. Schwartz HS, Springfield DS, Simon MA. Aneurysmal bone cyst: a review of 26 cases with emphasis on recurrence. Orthopedics. 1999;22(1):39–44.

27. Grier HE, Krailo MD, Tarbell NJ, et al. Addition of ifosfamide and etoposide to standard chemotherapy for Ewing's sarcoma and primitive neuroectodermal tumor of bone. N Engl J Med. 2003;348(8):694–701.
28. Hug EB, Fitzek MM, Liebsch NJ, et al. Locally challenging osteo- and chondrogenic tumors of the axial skeleton: results of combined proton and photon radiation therapy using three-dimensional treatment planning. Int J Radiat Oncol Biol Phys. 1995;31(3):467–76.
29. Indelicato DJ, Keole SR, Shahlaee AH, et al. Definitive radiotherapy for aneurysmal bone cysts in the pediatric population. Int J Radiat Oncol Biol Phys. 2010;78(3):S129.
30. Kamath R, Subramanian S, Prabhu K, et al. Stereotactic radiosurgery for benign tumors: integration into multidisciplinary management. J Neuro-Oncol. 2012;108(1):1–9.
31. Ye Y, Pringle LM, Lau AW, et al. TRE17/USP6 oncogene translocated in aneurysmal bone cyst induces matrix metalloproteinase production via activation of NF-kappaB. Oncogene. 2010;29(25):3619–29.
32. Lau AW, Pringle LM, Quick L, et al. TRE17/ubiquitin-specific protease 6 (USP6) oncogene translocated in aneurysmal bone cyst blocks osteoblastic maturation via an autocrine mechanism involving bone morphogenetic protein dysregulation. J Biol Chem. 2010;285(47):37170–80.
33. Lambin P, van Stiphout RG, Starmans MH, et al. Predicting outcomes in radiation oncology—multifactorial decision support systems. Nat Rev Clin Oncol. 2013;10(1):27–40.
34. Dormans JP, Hanna BG, Johnston DR, et al. Surgical treatment and recurrence rate of aneurysmal bone cysts in children. Clin Orthop Relat Res. 2004;421:205–11.

Vertebral Hemangioma

26

Kanika Sood Sharma and Shubhansha Jain

26.1 Introduction

Vertebral hemangiomas (VHs) are benign vascular tumors arising from the proliferation of blood vessels within the vertebral body. They are the most common tumors of the spinal axis, with a prevalence of 10–12% in the general population as identified in autopsy series and radiographic studies [1, 2]. Most VHs are discovered incidentally, as they are typically asymptomatic and detected during imaging for unrelated complaints. However, a small subset can become aggressive, leading to local pain, neurological deficits, and spinal instability due to cortical destruction or epidural extension. VHs can occur at any age but are most commonly diagnosed in middle-aged adults, with a peak incidence in the fifth decade of life. There is a slight female predominance (male: female ratio ~ 1:2) [3]. Aggressive vertebral hemangiomas (AVHs) may require multimodal management, including surgery, embolization, vertebroplasty, and radiotherapy (RT), particularly with advances in conformal and stereotactic techniques.

This chapter provides a comprehensive overview of VH, focusing on clinical features, imaging, management strategies, the role of radiotherapy, and evidence-based recommendations.

26.2 Clinical Presentation

VHs are mostly asymptomatic and do not require any intervention. However, a small subset becomes symptomatic, often termed "aggressive vertebral hemangiomas," accounting for less than 0.9–1.2% of all vertebral hemangiomas [3].

The clinical presentation of symptomatic VHs varies based on lesion location, size, and extent of spinal cord or nerve root compression. The most common

K. Sood Sharma (✉) · S. Jain
Dharamshila Narayana Superspeciality Hospital, Delhi, India

K. Sood Sharma (ed.), *Radiation Therapy for Benign Disorders*,
https://doi.org/10.1007/978-981-95-6635-8_26

symptom is localized back pain, which may result from expansion of the lesion causing mechanical stress or microfractures [4].

In aggressive cases, symptoms may escalate to neurological deficits, including radiculopathy, myelopathy, or paraparesis, due to epidural extension and spinal cord compression. Progressive lower limb weakness, gait instability, coordination issues, bowel/bladder dysfunction, and sensory disturbances are red flags for spinal cord compression. In rare cases, VHs may present acutely due to hemorrhage or pathological fracture. Rarely, bladder or bowel incontinence if autonomic pathways are involved. Thoracic spine involvement is most frequently associated with neurologic symptoms, followed by the lumbar and cervical spine [5].

26.3 Diagnosis and Imaging

Imaging plays a crucial role in the diagnosis and classification of VHs. Most of these tumors are accidental findings on routine radiographs. The histopathological characteristics of VHs form the basis for their imaging-based classification into typical, atypical, or aggressive. Typical VHs on plane radiographs may show vertically oriented striation due to thickened trabeculae known as the "corduroy cloth" or "jail bar" sign [6]. These striations develop when the vascular channels get intermingled with thickened vertical trabeculae (Fig. 26.1).

CT offers excellent delineation of internal bony architecture and shows classical features of thickening of vertical trabeculae, represented as areas of hyperdensities. These hyperdense areas look like dots on a hypodense background, hence termed as "polka dot sign" (Fig. 26.2) or salt and pepper appearance on axial image [6]. CT help is particularly helpful for evaluating cortical integrity and guiding percutaneous procedures.

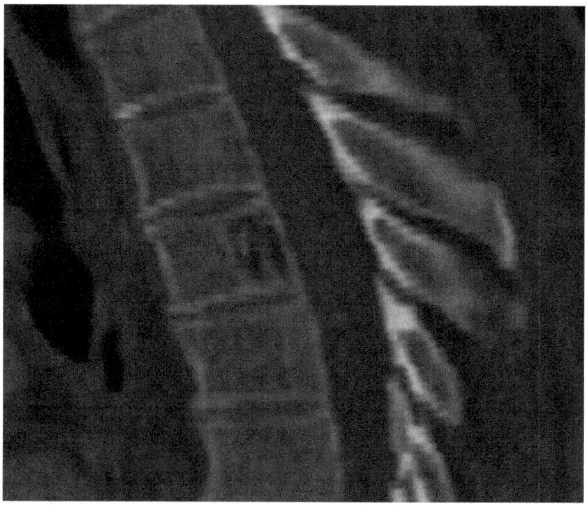

Fig. 26.1 Striations intermingled with the thickened vertebral trabeculae mimicking a corduroy cloth pattern. (Courtesy El Ouali et al. [6])

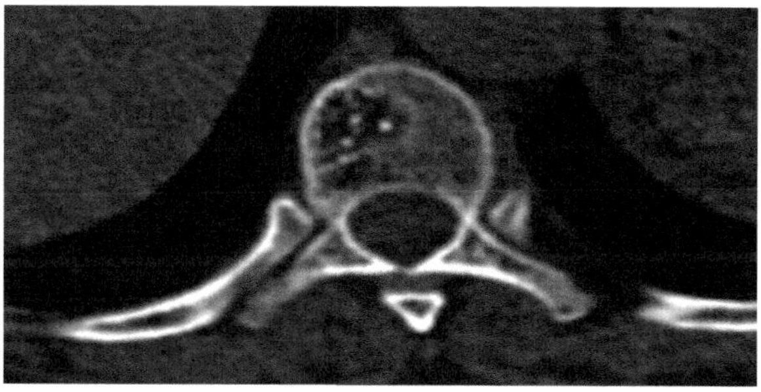

Fig. 26.2 Polka dot appearance in the left segment of the vertebral body. (Courtesy El Ouali et al. [6])

Atypical VHs may lack these classic signs, making diagnosis more challenging, and often require advanced imaging techniques for accurate characterization.

MRI is the most sensitive modality for identifying and characterizing VHs. Due to their high fat content, typical VHs appear hyperintense on both T1-weighted and T2-weighted images [7].

Aggressive VHs often show hypointensity on T1-weighted images and hyperintensity on T2-weighted images, reflecting reduced fat and increased vascularity or edema. MRI is essential for assessing soft tissue extension, epidural involvement, and spinal cord compression.

Typical VHs appear hyperintense on T1 images due to the fatty stroma & appear hyperintense on T2 images due to their vascular components. They may show a variable degree of enhancement; typically, lesions with a larger fatty component have a low enhancement pattern [7].

Atypical hemangiomas often exhibit a mixed, heterogeneous signal intensity pattern on imaging, which is attributed to inflammatory infiltration and a lack of fat within the lesion [8].

The aggressiveness of these hemangiomas correlates with a lower fat content and a predominance of vascular tissue. As the vascular component increases and fat decreases, the lesion tends to behave more aggressively [9–11]. Aggressive atypical hemangiomas are characterized by:

- Low signal intensity on T1-weighted MRI images and high signal intensity on T2-weighted images (Fig. 26.3a, b).
- Avid contrast enhancement, which may reveal cortical erosion and soft tissue stroma between the osseous trabeculae on CT scans.
- Additional features of aggressiveness include the presence of extradural soft tissue, expansion into the posterior elements, invasion of the spinal canal, and encroachment upon the spinal cord.

Histopathology Confirms diagnosis in atypical or aggressive cases, especially when surgery or biopsy is performed. These tumors are characterized by a mixture of various tissue components, including blood vessels of different sizes, adipocytes (fat cells), smooth muscle, fibrous tissue, hemosiderin (a blood breakdown pigment), interstitial edema, and remodeled bone. Macroscopically, VHs present as

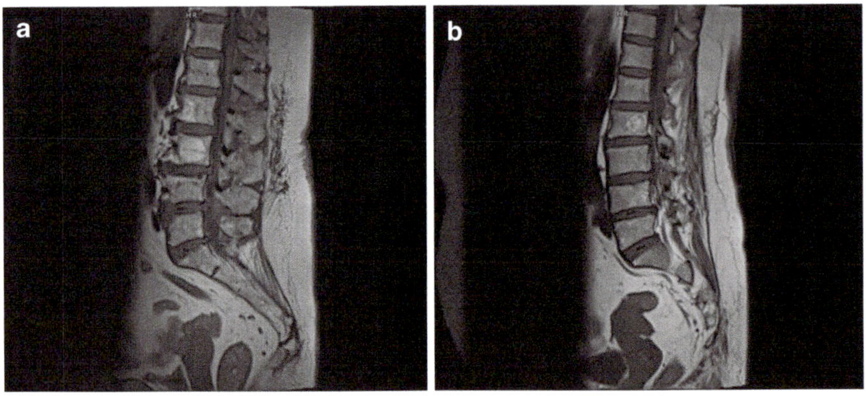

Fig. 26.3 (**a**, **b**) T1/T2 hyperintense lesion at L3 & L2 vertebrae, respectively, showing vertebral hemangioma. (Courtesy Dr. Shailendra Sharma, Department of Radiology, DNSH)

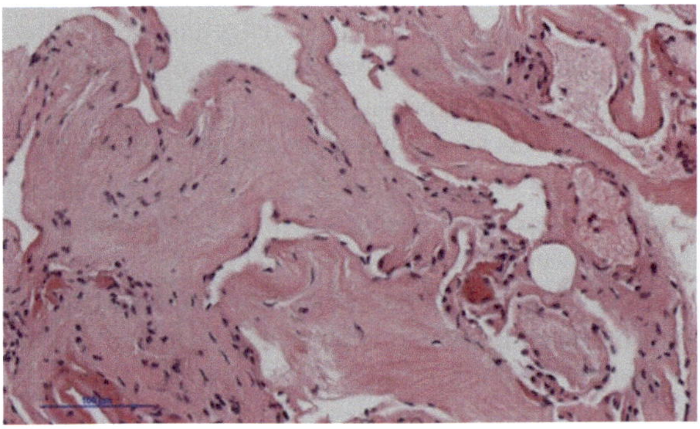

Fig. 26.4 Spinal hemangioma confirmed by hematoxylin and eosin staining, proliferation of small-caliber vessels within a fibrous stroma with surrounding bone. (Originally published in Insights Imaging (2016) McEvoy et al. [12])

soft, well-demarcated, dark red masses. They often contain sclerotic bony trabeculae and scattered blood-filled cavities, which give them a distinctive honeycomb appearance.

Microscopic Subtypes of Hemangiomas Based on the vascular composition, there are four main subtypes. The capillary hemangiomas, which comprise small, capillary-sized blood vessels. The cavernous hemangiomas are characterized by larger, dilated vascular spaces. The arteriovenous (AV) hemangiomas are composed of interconnected arterial and venous vessels, and venous hemangiomas consist of abnormal collections of veins [12] (Fig. 26.4).

Capillary and cavernous subtypes are the most common subtypes. These typically feature thin-walled blood vessels that are embedded in an edematous stroma with bony trabeculae that extend through the bone marrow space. In a study of 64 surgically treated VH cases, capillary hemangioma accounted for 50%, cavernous for 28%, and mixed form for 22%. Additional histological findings like secondary changes such as fibrous or adipose involution of bone marrow and remodeling of bone trabeculae may occur. Notably, the capillary and cavernous variants are typically linked with more favorable postoperative outcomes [2]. Table 26.1.

Table 26.1 Hemangioma Subtypes in VHs [2]

Subtype	Vascular composition	Prevalence in VHs	Prognosis
Capillary	Small, capillary-sized vessels	50%	Favorable outcomes
Cavernous	Large, dilated vascular spaces	28%	Favorable outcomes
Mixed	Features of both capillary/cavernous	22%	Variable
Arteriovenous	Interconnected arterial and venous nets	Rare	Not specified
Venous	Abnormal collections of veins	Rare	Not specified

Table 26.2 Enneking staging system for benign tumors [12]

Stage	Description
Stage I	Latent: Asymptomatic, slow-growing, low recurrence risk post-resection
Stage II	Active: Cortical thinning, defined borders, potential for growth
Stage III	Aggressive: Ill-defined borders, possible spinal canal extension, neurological involvement

Aggressive lesions, also termed "symptomatic VHs," are typically found in the thoracolumbar region and are more common in females (2:1 ratio). Pregnancy, especially in the third trimester, may exacerbate symptoms due to vascular engorgement and increased intra-abdominal pressure. The enneking staging system is the traditionally utilized system in management [13] (Table 26.2).

26.4 Management

The management of vertebral hemangioma is determined by clinical presentation, radiological features, and the presence or absence of neurological symptoms. Teferi et al. proposed a treatment algorithm for VHs based on their institutional experience and literature review [14] (Fig. 26.5).

Conservative Management Conservative treatment with observation and pain control are the mainstays of treatment for asymptomatic VH patients and those with mild-to-moderate pain, respectively [15]. Asymptomatic or minimally symptomatic VHs with no evidence of spinal instability or cord compression. Periodic clinical and radiological surveillance. There is no established protocol for the frequency of follow-up imaging, but it's usually done periodically to assess for change. While some VHs may show minor growth, they usually do so very slowly. This slow progression may not cause any symptoms and does not usually require treatment. In rare cases (around 1% of all lesions), they may become aggressive and cause symptoms due to bony expansion, extraosseous extension, or compression of the spinal cord.

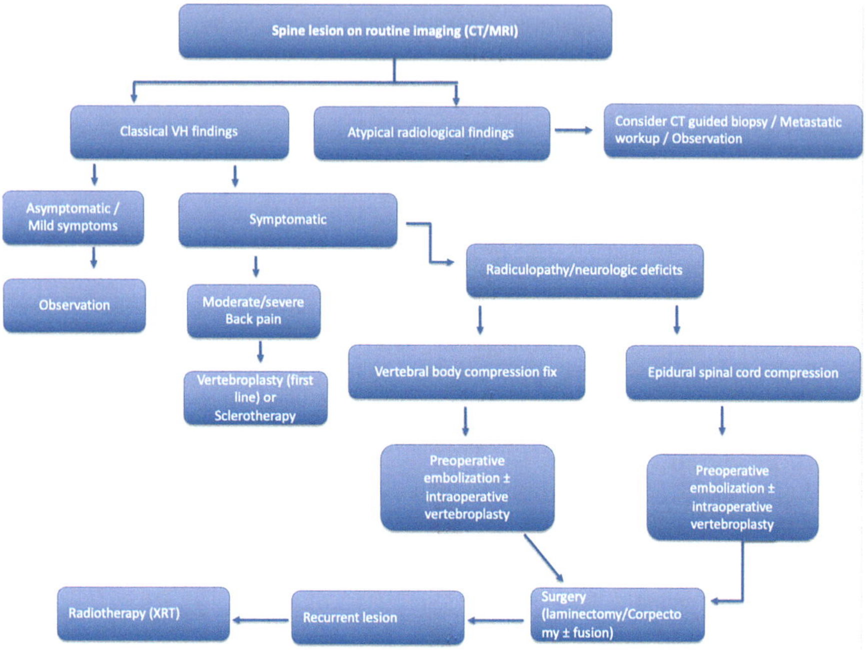

Fig. 26.5 Management algorithm for vertebral haemangioma based on imaging findings and symptom severity [14]

Surgery Surgery is indicated in progressive neurological deficit, spinal cord compression, or vertebral instability. The primary surgical goals remain neural decompression and spinal stabilization, with approach selection depending on tumor location and spinal involvement. VHs have been addressed with surgery since the 1950s. However, in the historic series, the mortality rate approached 11.5%, and neurological recovery rates ranged from 43% to 85%. The contemporary techniques combining decompressive laminectomy with procedures like vertebroplasty or preoperative embolization have improved outcomes, achieving near-complete neurological recovery and minimal mortality.

For ventral cord compression, corpectomy with anterior reconstruction may be employed, while dorsal compression is addressed via laminectomy. Occasionally surgery is challenging due to hypervascularity & bears the risk of significant intraoperative bleeding. Contemporary protocols often integrate multimodal strategies like preoperative embolization to reduce intraoperative bleeding or vertebroplasty to stabilize the bone and to reduce recurrence risk. Adjuvant RT to prevent tumor regrowth is also reserved for some cases. Combined approaches, such as laminectomy with intraoperative vertebroplasty, demonstrate reduced bleeding risks and enhanced spinal stability. These advancements have replaced traditional methods like standalone laminectomy, which carried higher mortality risks from exsanguination. Surgical decompression (laminectomy, vertebral body resection, spinal fusion) is often combined with preoperative transarterial embolization to reduce vascularity.

A retrospective study reviewed 75 VH cases managed from 2005 to 2022. Most patients were female, with a median age of 52. The majority of VHs were located in the thoracic spine (56–86%, depending on group). Among the 14 patients who underwent surgery, 93% were symptomatic—four with localized pain and nine with neurological deficits (numbness or paraparesis). Surgical procedures included decompression (13/14), vertebroplasty (2/14), and stabilization (5/14). Preoperative embolization (four cases) reduced median blood loss from 600 ml to 395 ml. Eight of nine patients with neurological deficits improved neurologically, and all had pain relief. Only one recurrence occurred (7% rate), with a median follow-up of 14.5 months. Complications were minimal, and three patients received adjuvant radiotherapy for residual tumor, remaining pain-free [14].

Embolization Embolization has established itself in a preoperative setting to reduce vascularity and blood loss and also to provide symptomatic relief in some cases. Most frequently, transarterial embolization with particles or coils is performed. In a protocol described by Berkefeld et al., preoperative endovascular embolization is routinely employed to minimize intraoperative hemorrhage in patients with aggressive hemangiomas causing neurologic deficits or focal symptoms. In their series, transarterial embolization using 150–250 micrometer polyvinyl alcohol (PVA) particles for targeted vascular occlusion. Rare combination with image-guided chemical ablation (e.g., ethanol) for lesions with complex angioarchitecture. While detachable coils and liquid embolics (e.g., Onyx®) are described, particulate agents remain preferred for balanced efficacy and procedural safety. This protocol reduces intraoperative blood loss by >70% compared to non-embolized cases, enabling safer tumor resection [16].

Percutaneous Vertebroplasty Percutaneous vertebroplasty (PVP) is a minimally invasive procedure that has proven effective for treating symptomatic VH in patients who do not respond to conservative medical management. It is indicated for pain relief in cases of vertebral body collapse or axial pain without significant epidural extension. Injection of polymethylmethacrylate (PMMA) cement into the vertebral body with fluoroscopic guidance is done under local anesthesia. Cement leakage into the spinal canal, venous filling, paravertebral soft tissue extravasation, and potential spinal cord injury are the known complications. In a retrospective cohort study by Gupta et al., 34 patients (mean age 36.91 years) had 38 vertebroplasties. Post-procedure outcome immediately revealed that 44.12% of the patients became asymptomatic, 38.23% improved significantly, 11.77% did not change, and 2.94% worsened from cement leakage leading to laminectomy. Pain reduction, enhanced activity, and reduced usage of analgesics at all follow-up points were observed. By 3 months, 76.47% were asymptomatic, and by 12 months, 90.9%. Of 16 patients followed up to 5 years, 87.5% remained asymptomatic with a single instance of deterioration. Complications were seen in 29.4% of the patients in the form of cement leakage into the epidural space (14.7%), venous filling (5.88%), paravertebral soft tissue extravasation (5.88%), and disc space filling (2.94%). Two patients only had symptomatic complications that needed surgical decompression; all the others were clinically silent [17].

Intralesional Ethanol Injection Ethanol sclerosis therapy involves the injection of highly concentrated ethanol directly into the hemangioma, inducing coagulative necrosis of the vascular endothelium and surrounding tissues, leading to irreversible vascular occlusion. It is performed under local or general anesthesia, guided by fluoroscopy or computed tomography (CT), and usually involves the slow injection of 10–15 mL of ethanol through a needle inserted via the pedicle. It is considered a viable and effective option for managing aggressive VHs, particularly when other treatments are unsuitable or have failed. It can be used independently or in combination with other treatments. Clinical outcomes from multiple case series and reports indicate that it can lead to significant improvement in symptoms, including pain relief and recovery from paralysis, with most patients experiencing good to excellent results. Complications include hypotension and arrhythmia during the injection, transient or delayed neurological deterioration, and, in some cases, delayed vertebral compression fractures—especially when large volumes of ethanol are used. Pre-injection of contrast medium is recommended to prevent inadvertent leakage into the spinal canal, which could lead to serious complications. The procedure's safety and efficacy are well-documented, but careful patient selection and meticulous technique are essential to minimize complications and optimize outcomes [18].

26.4.1 Radiotherapy (RT)

RT plays a pivotal role in the management of symptomatic and aggressive vertebral hemangioma, especially in patients who are poor surgical candidates. RT is non-invasive and effective for pain control, arresting tumor growth, and inducing regression. Radiation induces endothelial damage and thrombosis within the vascular channels of the hemangioma, leading to vessel obliteration, sclerosis, and reduction in lesion size and associated symptoms.

26.4.2 Indications for RT

- Symptomatic aggressive VHs with epidural extension or cord compression.
- Persistent pain unresponsive to conservative treatment.
- Recurrent lesion after surgery or embolization.
- Patients unfit for surgery.
- Adjuvant radiotherapy following partial excision or in light of residual disease. The recurrence rate is approximately 30–50% following subtotal resection, and this rate may be reduced by employing radiotherapy as an adjuvant therapy. Radiation may be given as an adjuvant in the case of a partial resection, where extensive tumor volume exists, or where pathological fracture has occurred.

26.4.3 Mechanism of Action

The radiobiological mechanisms underlying RT for spinal VH remain subject to ongoing debate. One prominent hypothesis identifies vascular endothelial cells as a key radiation-sensitive target, with vascular fibrosis—leading to impaired circulation and elimination of abnormal vessels—proposed as the primary therapeutic mechanism. Conversely, some researchers emphasize RT's anti-inflammatory effects at total doses around 20 Gy as the dominant factor. While SVH typically doesn't compromise vertebral stability, extensive bone involvement can result in pathological fractures. Post-treatment radiographic evidence of remineralization is uncommon, a finding consistent across multiple studies, including this investigation. This persistent lack of mineral restoration suggests bone remodeling may not be RT's primary mode of action in SVH management.

26.4.4 Radiation Techniques and Dosages

Earlier 2-dimensional tech or 3D CRT techniques were used to deliver the treatment, often utilizing posterior or parallel opposing fields with relatively higher weightage of the posterior beam. Now we use more advanced modalities such as intensity modulated radiation therapy (IMRT) and volumetric modulated arc therapy (VMAT).

Stereotactic radiosurgery (SRS) and stereotactic body radiation therapy (SBRT) are increasingly being used for VHs. These methods involve delivering high radiation doses per fraction with rapid dose fall off outside the target area. Accurate delineation of the clinical target volume (CTV) is critical, as steep dose gradients in SRS can lead to inadequate coverage of the planning target volume (PTV) and elevate the risk of toxicities to nearby structures. SRS and SBRT can now be administered using advanced systems such as the CyberKnife (CK). It delivers a highly focused beam with precision, allowing accurate targeting of the small or irregularly shaped lesion near critical structures like the spinal cord.

Simulation The patient is placed supine on the treatment couch for both simulation and treatment. Thermoplastic casts or vacuum cushions (e.g., VacLoc) are used to ensure comfort and reproducibility of positioning for each session. This is crucial for accuracy, especially when using advanced techniques like IMRT, VMAT, or SBRT, which require precise alignment. A high-resolution CT scan is obtained in the treatment position to define the anatomy and target volumes. MRI is often co-registered with the planning CT to better delineate the extent of the hemangioma, particularly in cases with epidural or soft tissue involvement. Image-guided radiotherapy (IGRT) techniques, such as cone-beam CT or kilovoltage imaging, are used to verify patient position before each treatment, minimizing setup errors.

26.4.5 Target Volume Delineation

Gross Tumor Volume (GTV): The visible hemangioma on imaging, typically defined on CT or MRI.
Clinical Target Volume (CTV): The entire affected vertebral body is usually included to ensure all microscopic disease is covered.
Planning Target Volume (PTV): The PTV margin is determined by type of immobilization, imaging employed for verification, and institutional protocols. The CTV plus a margin (commonly 3–5 mm) to account for setup variability and organ motion.

Dose Prescription and Fractionation Different dose schedules have been employed for VH. The schedules have moved to more hypofractionated being employed in the SBRT era. Conventional fractionation schedules provide good pain relief and tumor control while minimizing risk to the spinal cord. Dose ranges from 36 to 44 Gy in 18 to 22 fractions (e.g., 40 Gy in 20 fractions). Hypofractionated/SBRT: Shorter treatment courses with higher doses per fraction are effective & convenient, especially for patients with acute symptoms or requiring rapid pain relief. Dose ranges from 24–32 Gy in 3–5 fractions or a single fraction of SBRT (18–20 Gy) (Table 26.3)

Techniques—Historically, posterior or parallel-opposed (AP/PA) beams were used with reasonable results. However, the ability to spare neighboring organs at risk was limited, prohibiting dose escalations and hypofractionation. Modern techniques like intensity-modulated radiation therapy (IMRT) permit highly conformal dose distributions, sparing adjacent organs-at-risk. Volumetric modulated arc therapy (VMAT) further delivers treatment more quickly than IMRT while maintaining dose conformity. Stereotactic body radiation therapy further enables the delivery of high doses with rapid dose fall-off, ideal for sparing the spinal cord and surrounding tissue.

Table 26.3 Indication-based radiation approaches for vertebral hemangioma

Technique	Total Dose (Gy)	Fraction Size (Gy)	Fractions	Indication
3D-CRT/IMRT	30–40	1.8–2.5	15–20	Standard/aggressive lesions
SBRT/SRS	16–24	8–24	1–3	Small, focal, near spinal cord
Adjuvant RT	20–30	2–3	10–15	Post-surgery/residual disease

26.4.6 Dose Constraints and Organs at Risk

Spinal Cord—Strict dose constraints are applied to avoid radiation myelopathy (e.g., maximum dose typically kept below 45–50 Gy in conventional fractionation or 14–16 Gy in single fraction SBRT).

Other organs—kidneys, lungs, and esophagus, may also be considered depending on the vertebral level involved.

26.4.7 Results

A randomized clinical trial conducted by Marcin Miszczyk et al. compared CK hypofractionated rRT (25 Gy in 5 fractions over 2–3 days) with conventional RT fractionated (36 Gy in 18 fractions over 5 days/week) for painful VHs. Of the 74 evaluable patients, the CK group achieved significantly greater pain relief at 2 years (73.7% improvement vs. 50% improvement in the conventional arm, $p = 0.036$). Overall improvement was observed in 62.2% of cases, with 28.4% stable and 9.5% worsened. The CK arm median treatment time was almost half (13 days vs. 25 days). Both groups had a similar adverse events profile, with only mild adverse events reported.

Supporting evidence includes a case study where CK (24 Gy in 2 fractions) resolved opioid-resistant pain in a patient with a lumbar VH, enabling a return to normal activities. Other studies note high pain relief rates (80–90%) with CK or conventional RT, particularly at doses ≥34 Gy.

For VHs causing neurological deficits, conventional fractionation (e.g., 42–44 Gy) has also shown efficacy in symptom regression [Table 26.4]. These findings position CK hypofractionation as a safe, effective, and time-efficient alternative to conventional RT for painful VHs, while conventional regimens remain viable for cases requiring neurological symptom management [19].

B Pinar et al. performed an IORT in the case of an aggressive VH using a combination of intraoperative radiation therapy (IORT) and kyphoplasty, termed Kypho-IORT. In this case, a patient with progressive neurological deficits due to a T5 VH underwent unsuccessful embolization, followed by a combined procedure. Using a transpedicular approach, metallic sleeves guided the INTRABEAM miniature X-ray generator into the vertebral body, delivering a single 8 Gy dose at a 10 mm distance. After IORT, kyphoplasty with cement injection was performed for

Table 26.4 Comparison of clinical outcomes between CK and conventional treatment arms

Outcome	CK Arm ($n = 38$)	Conv. Arm ($n = 36$)	p-value
Pain improvement (SRAS)	73.7%	50%	0.036
Median NRS decrease	4 (IQR 1–5)	4 (IQR 1–5)	NS
Median % NRS reduction	59%	59%	NS
Treatment duration (median)	13 days	25 days	<0.05
Adverse events (any)	Rare	Rare	NS

stabilization. The patient experienced rapid neurological recovery and remained symptom-free with stable vertebral morphology and reduction in epidural mass at 30 months follow-up [20].

Pain relief may be achieved in 85–90% of cases. Neurological improvement is gradual and may be incomplete. Wang et al. reported in their retrospective study that RT is a safe and effective first-line treatment choice in aggressive VH cases, but in cases of severe spinal cord compression, neurological deterioration might be found after radiotherapy, which requires further surgical intervention [21]. A retrospective multicenter study was done by Hyde and co-authors from seven German institutions, encompassing 84 patients treated between 1969 and 2008 with symptomatic lesions of VH. The primary indication for RT was pain (97.6% of patients) and neurological deficit (28.6%). The study reported an overall patient response rate of 90.5% after a median follow-up period of 68 months [22].

Aksoy et al. evaluated 80 patients treated with RT for painful VHs and reported an overall pain response rate of 85%, with complete pain relief in 58.8% of patients. Neurological recovery following treatment for VHs tends to be gradual [23]. In a study by Aich et al. [24], RT provides clinical benefit in six patients presenting with neurological deficit. However, full recovery was not achieved, and it took over 2 years for significant improvement in muscle strength. Similarly, research conducted by Zhang et al. used CyberKnife stereotactic radiosurgery in 5 patients; 4 of them showed some degree of neurological improvement, but only after an average follow-up of one year [25]. One possible explanation for the limited or delayed neurological recovery could be the morphological changes seen in VH after RT. An optimal treatment plan aims to cover at least 95% of the target volume of the prescribed dose while maintaining dose heterogeneity within the range of −5% to +7%. Among the commonly used fractionation regimens, doses between 1.8 and 3 Gy per fraction are standard, with a threshold dose of 34 Gy generally considered effective for disease control. Ongoing studies (e.g., NCT02332408) are comparing conventional versus hypofractionated regimens to optimize pain relief and minimize side effects.

Toxicities: The acute toxicities include skin erythema, fatigue, and mild pain flare. Late toxicities, though rare, include fibrosis, vertebral fracture, and a very low risk of radiation-induced malignancy.

26.5 Summary

VHs are common benign vascular tumors of the spine, most often asymptomatic and incidentally detected. Aggressive or symptomatic cases, though rare, can cause significant morbidity due to pain, neurological deficits, and spinal instability. Management is tailored to clinical presentation and ranges from observation to surgery, embolization, vertebroplasty, and radiotherapy.

RT, especially with modern conformal and stereotactic techniques, has emerged as a cornerstone in the nonsurgical management of aggressive VHs. It provides effective symptom control, local disease stabilization, and a favorable safety profile.

Radiosurgery is a highly effective, non-invasive treatment for aggressive cases, particularly for patients unfit for surgery or with residual disease post-operatively.

A multidisciplinary approach, involving radiologists, neurosurgeons, and radiation oncologists, is essential for optimal patient care. Ongoing research and technological advances continue to refine the role of radiotherapy in VH management.

References

1. Rodallec MH, Feydy A, Larousserie F, Anract P, Campagna R, Babinet A, et al. Diagnostic imaging of solitary tumors of the spine: what to do and say. Radiographics [Internet] [cited 2025 Jun 5]. 2008;28(4):1019–41. https://pubmed.ncbi.nlm.nih.gov/18635627/
2. Pastushyn AI, Slin'ko EI, Mirzoyeva GM. Vertebral hemangiomas: diagnosis, management, natural history and clinicopathological correlates in 86 patients. Surg Neurol [Internet] Dec [cited 2025 Jun 4]. 1998;50(6):535–47. https://pubmed.ncbi.nlm.nih.gov/9870814/
3. Kato K, Teferi N, Challa M, Eschbacher K, Yamaguchi S. Vertebral hemangiomas: a review on diagnosis and management. J Orthop Surg Res., ISSN: 1749-799X. 19(1):310. https://doi.org/10.1186/s13018-024-04799-5.
4. Acosta FL, Sanai N, Chi JH, Dowd CF, Chin C, Tihan T, et al. Comprehensive management of symptomatic and aggressive vertebral hemangiomas. Neurosurg Clin N Am [Internet] Jan [cited 2025 Jun 4]. 2008;19(1):17–29. https://pubmed.ncbi.nlm.nih.gov/18156044/
5. Fox MW, Onofrio BM. The natural history and management of symptomatic and asymptomatic vertebral hemangiomas. J Neurosurg [Internet] [cited 2025 Jun 4]. 1993;78(1):36–45. https://pubmed.ncbi.nlm.nih.gov/8416240/
6. El Ouali I, Amalik S, Jerguigue H, Latib R, Omor Y. Vertebral hemangiomas: polka-dot and corduroy sign. Int J Clin Med Imaging. 2021;8:785.
7. Goldstein CL, Varga PP, Gokaslan ZL, Boriani S, Luzzati A, Rhines L, et al. Spinal hemangiomas: results of surgical management for local recurrence and mortality in a multicenter study. Spine (Phila Pa 1976) [Internet] May 1 [cited 2025 Jun 4]. 2015;40(9):656–64. https://pubmed.ncbi.nlm.nih.gov/26030216/
8. Gaudino S, Martucci M, Colantonio R, Lozupone E, Visconti E, Leone A, et al. A systematic approach to vertebral hemangioma. Skeletal Radiol [Internet] [cited 2025 Jun 4]. 2015;44(1):25–36. https://pubmed.ncbi.nlm.nih.gov/25348558/
9. Ross JS, Masaryk TJ, Modic MT, Carter JR, Mapstone T, Dengel FH. Vertebral hemangiomas: MR imaging. Radiology [Internet] [cited 2025 Jun 4]. 1987;165(1):165–9. https://pubmed.ncbi.nlm.nih.gov/3628764/
10. Hanrahan CJ, Christensen CR, Crim JR. Current concepts in the evaluation of multiple myeloma with MR imaging and FDG PET/CT. Radiographics [Internet] Jan [cited 2025 Jun 5]. 2010;30(1):127–42. https://pubmed.ncbi.nlm.nih.gov/20083590/
11. Laredo JD, Assouline E, Gelbert F, Wybier M, Merland JJ, Tubiana JM. Vertebral hemangiomas: Fat content as a sign of aggressiveness. Radiology [Internet] [cited 2025 Jun 5]. 1990;177(2):467–72. https://pubmed.ncbi.nlm.nih.gov/2217787/
12. McEvoy SH, Farrell M, Brett F, Looby S. Haemangioma, an uncommon cause of an extradural or intradural extramedullary mass: case series with radiological pathological correlation. Insights Imaging. 2016;7(1):87–98. https://doi.org/10.1007/s13244-015-0432-y. Epub 2015 Sep 18. PMID: 26385689; PMCID: PMC4729714
13. Enneking WF, Spanier SS, Goodman MA. A system for the surgical staging of musculoskeletal sarcoma. Clin Orthop Relat Res. 1980;153:106–20.
14. Teferi N, Chowdhury AJ, Mehdi Z, Challa M, Eschbacher K, Bathla G, Hitchon P. Surgical management of symptomatic vertebral heman-giomas: a single institution experience and literature review. Spine J. 2023;23(9):1243–54. https://doi.org/10.1016/j.spinee.2023.04.002. PMID: 37059306

15. Kato K, Teferi N, Challa M, Eschbacher K, Yamaguchi S. Vertebral hemangiomas: a review on diagnosis and management. J Orthop Surg Res [Internet] [cited 2025 Jun 4]. 2024;19(1):1–11. https://josr-online.biomedcentral.com/articles/10.1186/s13018-024-04799-5
16. Berkefeld J, Scale D, Kirchner J, Heinrich T, Kollath J. Hypervascular spinal tumors: Influence of the embolization technique on perioperative hemorrhage. Am J Neuroradiol [Internet] [cited 2025 Jun 5]. 1999;20(5):757–63. https://pubmed.ncbi.nlm.nih.gov/10369341/
17. Gupta AK, Phukan P, Bodhey N. Percutaneous vertebroplasty for the treatment of symptomatic vertebral hemangioma with long-term follow-up. Interdiscip Neurosurg. 2021;23:100968., ISSN 2214-7519. https://doi.org/10.1016/j.inat.2020.100968.
18. Tonosu J, Yamaguchi Y, Higashikawa A, Watanabe K. Ethanol sclerosis therapy for aggressive vertebral hemangioma of the spine: a narrative review. J Clin Med. 2023;12(12):3926. https://doi.org/10.3390/jcm12123926. PMID: 37373622; PMCID: PMC10298994
19. Miszczyk L, Tukiendorf A. Radiotherapy of painful vertebral hemangiomas: the single center retrospective analysis of 137 cases. Int J Radiat Oncol Biol Phys [Internet] Feb 1 [cited 2025 Jun 5]. 2012;82(2) https://pubmed.ncbi.nlm.nih.gov/21640516/
20. Pinar Sedeño B, et al. First reported treatment of aggressive hemangioma with intraoperative radiation therapy and kyphoplasty (Kypho-IORT). Clin Transl Radiat Oncol. 2017;2:19–22. https://doi.org/10.1016/j.ctro.2016.12.008/.
21. Wang B, Meng N, Zhuang H, Han S, Yang S, Jiang L, et al. The role of radiotherapy and surgery in the management of aggressive vertebral hemangioma: A retrospective study of 20 patients. Med Sci Monit [Internet] Sep 27 [cited 2025 Jun 5]. 2018;24:6840–50. https://pubmed.ncbi.nlm.nih.gov/30259906/
22. Heyd R, Seegenschmiedt MH, Rades D, Winkler C, Eich HT, Bruns F, et al. Radiotherapy for symptomatic vertebral hemangiomas: results of a multicenter study and literature review. Int J Radiat Oncol Biol Phys [Internet] [cited 2025 Jun 5]. 2010;77(1):217–25. https://pubmed.ncbi.nlm.nih.gov/19699592/
23. Aksoy RA, Aksu MG, Korcum AF, Genc M. Radiotherapy for vertebral hemangioma: the single-center experience of 80 patients. Strahlenther Onkol. 2022;198 https://doi.org/10.1007/s00066-022-01915-4.
24. Aich RK, Deb AR, Banerjee A, Karim R, Gupta P. Symptomatic vertebral hemangioma: treatment with radiotherapy. J Cancer Res Ther [Internet] [cited 2025 Jun 5]. 2010;6(2):199–203. https://pubmed.ncbi.nlm.nih.gov/20622368/
25. Zhang M, Chen YR, Chang SD, Veeravagu A. Cyber Knife stereotactic radiosurgery for the treatment of symptomatic vertebral hemangiomas: a single-institution experience. Neurosurg Focus. 2017;42(1):E13. https://doi.org/10.3171/2016.9.FOCUS16372.

Heterotopic Ossification

27

Kuldeep Sharma, Mohit Kadian, and Swarnita Sahu

27.1 Introduction

Heterotopic ossificans (HO) is the formation of mature lamellar bone in the soft tissues. The word heterotopic has been derived from the ancient Greek language, where "hetero" and "topos" mean "other" and "placement/place." It is also known as neurogenic osteoma, heterotopic calcification, neurogenic ossifying fibro myopathy, paraosteoarthropathy, myositis ossificans, periarticular new bone formation and periarticular ectopic ossification [1]. It was first described in 1692 by a French physician named Patin who termed it as myositis ossificans progressiva [2]. Later in 1918, during the World War I, Dejerine and Ceilier elaborated this condition in soldiers as a consequence of military wounds [3] describing it as para-osteoarthropathy. It was found to be one of the reason for long-term morbidity in injured service personnel [4]. The prevalence of HO is gradually seen more among the military soldiers because of the availability of immediate medical care and better rehabilitation programs leading to their long-term survival even after severe injuries to the extremities [5]. Impaired wound healing and bacterial colonization are the few wound-related factors that are responsible for the development of HO in this population. This condition leads to the disturbance in local microvasculature, making the soft tissues hypoxic and acidic, which further modulates the cell lineages in the soft tissues.

K. Sharma (✉) · M. Kadian · S. Sahu
Radiation Oncology, Venkateshwar Hospital, New Delhi, India
e-mail: dr_kuldeepsharma@yahoo.co.in;
mohit.kadian@venkateshwarhospitals.com; swarnita.sahu@venkateshwarhospitals.com

K. Sood Sharma (ed.), *Radiation Therapy for Benign Disorders*,
https://doi.org/10.1007/978-981-95-6635-8_27

27.2 Epidemiology

HO can broadly be classified into genetic or nongenetic type (neurogenic and traumatic). While the genetic type of HO mostly affects the children [6], the more common nongenetic type affects the young adults, mostly men in their second and third decades [7].

27.2.1 Types

1. Genetic
   - Fibrodysplasia ossificans progressiva (FOP): It is a rare condition caused by ACVR1/ALK2 mutations, which can either be spontaneous or caused by autosomal dominant transmission. It first presents in childhood either spontaneously or after trauma. Multiple congenital anomalies (like abnormalities in the first toe, digits of hands, and cervical spine) are also associated with FOP. It is characterized by progressive ossification of tendon, muscles, and ligaments. It gradually progresses by early adulthood leading to ankyloses of all the major joints of the axial and the appendicular skeleton [8]. Biopsies or any kind of surgical intervention should be avoided in this condition, as it may lead to further progression of the disease. FOP generally appears as well-circumscribed areas of HO in radiographs. There is no definitive treatment for FOP; rather, it is managed symptomatically.
   - Progressive osseous heteroplasia (POH) and Albright's hereditary osteodystrophy (AHO): It is related to mutations in GNAS1 gene, which can again be either spontaneous or by autosomal dominant transmission. It is also a rare condition starting from infancy, initially causing dermal HO and gradually progressing to the deeper tissues [9]. POH appears as a cocoon-like web of HO in radiographs. There is again no cure for this condition except for supportive and rehabilitative care.
2. Neurogenic:

Neurogenic HO is usually seen after any type of insult to central nervous system, mostly after major head or spinal trauma. The most common joint involved is hip followed by shoulder and elbow [10]. Other less common causes associated with HO are epidural abscess, tetanus, meningitis, brain tumors, subarachnoid hemorrhage, myelitis, and encephalitis.

3. Traumatic:

The most common injuries are fractures, dislocations, burns, and operative procedures. In cases of trauma, HO usually occurs around joints but has also been reported in the soft tissues, located away from the joints [11]. The most commonly affected joint is the hip either after its fracture and open reduction internal fixation or after total hip arthroplasty (THA). Other sites are shoulder, knee, ankle, and temporomandibular joint.

27.3 Pathophysiology

The process of normal bone formation comprises a signaling pathway (chemical mediators), which triggers the osteoprogenitor cells (capable of being differentiated into bone-forming osteoclasts) in an environment conducive for osteogenesis. The process of osteogenesis along with the osteoclast resorption enables the skeletal system to adapt to normal physiological processes (growth or increase in physical activity) allowing a slow metabolic turnover of normal bone [12].

The exact pathophysiology of HO is still unclear. A per Kirsch, the pathological bone formation in HO is due to the molecular mechanisms involved in normal bone formation, present in extra-skeletal sites (soft tissue, cartilage, blood vessels, and muscles). It has been recently reported that an acidic environment is capable of reprogramming pluripotent cells from one lineage to another [13]. Some studies have demonstrated the role of released chemokines, inflammatory cytokines (like human monocyte chemotactic protein 1, IL-10, and IL-6) and proteins (macrophage inflammatory protein, interferon inducible protein) after penetrating injuries to the extremities [14]. All these biochemical imbalances can lead to the development of HO as a result of localized and systemic hyper-inflammatory response to the index injury. The ability of progenitor cells from the extra-skeletal tissues to be capable of differentiating into osteoprogenitor cells (osteoblastic cells), further boosts new bone formation [15].

27.4 Clinical Presentation

It usually presents as an incidental finding on an X-ray, which is usually evident around six weeks after the traumatic insult [16]. Bone scan can detect HO as early as three weeks after trauma. When symptomatic, it presents as decreased range of motion associated with localized warmth, mild edema, and erythema gradually leading to complete bony ankyloses in later stages [17]. It can be radiologically classified in two different ways depending on the anatomic location. First is Broker classification [18] and other is Hasting's and Graham Classification [19] (Tables 27.1 and 27.2).

Table 27.1 Broker classification system for hip

I	Islands of bone within soft tissues of the hip
II	Bone spurs in the pelvis or femur (with >/= 1 cm gap between the opposing bony surfaces)
III	Bone spurs within the pelvis or femur (with <1 cm gap between the opposing bony surfaces)
IV	Ankyloses of the hip

Table 27.2 Hastings and Graham classification for elbow

I	Radiographic evidence without functional deficit
IIA	Radiographic evidence with limitation in flexion-extension axis
IIB	Radiographic evidence with limitation in pronation-supination axis
IIIA	Ectopic bone formation and ankyloses of joint in flexion-extension axis
IIIB	Ectopic bone formation and ankyloses of joint in pronation-supination axis
IIIC	Ectopic bone formation and ankyloses of joint in flexion-extension and pronation-supination axis

27.5 Risk Factors

1. Traumatic Spinal-Cord or Brain Injuries:

It accounts for 10–53% of the HO. It occurs a few months after injury and progresses over next few years. The exact correlation between nervous system and bone formation is unknown but studies have shown that the peripheral neurotransmitters can affect the osteoblast formation. The severity of HO depends on the severity and the level of spinal cord injury, with cervical and thoracic level injuries being more severe. Patients with low-thoracic or high-cervical cord injuries are more prone to develop this condition. Patients with severe spasticity, impaired cognition, pneumonia, tracheostomy, and urinary tract infections are at higher risk. HO tends to appear caudal to the level of injury (most common being the hip) in cases of spinal cord injuries, while it can occur anywhere in the body (hip, knee, elbow, or shoulder) in case of traumatic brain injuries [20].

2. Thermal Injuries:

The extent of burn is directly related to the risk of developing HO, which usually occurs in cases affecting >20% of the body surface area. The other risk factors are being male sex and having full thickness burn or burn near a joint. The elbow is the most common joint affected, followed by shoulder and hip [21].

Scar contractures can easily be confused with HO. X-rays and clinical examination can help distinguish between them. Palpation of a locking sensation on extension/flexion of a joint usually indicates HO in such cases.

3. Surgical Trauma

Around 40 percent postoperative cases of acetabular fractures/hip arthroplasty develop HO to some extent. The most common risk factors in such cases are male gender, history of prior surgery at same site, history of ankyloses spondylitis, extended ischemia time, use of cemented implants, type of approach, concomitant nerve injury, delayed internal fixation and use of bone graft or its substitutes [22].

27.6 Diagnosis

27.6.1 Radiology

Radiographs are usually the most common modality for diagnosis of HO. The classic picture is appearance of well-demarcated radio-dense mass with a zonal ossification process also known as eggshell calcification (Fig. 27.1a, b). Early stages show flocculent opacities without any zonal demarcation. It usually appears in soft tissue but may attach to bony surface sometimes (paraosteal HO). The attachment to the bone is usually focal but can also be broad-based. In some cases of paraosteal HO, the periosteal reaction may obscure the classic radiographic picture of HO. HO along the tendons and ligaments has a different radiological appearance, which usually follows the anatomy of affected structure.

Apart from plain radiographs, CT (computed tomographs) scans have a characteristic appearance showing the zonal maturation of the lesion [23]. It shows a low-density mass in early HO, but the appearance can be more characteristic after the appearance of peripheral calcification at a later stage in follow-up CT. Although CT scans are not used routinely for diagnosis, but it is a useful tool in preoperative planning for having a better visualization of the lesion along with the 3-dimensional exact measurements and relationship with adjacent anatomic structures.

MRI shows a variable appearance, depending on the stage of maturation. In early stages, there is presence of fluid-filled areas because of hemorrhage. Central enhancement of contrast sometimes makes it difficult to differentiate it from soft tissue sarcoma. As the HO matures, the appearance of zonal enhancement of contrast helps in differentiating it from sarcoma.

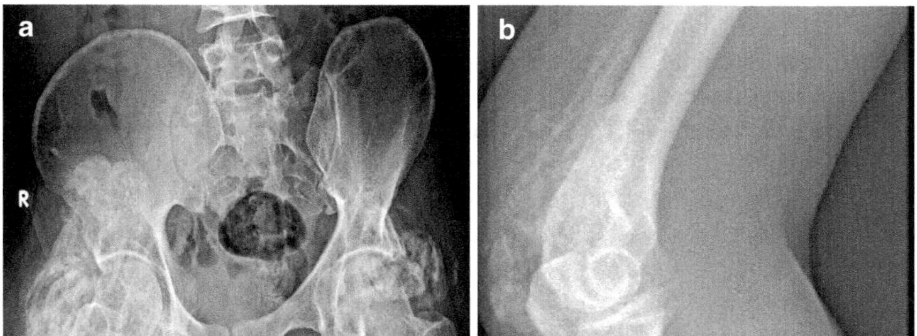

Fig. 27.1 A young adult who had polytrauma in a road traffic accident. (**a**) Heterotopic ossificans with zonal maturation of the lesion in bilateral hip joint (Rt > Lt). (**b**) Early phase of HO showing flocculant opacities

Other less commonly used diagnostic modalities are PET (positron emission tomography) [24], Single positron emission imaging [25], Raman spectroscopy, near-infrared imaging and ultrasonography.

27.6.2 Pathology

Early lesions of HO are hypercellular with very little bone matrix, while the advanced lesions show prominent bone formation with zonal ossification, which is the hallmark of HO. It is well circumscribed by thick blood vessels forming a fibrous pseudo-capsule.

HO can be confused with extra-skeletal sarcoma or osteosarcoma. A gradual change of woven bone to mature bone often helps in distinguishing HO from extra-skeletal sarcoma. Another differentiating feature of HO is that it does not show any nuclear atypia [26].

27.7 Management

It can be divided into prophylaxis and treatment depending on the stage at which the patient presents. Most of the current studies are confined to management of nongenetic forms [27].

A. Prophylaxis
   1. NSAID—Non-steroidal anti-inflammatory drugs are the most commonly used agents for prophylaxis. The gold standard is Indomethacin (25 mg thrice daily for up to 6 weeks) used in the postoperative period. Recently, COX-2 inhibitors are preferred over non-selective NSAIDs due to better GI (gastrointestinal) side-effect profile. NSAIDs are also known to cause non-union in fracture healing [28].
   2. Bisphosponates—These have antiresorptive mechanisms, which induce osteoclast apoptosis and hence inhibit calcification. While some authors say it is effective for prevention of HO, others do not support this [29, 30].
   3. Radiation Therapy—It has emerged as an effective modality. It is an alternative to Indomethacin as it eliminates the risk of GI toxicity and non-union of fractures associated with the use of NSAIDs. It is, however, costlier than the conventional NSAIDs, has its own radiation-induced side effects but can be considered in properly selected cases [31]. Experiments led by Caven and Urist [32] in 1971 suggested that the osteoprogenitor cells present in the early phase of HO are radiosensitive due to their high mitotic rate and are thus inhibited by radiation. Radiation is not effective once HO sets in as the proportion of radio-resistant or the mature cells increases [33]. This makes the timing of radiotherapy in postoperative cases a very crucial factor in the prophylaxis of HO. The limited time interval between surgery and postoperative radiotherapy usually becomes an obstacle in timely delivery of

Table 27.3 Important studies regarding radiotherapy in HO

Authors	Conclusion
Coventry et al. 1981 [34]	RT is effective for HO
Lo et al. 1988 [35]	Single fraction [7 Gy (Gray)] is effective
Pelligrini et al. 1992 [36]	Single fraction is similar to fractionated RT
Gregoritch et al. 1994 [37]	Preoperative RT is similar to postoperative RT
Pakos et al. 2004 [38]	RT is more effective than NSAIDS

radiotherapy. The most important being the difficulty in sequencing and transportation of the patient to a radiation facility just after surgery when mobilization of the operated area is restricted due to pain and postoperative care is being still ongoing.

Few important studies regarding the role of radiotherapy in HO have been reported in the literature (Table 27.3):

Most of the studies are conducted on patients with hip arthroplasty, and the results have been extrapolated from those studies for other sites [39]. Low-dose radiotherapy has been studied for prevention of occurrence and recurrence of HO. Doses usually range from 4 Gy to 8 Gy, which are given either 24 hours before surgery or 72 hours after surgery. Higher doses have not proven to provide any extra benefit [31] while having higher potential for adverse effects. The current standard practice is single-fraction radiotherapy of 7 Gy or 8 Gy delivered within 24 hours preoperatively or 72 hours postoperatively. Another common regimen is dose of 17.5 Gy (3.5 Gy for 5 daily fractions) delivered in the postoperative period to the patients with high risk factors [40].

HO usually develops between the head of femur and pelvis, involving the greater trochanter of the femur to the ilium and/or the lesser trochanter of the femur to the ischium. This has to be considered while planning radiation fields for treatment. The treatment portals are marked from 3 cm above the acetabulum to 3 cm below the lesser trochanter. The upper third of the implant (if present) shaft is also included. The surrounding soft tissues should be shielded, allowing a margin of 1.5–2 cm from the bone and the prior areas of HO, if any [41]. Most of the prosthesis used in HO are cementless with porous surfaces allowing bony ingrowth for fixation of prosthesis. Studies have shown that radiotherapy may inhibit the bony ingrowth leading to failure of the prosthesis. Hence, shielding of the prosthesis are also advised by the authors [42]. Thus, the target volume being treated by conformal techniques should include the whole joint along with typical locations of HO with a margin of 1–2 cm [43].

Since most of the patients of HO are young adults of productive age group, it is important to consider treatment related adverse effects related to radiotherapy. The most concerning side effect of radiotherapy is carcinogenesis even though there are no documented cases [44]. Thus, it is advisable to always prescribe the lowest possible dose effective for a particular disease and to reduce exposure of uninvolved organs to the minimum. Reduction in sperm count and radiation-induced hereditary effects are the other potential concerns. Dose of 1.2 Gy or more is considered to cause permanent azoospermia [45]. Trochanteric nonunion or prosthesis failure are also other potential side effects that can occur in cases where the prosthesis or the osteotomy sites are not properly shielded [46]. Studies have revealed that pre- or postoperative radiotherapy can prevent HO by about 90% after hip replacement surgeries [47].

B. Treatment
   1. Physical Therapy: Definitive measures are lacking. While few recommend physical therapy to increase range of movements and decrease risk of contractures [48], other studies caution against it as passive exercises could increase inflammation that can further aggravate development of HO.
   2. Surgery: Complete resection of HO is rarely possible; incomplete surgeries are associated with recurrences. Unlike neoplastic lesions, HO is known to invade natural anatomic boundaries and hence can encase neurovascular bundles post-surgery [49]. Soft tissue coverage becomes another challenge in surgeries of HO resulting from burn injuries in view of scarring, relative laxity of surrounding soft tissue injury, and tenuous skin grafts.

27.8 Conclusion

HO is an entity that leads to lot of morbidity in cases of surgical and physical trauma. Prompt and accurate diagnosis and initiation of timely preventive and treatment measures are the key management strategies currently. The main treatment is either medical or radiotherapy. The surgical option is reserved only for advanced symptomatic cases who have failed other conservative management. Good functional outcome with limited risk of recurrence has been observed in cases where surgery is combined with other preventive measures (COX2 inhibitors/radiotherapy).

27.9 Future Direction

In future, the incidence of HO can be reduced by research focusing on better understanding of pathophysiology, prevention, and treatment of HO. The use of NSAIDs, radiotherapy, and surgery for prevention and treatment of HO has its own limitations, demanding the need of development of better modalities.

Bone morphogenetic protein (BMP) inhibitors and nuclear retinoic acid receptor-gamma (RARγ) agonists are being studied as new targets to address the pathological processes of HO formation [50]. The ongoing studies look forward to reshape the future of HO management.

Bibliography

1. Sawyer JR, Myers MA, Rosier RN, et al. Heterotopic ossification: clinical and cellular aspects. Calcif Tissue Int. 1991;49:208–15.
2. Geschickter CF, Maseritz I. Myositis ossificans. J Bone Joint Surg Am. 1938;20:661–74.
3. Khalaf ibn 'Abbās AQ. Albucasis: on surgery and instruments. Translated by Spink MS and Lewis GL. Berkeley: University of California Press, 1973.
4. Dougherty PJ, McFarland LV, Smith DG, et al. Multiple traumatic limb loss: a comparison of Vietnam veterans to OIF/OEF servicemembers. J Rehabil Res Dev. 2010;47:333–48.
5. Brown KV, Clasper JC. The changing pattern of amputations. J R Army Med Corps. 2013;159:300–3.
6. Sankar R, Gowrishankar K, Viswanathan S. Genetic disorders with heterotopic ossificans. Indian J Orthop. 2015;49(3):361–4. https://doi.org/10.4103/0019-5413.156228. PMID: 26015640; PMCID: PMC4443422.
7. Dorfman HD, Czerniak B. Bone tumors. Maryland Heights, MO: Mosby; 1998.
8. Cohen RB, Hahn GV, Tabas JA, et al. The natural history of heterotopic ossification in patients who have fibrodysplasia ossificans progressiva. A study of forty-four patients. J Bone Joint Surg Am. 1993;75:215–9.
9. Shore EM, Ahn J, Jan de Beur S, et al. Paternally inherited inactivating mutations of the GNAS1 gene in progressive osseous heteroplasia. N Engl J Med. 2002;346:99–106.
10. Garland DE, Blum CE, Waters RL. Periarticular heterotopic ossification in head-injured adults. Incidence and location. J Bone Joint Surg Am. 1980;62:1143–6.
11. Garland DE. A clinical perspective on common forms of acquired heterotopic ossification. Clin Orthop Relat Res. 1991;263:13–29.
12. Chalmers J, Gray DH, Rush J. Observations on the induction of bone in soft tissues. J Bone Joint Surg Br. 1975;57:36–45.
13. Kaplan FS, Glaser DL, Hebela N, et al. Heterotopic ossification. J Am Acad Orthop Surg. 2004;12:116–25.
14. Evans KN, Forsberg JA, Potter BK, et al. Inflammatory cytokine and chemokine expression is associated with heterotopic ossification in high-energy penetrating war injuries. J Orthop Trauma. 2012;26:e204–13.
15. Davis TA, O'Brien FP, Anam K, et al. Heterotopic ossification in complex orthopaedic combat wounds: quantification and characterization of osteogenic precursor cell activity in traumatized muscle. J Bone Joint Surg Am. 2011;93:1122–31.
16. Orzel JA, Rudd TG. Heterotopic bone formation: clinical, laboratory, and imaging correlation. J Nucl Med. 1985;26(125):132.
17. Xu Y, Huang M, He W, He C, Chen K, Hou J, Huang M, Jiao Y, Liu R, Zou N, Liu L, Li C. Heterotopic ossification: clinical features, basic researches, and mechanical stimulations. Front Cell Dev Biol. 2022;10:770931. https://doi.org/10.3389/fcell.2022.770931. PMID: 35145964; PMCID: PMC8824234.
18. Brooker AF, Bowerman JW, Robinson RA, Riley LH Jr. Ectopic ossification fol lowing total hip replacement. Incidence and a method of classification. J Bone Joint Surg Am. 1973;55(8):1629–32.
19. Hastings H 2nd, Graham TJ. The classification and treatment of heterotopic ossification about the elbow and forearm. Hand Clin. 1994;10(3):417–37.
20. Sullivan MP, Torres SJ, Mehta S, Ahn J. Heterotopic ossification after central nervous system trauma: a current review. Bone Joint Res. 2013;2(3):51-57. Epub 2013 Mar 1.
21. Medina A, Shankowsky H, Savaryn B, Shukalak B, Tredget EE. Characterization of heterotopic ossification in burn patients. J Burn Care Res. 2014;35(3):251–6.
22. Chen HC, Yang JY, Chuang SS, Huang CY, Yang SY. Heterotopic ossification in burns: our experience and literature reviews. Burns. 2009;35(6):857–62. Epub 2009 May 29.
23. McCarthy EF, Sundaram M. Heterotopic ossification: a review. Skeletal Radiol. 2005;34(10):609–19.

24. Kransdorf MJ, Meis JM, Jelinek JS. Myositis ossificans: MR appearance with radiologic-pathologic correlation. AJR Am J Roentgenol. 1991;157(6):1243–8.
25. Deryk S, Goethals L, Vanhove C, et al. Imaging characteristics of heterotopic mesenteric ossification on FDG PET and Tc-99m bone SPECT. Clin Nucl Med. 2008;33(7):496–9.
26. Cocks M, Mohan A, Meyers CA, et al. Vascular patterning in human heterotopic ossification. Hum Pathol. 2017;63:165–70.
27. Winkler S, Wagner F, Weber M, et al. Current therapeutic strategies of heterotopic ossification––a survey amongst orthopaedic and trauma departments in Germany. BMC Musculoskelet Disord. 2015;16:313.
28. Ritter MA, Sieber JM. Prophylactic indomethacin for the prevention of heterotopic boneformationfollowingtotalhiparthroplasty. Clin Orthop Relat Res. 1985;196:217–25.
29. Crane NJ, Elster EA. Vibrational spectroscopy: a tool being developed for the noninvasive monitoring of wound healing. J Biomed Opt. 2012;17(1):010902.
30. Shafer DM, Bay C, Caruso DM, Foster KN. The use of eidronate disodium in the prevention of heterotopic ossification in burn patients. Burns. 2008;34(3):355–60. Epub 2007 Sep 14.
31. Popovic M, Agarwal A, Zhang L, et al. Radiotherapy for the prophylaxis of heterotopic ossification: a systematic review and meta-analysis of published data. Radiother Oncol. 2014;113(1):10–7.
32. Cooley LM, Goss RJ. The effects of transplantation and x-irradiation on the repair of fractured bones. Am J Anat. 1958;102:167–81.
33. Craven PL, Urist MR. Osteogenesis by radioisotope labelled cell populations in implants of bone matrix under the influence of ionizing radiation. Clin Orthop Relat Res. 1971;76:231–3.
34. Helal BM. C OVENTRY (Ed.) The 1981 year book of orthopedics. Br J Sports Med. 1982;16:90.
35. Lo TC, Healy WL, Covall DJ, et al. Heterotopic bone forma tion after hip surgery: prevention with single-dose postoper ative hip irradiation. Radiology. 1988;168:851–4.
36. Pellegrini VD Jr, Konski AA, Gastel JA, et al. Prevention of heterotopic ossification with irradiation after total hip arthro plasty. Radiation therapy with a single dose of eight hundred centigray administered to a limited field. J Bone Joint Surg Am. 1992;74:186–200.
37. Seegenschmiedt MH, Keilholz L, Martus P, et al. Prevention of heterotopic ossification about the hip: final results of two randomized trials in 410 patients using either preoperative or postoperative radiation therapy. Int J Radiat Oncol Biol Phys. 1997;39:161–71.
38. Pakos EE, Ioannidis JP. Radiotherapy vs. nonsteroidal anti inflammatory drugs for the prevention of heterotopic ossifica tion after major hip procedures: a meta-analysis of random ized trials. Int J Radiat Oncol Biol Phys. 2004;60:888–95.
39. Mishra MV, Austin L, Parvizi J, Ramsey M, Showalter TN. Safety and efficacy of radiation therapy as secondary prophylaxis for heterotopic ossification of non-hip joints. J Med Imaging Radiat Oncol. 2011;55(3):333–6.
40. Reinartz G, Eich HT, Pohl F; German Cooperative Group on Radiotherapy for Benign Diseases (GCG-BD). DEGRO practical guidelines for the radiotherapy of non-malignant disorders - part IV: symptomatic functional disorders. Strahlenther Onkol. 2015;191(4):295–302. https://doi.org/10.1007/s00066-014-0789-8. Epub 2014 Dec 9.
41. Lee A, Maani EV, Amin NP. Radiation Therapy for Heterotopic Ossification Prophylaxis. [Updated 2022 Oct 3]. In.
42. Konski A, Weiss C, Rosier R, et al. The use of postoperative irradiation for the prevention of heterotopic bone after total hip replacement with biologic fixation (porous coated) pros thesis: an animal model. Int J Radiat Oncol Biol Phys. 1990;18:861–5.
43. Pakos EE, Ioannidis JP. Radiotherapy vs. nonsteroidal anti-inflammatory drugs for the prevention of heterotopic ossification after major hip procedures: a meta-analysis of randomized trials. Int J Radiat Oncol Biol Phys. 2004;60(3):888–95. https://doi.org/10.1016/j.ijrobp.2003.11.015.
44. Sheybani A, TenNapel MJ, Lack WD, et al. Risk of radiation-induced malignancy with heterotopic ossification prophylaxis: a case control analysis. Int J Radiat Oncol Biol Phys. 2014;89(3):584–9.

45. Kim JH, Chu FC, Woodard HQ, et al. Radiation-induced soft-tissue and bone sarcoma. Radiology. 1978;129:501–8.
46. Coventry MB, Scanlon PW. The use of radiation to discourage ectopic bone. A nine-year study in surgery about the hip. J Bone Joint Surg Am. 1981;63:201–8.
47. Seegenschmiedt MH, et al. Radiation prophylaxis for heterotopic ossification about the hip joint—a multicenter study. Int J Radiat Oncol Biol Phys. 51(3):756–65.
48. Aronen JG, Garrick JG, Chronister RD, McDevitt ER. Quadriceps contusions: clinical results of immediate immobilization in 120 degrees of knee flexion. Clin J Sport Med. 2006;16(5):383–7.
49. Pavey GJ, Polfer EM, Nappo KE, Tintle SM, Forsberg JA, Potter BK. What risk factors predict recurrence of heterotopic ossification after excision in combat-related amputations? Clin Orthop Relat Res. 2015;473(9):2814–24.
50. Hwang CD, Pagani CA, Nunez JH, Cherief M, Qin Q, Gomez-Salazar M, Kadaikal B, Kang H, Chowdary AR, Patel N, James AW, Levi B. Contemporary perspectives on heterotopic ossification. JCI Insight. 2022;7(14):e158996. https://doi.org/10.1172/jci.insight.158996. PMID: 35866484; PMCID: PMC9431693.

Pigmented Villonodular Synovitis

28

Adhar Amritt and Supriya Mallick

28.1 Introduction

Pigmented villonodular synovitis (PVNS) is a rare, benign yet locally aggressive proliferative condition affecting synovial tissue. It was first described in 1941 by Jaffe, Lichtenstein, and Sutro as "pigmented villonodular synovitis, bursitis, and tenosynovitis" [1]. This disease is characterized by hyperplasia of the synovium, often associated with hemosiderin deposition, lipid-laden macrophages, multinucleated giant cells, and chronic inflammation. The annual incidence is less than 2 cases per million population [2]. The clinical manifestations of PVNS include joint swelling, pain, stiffness, and occasionally mechanical symptoms such as locking or giving way. The knee is the most affected joint, followed by the hip, ankle, and shoulder. The typical age distribution is in the third to fourth decade.

PVNS exists in two main forms as described by Granowitz [3]:

- "Localized PVNS": Involves discrete nodular masses, typically within the synovium.
- "Diffuse PVNS": Involves widespread proliferation of the synovium, often encasing the joint and invading periarticular structures.

A. Amritt
Department of Radiation Oncology, National Cancer Institute-Jhajjar, All India Institute of Medical Sciences, New Delhi, India

S. Mallick (✉)
Department of Radiation Oncology, All India Institute of Medical Sciences, New Delhi, India

Department of Radiation Oncology, National Cancer Institute-Jhajjar, All India Institute of Medical Sciences, New Delhi, India

K. Sood Sharma (ed.), *Radiation Therapy for Benign Disorders*,
https://doi.org/10.1007/978-981-95-6635-8_28

While the exact etiology remains unclear, PVNS is thought to result from an abnormal inflammatory or neoplastic process driven by chromosomal translocations leading to overexpression of colony-stimulating factor 1 (CSF1) [4, 5].

28.2 Diagnosis

Diagnosis of PVNS often involves a combination of clinical evaluation, imaging, and histopathological analysis. Most common presenting symptoms include pain and swelling around joints, which is intermittent and often long standing.

Imaging: MRI is the gold standard for diagnosing PVNS, showing characteristic findings such as hemosiderin deposition (blooming artifact on gradient echo sequences), joint effusion, and synovial thickening [6].

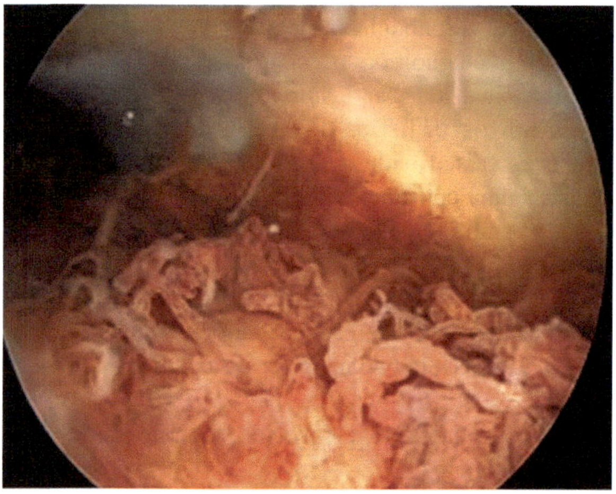

Fig. 28.1 Still image from video of knee arthroscopy performed because of suspected synovitis. Multiple reddish brown frondlike or villous synovial projections are noted throughout the visualized joint

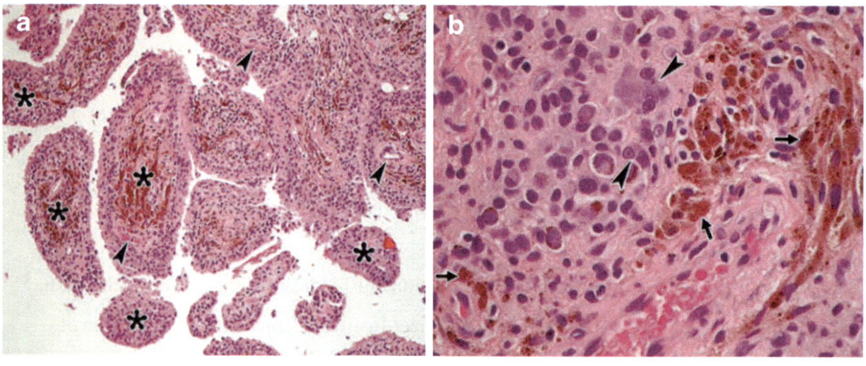

Fig. 28.2 (**a**)100X, H-E show villous architecture (*) and hypervascularity (arrowheads) of synovium (**b**) 400X, H-E stain, multinucleated giant cells (arrowheads) and monomorphic population of round cells among fibrous stroma and multiple vascular channels. Brown pigment (hemosiderin), intra- and extracellularly (arrows). (Used with permission [8])

Arthrocentesis/Arthrogram (Fig. 28.1): Macroscopically there is proliferation of synovium and presence of brownish villi.

Histopathology: Biopsy reveals multinucleated giant cells, hemosiderin-laden macrophages (Fig. 28.2a), and mononuclear stromal cells (Fig. 28.2b), confirming the diagnosis [7].

28.3 Management of PVNS

28.3.1 Surgical Treatment

The primary treatment for PVNS is surgical resection of the affected synovium either through arthroscopic or open techniques.

Hence, surgery alone has a significant recurrence rate, particularly for diffuse PVNS, with rates reported to be as high as 40% to 60% in some studies. Challenges include complete removal of synovial tissue and the potential for postoperative complications such as joint stiffness and instability [9, 10].

28.3.2 Role of Radiotherapy

Radiotherapy has emerged as an effective adjunctive treatment for PVNS, particularly in cases of incomplete surgical resection, recurrent disease, or contraindications to surgery. Both external beam radiotherapy (EBRT) and intra-articular radioactive synovectomy have been used in the management of PVNS [11].

A. *Mechanism of Radiotherapy in PVNS*
   Radiotherapy exerts its effects by targeting the proliferative synovial tissue, inducing DNA damage that inhibits cellular replication and reduces inflammation. The anti-inflammatory effects of radiotherapy also contribute to symptom relief.
B. *Techniques of Radiotherapy*:
   (a) External Beam Radiotherapy (EBRT): EBRT typically involves the delivery of a moderate dose of radiation over several fractions to minimize toxicity to surrounding tissues [12].
   Acceptable dose fractionations used—35Gy/15# or 40 Gy/20# or 45 Gy/25# [11].
   CTV = Entire PVNS mass (Fig. 28.3) or whole synovial space [13].
   PTV = 5 mm or immobilization specific margin.
   Advanced techniques such as intensity-modulated radiotherapy (IMRT) or proton therapy may be employed to improve precision and reduce dose to adjacent structures.
   (b) Radiosynoviorthesis (Radioactive Synovectomy):
   - Involves the intra-articular injection of radioactive isotopes such as yttrium-90, rhenium-186, or erbium-169 [14].
   - Particularly useful for patients with contraindications to surgery or those with small, localized disease recurrence.

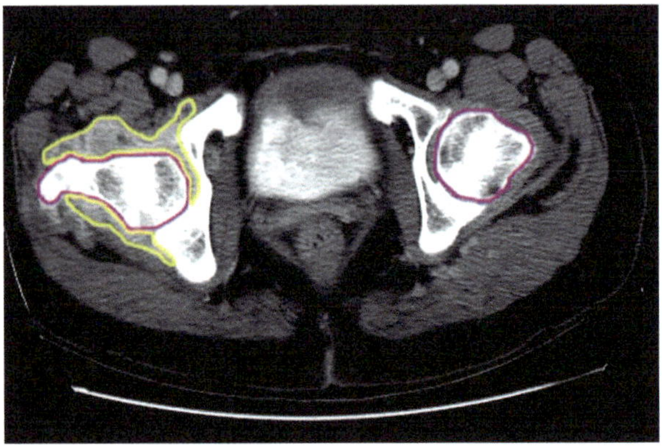

Fig. 28.3 Residual disease (yellow) and right femur (pink)

C. *Indications for Radiotherapy*

- Postoperative treatment for incomplete resection.
- Recurrent PVNS after one or more surgeries [15].
- Primary treatment in patients who are not surgical candidates.

D. *Outcomes and Efficacy*
Multiple studies have demonstrated the efficacy of radiotherapy in reducing recurrence rates and improving functional outcomes (Table 28.1). For instance, recurrence rates after combined surgery and radiotherapy are reported to be significantly lower compared to surgery alone. Symptomatic relief, including reduced pain and swelling, is observed in most patients undergoing radiotherapy [31].

E. *Potential Complications*
While generally well-tolerated, radiotherapy can have potential side effects, including:
- Radiation-induced joint stiffness.
- Skin changes or fibrosis in the treated area.
- Rarely, secondary malignancies in the irradiated field, though this is exceedingly rare with modern techniques and doses [12, 32].

Table 28.1 Review of literature and relevant studies for post-operative RT

Author	Site	Year	Total (RT)	Median dose (Gy)	Median F/up	Recurrence
Sun et al. [16]	Hip	2022	16(8)	10–30	24 mos	0(LC-100%)
Chien et al. [17]	Knee	2021	24(14)	35(20–40)	72 mos	10/249(LC-95%)
Al-Hajri et al. [18]	Knee	2021	5(5)	30–36	54 mos	0(LC-100%)
Yang et al. [19]	TMJ	2019	1(1)	40	24 mos	0(LC-100%)
Duan et al. [20]	Knee	2018	1(1)	30/15#	36 mos	1(LC-100%)
Serra et al. [21]	Shoulder	2017	1(1)	40/20#	12 mos	0(LC-100%)
Mollon et al. [22]	Knee	2015	630(123)	30Gy/15#	60 mos	14/123(LC-88.6%)
Li et al. [23]	Knee	2015	28(26)	20–30	54 mos	0(LC-100%)
Joshi et al. [11]	TMJ	2015	71(8)	35	18 mos	2(LC-68%)
de Carvalho et al. [24]	Knee	2012	8(8)	20(10–39.6)	100 mos	1(LC-92.5%)
Park et al. [25]	Knee	2012	23(23)	20(12–34)	96 mos	0(LC-100%)
Griffin et al. [26]	Knee	2011	50(50)	39.8	94 mos	3(LC-94%)
Li et al.	Hip	2011	1(1)	35	24 mos	1(LC-0%)
Horoschak et al. [27]	Knee	2009	18(18)	34	46 mos	4(LC-75%)
Berger et al. [13]	Knee	2007	7(7)	40(30–50)	29 mos	0(LC-100%)
Lee et al.	Foot ankle	2005	7(7)	35	24 mos	0(LC-100%)
O'Sullivan et al. [28]	Knee	2005	41(41)	35(28–50)	77 mos	1(LC-98%)
Blanco et al. [29]	Knee	2001	22(22)	26Gy	33 mos	LC- 86%
Kotwal et al. [30]	Knee	2000	14(14)	20	NA	14/14(100%)

28.4 Future Perspectives and Research Directions

Emerging therapies targeting the molecular pathogenesis of PVNS are being explored, such as:

Tyrosine kinase inhibitors (e.g., Vimseltinib, an FDA approved CSF1R inhibitor, Pexidarinib, Nilotinib, Imatinib).
Monoclonal antibody to CSF1R inhibitor (Emactuzumab).

These agents may complement or, in some cases, replace traditional modalities like surgery and radiotherapy. Research into optimizing radiotherapy techniques to further minimize toxicity while maintaining efficacy continues to evolve, with advances in imaging and treatment planning [33, 34].

28.5 Conclusion

Pigmented villonodular synovitis is a challenging condition requiring a multidisciplinary approach for optimal management. While surgery remains the cornerstone of treatment, radiotherapy provides a valuable adjunctive or alternative therapy, particularly in diffuse or recurrent cases. Therefore, the integration of novel molecular therapies and advanced radiotherapy techniques holds a definite promise for improving outcomes for patients with this rare debilitating condition

References

1. Larmon WA. Pigmented villonodular synovitis. Med Clin North Am [Internet]. 1965;49(1):141–50. Available from: https://linkinghub.elsevier.com/retrieve/pii/S0025712516333569.
2. Mendenhall WM, Mendenhall CM, Reith JD, Scarborough MT, Gibbs CP, Mendenhall NP. Pigmented villonodular synovitis. Am J Clin Oncol. 2006:548–50.
3. Granowitz SP, Mankin HJ. Localized pigmented villonodular synovitis of the knee report of five cases. J Bone Joint Surg. 1967;49(1):122–8.
4. Jaffe Henry L Tumors and tumorous conditions of the bones and joints. Cancer. Philadelphia; 1959 January/February.
5. West RB, Rubin BP, Miller MA, Subramanian S, Kaygusuz G, Montgomery K, et al. A landscape effect in tenosynovial giant-cell tumor from activation of CSF1 expression by a translocation in a minority of tumor cells [Internet]. 2005. Available from: https://doi.org/10.1073/pnas.0507321103
6. Narváez JA, Narváez J, Aguilera C, De Lama E, Portabella F. MR imaging of synovial tumors and tumor-like lesions. Eur Radiol. 2001;11(12):2549–60.
7. Flandry F. Diagnostic features of diffuse pigmented villonodular synovitis of the knee. Clin Orthop Relat Res. 1994;(298):212–20.
8. Garner HW, Ortiguera CJ, Nakhleh RE. Best cases from the AFIP pigmented villonodular synovitis. Vol. 28, Radiographics. 2009. pp. 1519–23.
9. Byers PD, Cotton RE, Deacon OW, Lowy M, Newman PH, Sissons HA, et al. The diagnosis and treatment of pigmented villonodular synovitis. J Bone Joint Surg Br. 1968;50(2):290–305.
10. Sharma H, Rana B, Mahendra A, Jane MJ, Reid R. Outcome of 17 pigmented villonodular synovitis (PVNS) of the Knee at 6 years mean follow-up. Knee. 2007;14(5):390–4.
11. Joshi K, Huang B, Scanga L, Buchman C, Chera BS. Postoperative radiotherapy for diffuse pigmented villonodular synovitis of the temporomandibular joint. Am J Otolaryngol. 2015;36(1):106–13.
12. Heyd R, Micke O, Berger B, Eich HT, Ackermann H, Seegenschmiedt MH. Radiation therapy for treatment of pigmented villonodular synovitis: results of a national patterns of care study. Int J Radiat Oncol Biol Phys. 2010;78(1):199–204.
13. Berger B, Ganswindt U, Bamberg M, Hehr T. External beam radiotherapy as postoperative treatment of diffuse pigmented villonodular synovitis. Int J Radiat Oncol Biol Phys. 2007;67(4):1130–4.
14. Sun H, Ju XD, Huang HJ, Zhang X, Wang JQ. Clinical outcomes of endoscopic synovectomy with adjuvant radiotherapy of pigmented villonodular synovitis of the hip: a case series of single center. BMC Musculoskelet Disord 2022;23(1).

15. Chien JC, Wei YP, Chen CY, Hsiang WH, Wang YY, Liu WS, et al. Long-term functional outcomes of diffuse pigmented villonodular synovitis of knee: the role of adjuvant radiotherapy. Medicine (United States). 2021;100(12):E23794.
16. Al-Hajri T, Al-Madailwi K, Riromar J. Postoperative radiotherapy for pigmented villonodular synovitis (PVNS): Case series and literature review. J Radiother Pract. 2023;22.
17. Yang X, Sun Y, Yu W, Fu J. Pigmented villonodular synovitis of the temporomandibular joint: case report and the literature review for postoperative radiotherapy. J Radiol Case Rep. 2019;13(8):31–9.
18. Duan Y, Qian J, Chen K, Zhang Z. Necessity of adjuvant postoperative radiotherapy for diffuse pigmented villonodular synovitis of the knee. Vol. 97, Medicine (United States). Lippincott Williams and Wilkins; 2018.
19. Serra TQ, Morais J, Goncalves Z, Agostinho F, Melo G, Henriques M. An unusual case of diffuse pigmented villonodular synovitis of the shoulder: a multidisciplinary approach with arthroscopic synovectomy and adjuvant radiotherapy. Eur J Rheumatol. 2017;4(2):142–4.
20. Mollon B, Lee A, Busse JW, Griffin AM, Ferguson PC, Wunder JS, et al. The effect of surgical synovectomy and radiotherapy on the rate of recurrence of pigmented villonodular synovitis of the knee. Bone Joint J. 2015;97:550–7.
21. Li W, Sun X, Lin J, Ji W, Ruan D. Arthroscopic synovectomy and postoperative assisted radiotherapy for treating diffuse pigmented villonodular synovitis of the knee: an observational retrospective study. Pak J Med Sci. 2015;31(4):956–60.
22. De Carvalho LH, Soares LFMH, Gonalves MBJ, Temponi EF, De Melo SO. Long-term success in the treatment of diffuse pigmented villonodular synovitis of the knee with subtotal synovectomy and radiotherapy. Arthroscopy. 2012;28(9):1271–4.
23. Park G, Kim YS, Kim JH, Lee SW, Song SY, Choi EK, et al. Low-dose external beam radiotherapy as a postoperative treatment for patients with diffuse pigmented villonodular synovitis of the knee. Acta Orthop. 2012;83:256–60.
24. Griffin AM, Ferguson PC, Catton CN, Chung PWM, White LM, Wunder JS, et al. Long-term outcome of the treatment of high-risk tenosynovial giant cell tumor/pigmented villonodular synovitis with radiotherapy and surgery. Cancer. 2012;118(19):4901–9.
25. Horoschak M, Tran PT, Bachireddy P, West RB, Mohler D, Beaulieu CF, et al. External beam radiation therapy enhances local control in pigmented villonodular synovitis. Int J Radiat Oncol Biol Phys. 2009;75(1):183–7.
26. O'sullivan B, Cummings B, Catton C, Bell R, Davis A, Fornasier V, et al. Outcome following radiation treatment for high-risk pigmented villonodular synovitis. Int J Radiat Oncol Biol Phys. 1995;32.
27. Blanco CER, Leon HO, Guthrie TB. Combined partial arthroscopic synovectomy and radiation therapy for diffuse pigmented villonodular synovitis of the knee. Arthroscopy. 2001;17(5):527–31.
28. Kotwal P, Gupta V, Malhotra R. Giant-cell tumour of the tendon sheath.Is radiotherapy indicated to prevent recurrence after surgery? J Bone Joint Surg Br. 2000;82(4):571–3.
29. Kat S, Kutz R, Elbracht T, Weseloh G, Kuwert T. Radiosynovectomy in pigmented villonodular synovitis. Nuklearmedizin. 2000;39:209.
30. Cherian Philips A, Karineravanda Machaiah P. Management of recurrent diffuse pigmented villonodular synovitis: a case report. J Surg Res (Houst) [Internet]. 2024;7(4). Available from: https://www.fortunejournals.com/articles/management-of-recurrent-diffuse-pigmented-villonodular-synovitis-a-case-report.html
31. Ajith K, Thilak L, Rathnadevi R, Subathira B. Unveiling the role of radiotherapy in managing pigmented Villonodular synovitis (PVNS): a unique case analysis. Apollo Medicine [Internet]; 2024 Oct 5; Available from: https://journals.sagepub.com/doi/10.1177/09760016241284354

32. Mazonakis M, Tzedakis A, Lyraraki E, Damilakis J. Organ-specific radiation-induced cancer risk estimates due to radiotherapy for benign pigmented villonodular synovitis. Phys Med Biol. 2016;61(17):6400–12.
33. Cassier PA, Italiano A, Gomez-Roca CA, Le Tourneau C, Toulmonde M, Cannarile MA, et al. CSF1R inhibition with emactuzumab in locally advanced diffuse-type tenosynovial giant cell tumours of the soft tissue: a dose-escalation and dose-expansion phase 1 study. Lancet Oncol. 2015;16(8):949–56.
34. Brahmi M, Vinceneux A, Cassier PA. Current systemic treatment options for tenosynovial giant cell tumor/pigmented villonodular synovitis: targeting the CSF1/CSF1R axis. Vol. 17, Current treatment options in oncology. Springer New York LLC; 2016. pp. 1–9.

Refractory Inflammatory Conditions of Bone and Soft Tissue

29

Himanshu Joshi

29.1 Background

Refractory inflammatory musculoskeletal conditions such as epicondylitis humeri (tennis or golfer's elbow), plantar fasciitis, and achillodynia are common and debilitating. These disorders are typically associated with repetitive strain and microtrauma, resulting in chronic localized pain and functional limitations. The prevalence of epicondylitis humeri alone is about 1.7% in the general population [6].

Tendinopathies are conditions that affect the tendons due to overuse and lead to pain, stiffness, and difficulty with movement. Similarly, enthesopathies affect at the spot where tendons or ligaments attach to bone, often causing long-lasting discomfort. These issues may not seem serious at first, but they can become stubborn and significantly interfere with daily life.

Standard treatments are conservative, including physical therapy, NSAIDs, corticosteroid injections, orthotic etc. While effective in many, a subset of patients remains symptomatic despite these conservative measures, leading to consideration of different options [1, 3].

Low-dose radiotherapy (LDRT) has a long history in Europe as a treatment for benign musculoskeletal conditions. Its anti-inflammatory effects, low toxicity, and cost-effectiveness make it an appealing noninvasive option for selected refractory cases [2, 4]. Despite limited adoption in other regions, there is robust data from Europe, supporting its safety and efficacy.

H. Joshi (✉)
DNB Radiation Oncology, DrNB Medical Oncology SR, Metro Hospital, Preet Vihar, New Delhi, India

K. Sood Sharma (ed.), *Radiation Therapy for Benign Disorders*,
https://doi.org/10.1007/978-981-95-6635-8_29

29.2 Pathogenesis

Chronic tendinopathies and enthesopathies result from repetitive mechanical overuse and a failed healing response. Pathologically, these disorders are less about acute inflammation and more about degenerative processes. Histological studies describe angiofibroblastic hyperplasia, an abnormal proliferation of fibroblasts accompanied by irregular collagen fibers and increased vascularization. Rather than classic signs of inflammation, such as dense infiltration by immune cells, the tissue exhibits signs of ongoing remodeling and breakdown, which explains why conventional anti-inflammatory therapies often fall short [8].

Epicondylitis humeri involves overuse of the forearm extensors or flexor tendons, leading to localized inflammation and degeneration at the lateral or medial epicondyle. Plantar fasciitis follows a similar pattern at the heel, often resulting in a calcaneal spur. Achillodynia involves chronic inflammation at the Achilles tendon insertion [1, 7].

Low-dose radiotherapy (LDRT) intervenes in this pathological cycle through a range of cellular and molecular mechanisms. As illustrated in Fig. 29.1, radiobiological studies have shown that low doses of ionizing radiation (0.5–1 Gy) exert immunomodulatory effects rather than cytotoxic ones [2, 7]. There is reduced expression of pro-inflammatory cytokines (e.g., TNF-α, IL-1β), inhibition of leukocyte adhesion to vascular endothelium, and promotion of apoptosis in endothelial cells and macrophages. These effects result in a net reduction in inflammation and pain perception [2].

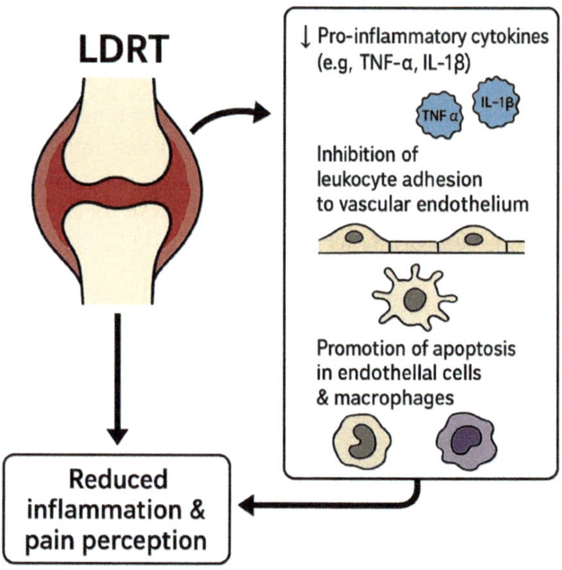

Fig. 29.1 Mechanism of inflammation at the bone–tendon interface and its modulation by low-dose radiotherapy. LDRT reduces cytokine expression, inhibits immune cell adhesion, and promotes apoptosis of inflammatory cells, resulting in reversal of the inflammatory cascade and pain relief

Interestingly, the analgesic effect is often delayed, peaking several weeks after completion of therapy. Patients typically report improvement several weeks after treatment, indicating that the mechanism is likely tied to gradual modulation of chronic inflammation rather than rapid tissue alteration [2, 4].

29.3 Role of Radiation Therapy

LDRT has been used effectively in a range of refractory musculoskeletal conditions:

- *Epicondylitis humeri*: In a study of 138 elbows treated using linear accelerators, Hautmann et al. reported a significant decrease in pain scores (NRS reduced from 7 to 0 at 24 months), with 64.6% achieving complete or near-complete relief [6].
- *Plantar fasciitis*: In a prospective study of 171 patients, Badakhshi et al. observed marked pain relief in 67.3% of patients at 3 months and sustained benefit in 61.4% at a mean of 54 months [3].
- *Heel spur syndrome*: Micke et al. conducted a patterns-of-care analysis of over 7900 patients and found pain reduction in 70% of patients for at least 3 months, with 65% reporting persistent benefit [1].
- *Achillodynia*: Ott et al. showed long-term pain reduction in both 0.5 and 1.0 Gy groups, with up to 95% experiencing symptomatic improvement at 2 years [7].

A well-structured and adequately timed course of conservative management forms the cornerstone of initial treatment in these conditions. This typically includes rest, physiotherapy focused on tendon offloading and eccentric exercises, use of orthotic devices like braces or insoles, oral NSAIDs, local corticosteroid injections, extracorporeal shockwave therapy, and cryotherapy. Despite these approaches, a subset of patients fails to achieve satisfactory symptom relief, particularly those with chronic or recurrent presentations, prompting consideration of radiotherapy as a noninvasive alternative.

Low-dose radiotherapy is primarily indicated for patients with chronic musculoskeletal conditions such as epicondylitis, plantar fasciitis, or achillodynia who continue to experience symptoms for more than six months despite adequate trials of conservative therapy. Candidates are typically older adults (preferably above 40 years of age), as the long-term risks of radiation are lower in this population. LDRT is particularly suited for patients who are unfit for surgery due to comorbidities or those who decline invasive interventions. It also serves as an effective alternative when repeated corticosteroid injections or other pharmacological options have failed to provide lasting relief.

The benefits of LDRT are multifaceted. It is a non-invasive, outpatient procedure that does not require anesthesia or hospitalization, making it convenient and well-tolerated. The therapy has an excellent safety profile with minimal side effects, and robust clinical data support its ability to provide durable pain relief in a substantial proportion of patients. Moreover, LDRT can reduce dependence on long-term analgesics and help defer or avoid surgical procedures, making it a cost-effective and patient-friendly option for refractory cases.

Limitations include lack of standardization across countries, concerns over long-term risks in younger patients, and hesitation due to unfamiliarity with RT in non-malignant settings [1].

29.4 Radiation Technique

Modality: Most institutions use either orthovoltage units or linear accelerators (6 MV). Hautmann et al. confirmed linear accelerators are equally effective [6].

Positioning: Supine for elbows, prone for heels. Immobilization using cushions or Vacloc devices or thermoplastic molds is used to ensure reproducibility.

Field Design: Typically, two opposed lateral fields or a single direct beam. Margins include the affected enthesis with appropriate shielding.

Dose & Fractionation:

The most widely accepted regimen for low-dose radiotherapy (LDRT) in benign musculoskeletal conditions is 6 fractions of 1.0 Gy each, typically delivered three times a week over two weeks, resulting in a total dose of 6 Gy. This standard fractionation has demonstrated consistent efficacy and safety across multiple large studies, including those by Micke et al., Niewald et al., and Hautmann et al. [4–6]. The simplicity and reproducibility of this schedule have contributed to its broad acceptance in European clinical practice.

An alternative regimen of 12 fractions of 0.5 Gy, also totaling 6 Gy, has been explored in randomized trials to assess whether more extended, lower-dose fractionation might confer added benefit. However, results showed no statistically significant improvement in pain outcomes compared to the standard 6 × 1 Gy schedule, suggesting that dose fractionation should prioritize convenience and compliance unless specific patient factors warrant modification [5].

Re-irradiation may be considered in patients with partial or recurrent symptoms after an adequate interval, typically 8 to 12 weeks, following the initial course. The cumulative dose in such cases still remains well within safety limits due to the inherently low biological effectiveness of the regimens used.

Overall, the prescribed LDRT dose schedule balances efficacy with safety, providing durable symptomatic relief while minimizing any risk of toxicity.

Treatment Planning Simulation using X-rays or CT (rarely). Simple 2D planning suffices in most cases.

Due to low total doses, adjacent critical structures rarely require formal constraints, though unnecessary exposure should be avoided.

29.5 Toxicity Profile and Strategies to Minimize Risks

Across all reviewed studies, LDRT exhibited an excellent safety profile:

- No acute or chronic toxicity observed in over 700 patients in prospective and retrospective studies [2, 3].
- No significant skin reactions, fibrosis, or radiation-induced malignancy reported, even with long-term follow-up [6, 7].

Risk minimization strategies include:
- Limiting repeat courses unless strongly indicated.
- Avoiding use in pediatric or young adult patients.
- Using precise field margins and shielding to minimize scatter.

The overall benefit-to-risk ratio is highly favorable, particularly in older adults with disabling chronic pain [1].

29.6 Review of Literature and Case Studies

Over the past two decades, several well-designed prospective and randomized studies have helped shape the evidence base for the use of low-dose radiotherapy (LDRT) in benign inflammatory musculoskeletal conditions. These studies not only demonstrate clinical efficacy and safety but also provide insight into real-world practices around radiation planning, dose schedules, and equipment used.

One of the largest and most comprehensive datasets comes from Micke et al. (2018), who conducted a prospective multicenter study involving 703 patients with conditions such as plantar fasciitis, epicondylitis, and calcaneodynia. Patients received 6 Gy total dose, typically in 6 fractions of 1 Gy each. The study observed significant long-term pain relief in over 58% of patients, and no acute or late toxicities were reported [2].

In an earlier patterns-of-care analysis, Micke et al. (2004) had already noted that the most widely used techniques across Germany included orthovoltage therapy and conventional linear accelerators. Treatment planning was often done without 3D imaging, and delivery was via direct fields to the symptomatic site. The standard protocol remained 6 × 1 Gy [1].

Badakhshi and Buadch (2014) reported outcomes in 171 patients with plantar fasciitis treated using LDRT with total doses of 6 Gy. They emphasized that patients were treated with either orthovoltage or megavoltage machines, depending on local availability. Their follow-up results confirmed that more than 60% of patients maintained durable pain relief for over four years [3].

Niewald et al. (2012) conducted a pivotal randomized controlled trial comparing a standard dose of 6 × 1 Gy with a very low dose of 6 × 0.1 Gy in patients with painful heel spurs. Patients were treated using lateral opposing 4–6 MV photon beams, delivered on conventional LINACs. The trial clearly demonstrated the superiority of the standard 6 Gy regimen in terms of pain relief and quality of life. Importantly, no toxicity was observed even at one year of follow-up, reinforcing the safety of such low-dose exposures [4].

To test whether further dose fractionation could improve outcomes, Prokein et al. (2017) ran another randomized multicenter trial comparing 6 × 1 Gy vs. 12 × 0.5 Gy. Patients were treated with external beam radiotherapy using either orthovoltage or LINAC machines. The study found no statistically significant difference in outcomes between the two fractionation schedules, suggesting that increasing the number of fractions while keeping the dose constant may not enhance efficacy [5].

In a focused investigation on epicondylitis humeri, Hautmann et al. (2019) specifically evaluated patients treated with modern linear accelerators. This study involved 138 elbows and used 6 MV photons, with pain evaluated using a numeric rating scale (NRS). The results were striking: median pain scores dropped from 7 (baseline) to 0 at 12 and 24 months post-treatment. Importantly, no radiation-related toxicity was reported, validating the effectiveness of LINAC-based LDRT for this indication [6].

Ott et al. (2015) similarly explored the role of fractionation in achillodynia. Patients were randomized to receive either 6 × 0.5 Gy or 6 × 1.0 Gy using orthovoltage equipment. Long-term outcomes showed high response rates in both arms, with over 95% of patients reporting sustained pain reduction at 2 years. Once again, toxicity was negligible, underscoring LDRT's suitability for chronic tendinopathies [7].

Miszczyk et al. (2015) added further validation with a prospective analysis of patients suffering from epicondylitis humeri. They reported significant pain reduction and functional improvement using a standard 6 Gy regimen, although the technical details of delivery were less emphasized in their study [8].

Across all these trials, certain consistent patterns emerge:

- Most treatments were delivered using either orthovoltage units (100–250 kV) or 6 MV LINACs.
- No advanced techniques such as IMRT or IGRT were required or used, given the superficial location of the targets and the low doses involved.
- Patient positioning was straightforward (supine or prone), and immobilization was typically achieved with foam pads or wedges.
- Field design involved either direct single fields or lateral opposing beams without complex planning.

Collectively, the literature affirms that LDRT is not only effective but also practical. The simplicity of planning, minimal resources required, and excellent safety profile make it an appealing option, especially for patients with refractory symptoms and limited alternatives.

Table 29.1 Summary of key studies on LDRT in musculoskeletal pain

Study	Condition	Dose/Fractions	Outcome
Micke et al. (2004) [1]	Heel spur (PCS study)	6 Gy total	70% pain relief; 65% sustained
Micke et al. (2018) [2]	Mixed cohort (703 pts)	6 Gy total	58.4% good long-term response
Badakhshi et al. (2014) [3]	Plantar fasciitis	6 Gy total	61.4% with long-term benefit
Niewald et al. (2012) [4]	Heel spur (RCT)	6 Gy vs 0.6 Gy	6 Gy group superior in pain & QoL
Prokein et al. (2017) [5]	Heel spur	6 × 1 Gy vs 12 × 0.5 Gy	No added benefit with 12 × 0.5 Gy
Hautmann et al. (2019) [6]	Epicondylitis humeri	6 Gy with LINAC	64.6% pain-free at 12 months
Ott et al. (2015) [7]	Achillodynia	0.5 Gy vs 1.0 Gy	95% long-term response
Miszczyk et al. (2015) [8]	Epicondylitis	Various	Significant pain reduction

A summary of these clinical trials, including their target conditions, dose regimens, and reported outcomes, is provided in Table 29.1.

29.7 Future Directions

Despite its demonstrated effectiveness in refractory inflammatory conditions of bones and soft tissue, low-dose radiotherapy (LDRT) remains underutilized globally. Moving forward, several key areas warrant attention to optimize its clinical utility and broaden its adoption.

One major goal is the standardization of treatment protocols. While most studies, including those by Micke et al. [2] and Niewald et al. [4], used the 6 × 1 Gy regimen, other schedules like 12 × 0.5 Gy have also been explored. However, trials such as Prokein et al. [5] found no additional benefit with extended fractionation. Future comparative trials can help determine whether dose schedule or energy modality (orthovoltage vs. LINAC) impacts long-term outcomes.

There is also potential to expand LDRT's use to other chronic enthesopathies beyond epicondylitis and plantar fasciitis. Given its anti-inflammatory mechanism—primarily immunomodulation rather than cytotoxicity—it may benefit conditions like trochanteric bursitis or frozen shoulder. These indications remain unexplored in clinical trials but share similar underlying pathology.

Though techniques such as IMRT and IGRT are not currently used in these scenarios, technological advances may one day enable more precise delivery in anatomically complex or deep-seated sites, should the indications evolve.

Personalized medicine may also shape the future of LDRT. Currently, patient selection is empirical. Identifying clinical or molecular markers predictive of response—such as duration of symptoms or imaging characteristics—could refine patient stratification and improve outcomes.

Finally, wider international acceptance remains to be achieved. Studies like those by Hautmann et al. [6] and Ott et al. [7] provide strong safety data, yet clinical adoption outside Europe is limited. Health economic studies are needed to quantify LDRT's cost-effectiveness in comparison to surgery, repeated injections, or long-term pharmacotherapy.

With more robust trials, clearer guidelines, and interdisciplinary awareness, LDRT has the potential to become an integral part of evidence-based care for chronic musculoskeletal pain.

29.8 Conclusion

Low-dose radiotherapy is a valuable treatment for refractory inflammatory bone and soft tissue conditions, offering safe, sustained pain relief with minimal side effects. Evidence from high-quality trials and prospective studies supports its role in cases unresponsive to conventional therapy. As awareness and confidence grow among clinicians, LDRT has the potential to become a mainstream option in the multidisciplinary management of chronic musculoskeletal pain.

References

1. Micke O, et al. Radiotherapy in painful heel spur syndrome: patterns of care in Germany. Int J Radiat Oncol Biol Phys. 2004;58(3):828–43.
2. Micke O, et al. Radiotherapy for calcaneodynia and other musculoskeletal pain: results of a prospective study. Radiat Oncol. 2018;13:71.
3. Badakhshi H, Buadch V. Low dose radiotherapy for plantar fasciitis. Foot. 2014; https://doi.org/10.1016/j.foot.2014.07.005.
4. Niewald M, et al. Radiation therapy in plantar fasciitis: standard vs low dose. Int J Radiat Oncol Biol Phys. 2012;84(4):e455–62.
5. Prokein B, et al. Radiotherapy of painful heel spur: randomized multicenter trial. Strahlenther Onkol. 2017;193(6):483–90.
6. Hautmann MG, et al. Radiotherapy of epicondylitis humeri with linear accelerator. Strahlenther Onkol. 2019;195(4):343–51.
7. Ott OJ, et al. Radiotherapy for benign achillodynia: Erlangen dose optimization trial. Strahlenther Onkol. 2015;191(12):979–84.
8. Miszczyk L, et al. An evaluation of radiotherapy effectiveness for epicondylitis humeri. Ortop Traumatol Rehabil. 2015;17(5–6):471–9.

Ventricular Arrythmias and Prevention of Restenosis in CAD

30

Saurabha Kumar, Deepak Padmanabhan,
and Ann Christy Saju

30.1 Ventricular Arrythmias

30.1.1 Background

Ventricular tachycardia is defined as cardiac arrhythmia of three or more consecutive complexes originating in the ventricles at a rate greater than 100 bpm (cycle length: <600 ms). The types of VT are sustained: VT >30 s or requiring termination due to hemodynamic compromise in <30 s, non-sustained/unsustained: ≥3 beats, terminating spontaneously, monomorphic, polymorphic, and bidirectional. Ventricular tachycardia is a result of previous ischemic heart disease most commonly but also could be as a result of congenital heart disease, nonischemic cardiomyopathy, and a few hereditary cardiac conditions [1].

Cardiovascular disease (CVD) is the leading cause of death and disability-adjusted life years in the world. In India the burden is higher, as Indians present a decade earlier with CVD and are prone to develop CVD due to various demographic and biological reasons [2]. These higher CVD risks are a predisposition for ventricular arrhythmias following scarring of the cardiac musculature.

Stereotactic body radiotherapy is established as the standard of care in cancer treatment for lung, prostate, and various brain tumors. Delivering very high doses of radiation with ablative potential is harnessed as an alternative to surgery or other

S. Kumar (✉) · A. C. Saju
Department of Radiation Oncology, Mazumdar Shaw Medical Centre, Narayana Health City, Bangalore, India
e-mail: saurabha.kumar.dr@narayanahealth.org; annchristy.saju.dr@narayanahealth.org

D. Padmanabhan
Department of Electrophysiology, Narayana Institute of Cardiac Sciences, Narayana Health City, Bangalore, India
e-mail: deepak.padmanabhan.dr@narayanahealth.org

K. Sood Sharma (ed.), *Radiation Therapy for Benign Disorders*,
https://doi.org/10.1007/978-981-95-6635-8_30

ablation procedures like RF ablation or microwave ablation (MWA). Delivered with submillimeter accuracy using modern equipment, it's emerging in various cancer treatment strategies as a noninvasive procedure. Sharma et al. ablated a Hanford-Sinclair mini swine heart with a 25 Gy single fraction with the CyberHeart system to various targets within the heart and later evaluated it with electroanatomic voltage mapping and subsequent pathology of the specimens. He proved that noninvasive cardiac channel blocks should be feasible with minimal damage to adjacent nonirradiated tissue. In 2014, the Stanford University team successfully treated a 72-year-old patient with refractory VT with 25Gy single fraction SBRT. The patient had a considerable decrease in the number of episodes of VT following the ablation, 562 prior to treatment to 52 in the 9 months after SBRT.

30.1.2 Pathogenesis

Ventricular arrhythmias include triggered, automatic, and re-entrant rhythms that involve the ventricular muscle, the conduction system distal to the His bundle, or a combination of both tissues. Myocardial scar post-myocardial infarct is the most common cause of ventricular arrhythmias, although it can occur without observable structural abnormalities. The mechanism is most often a re-entry circuit in a region of healed myocardial infarction (MI). In these areas, gap junctions are often disrupted, leading to slow and disorderly conduction by surviving cardiomyocytes. Ventricular arrhythmia can be symptomatic and may ultimately lead to left ventricular dysfunction, subsequently to hemodynamic collapse with syncope or sudden death.

Various pathological sample analysis of heart samples post-SBRT have been able to identify acute effects such as sub-endothelial necrosis with a rim of fibrosis, cellular vacuolization of the myocytes, and vascular changes with myointimal thickening with prominence of endothelial cells. These immediate changes probably lead to immediate conduction blocks before the onset of Fibrosis [3].

30.1.3 Role of Radiation Therapy

Implantable cardioverter-defibrillators (ICDs) can effectively terminate VT episodes thus reducing the risk of sudden death. Heart failure is quite common despite well-functioning ICDs, and each shock will reduce the quality of life. Anti-arrhythmic medication is administered to 18% to 30% of ICD patients with spontaneous VT even when they have an ICD implanted. Antiarrhythmic drugs have poor efficacy, and VT can still be triggered. Catheter ablation is shown to give good results with termination of further VT episodes to as low as 10% in a few studies [4]. But in multicentric reports, recurrence can be as high as 50% at 6 months [5].

Recurrence could be the result of coexisting VT circuits, new circuits developing post ablation or deeper situated circuits that wouldn't be amenable to the standard procedure. Deep/inaccessible circuits could be made accessible with the help of combined endocardial and epicardial approach. Other radical approaches being used are surgical sympathetic denervation, transcoronary ethanol injection, and catheter ablation with an extendable needle.

SBRT for VT is a noninvasive approach to the problem that could achieve results in patients who have failed the first line of treatment and in patients who are not medically fit to undergo the invasive procedure. Also, in situations where the risk of doing the procedure is very high, as in a cardiac thrombus within the ventricle obscuring the target circuit. SBRT for VT is currently being tried in clinical trial settings alone in patients who have failed multiple catheter ablation procedures and in heart failure.

30.1.4 Radiation Technique

In cardiac SBRT, one of the most important criteria is to identify the site of the arrhythmic focus. Structural imaging is done with computer tomography that can be ECG-gated to check the wall thinning in the different phases of ECG. Cardiovascular MRI is used to identify the scarred myocardium and normal cardiac tissue that will aid in demarcating the target. Metabolic imaging can be used along to delineate the hypoxic myocardium by single photon emission computed tomography (SPECT) or 18-fluorodeoxyglucose positron emission tomography (PET) imaging. Cardiac mapping is done with the use of electrodes in the ventricle that can delineate the zone or region that is arrhythmogenic and can be extrapolated on the CT scan/cardiac MRI. Noninvasive mapping is done using an electromagnetic vest that can collect the signals with ECG leads and project the lesion to the corresponding wall [6].

Planning CT scan is done with respiratory motion management using 4D CT or breath-hold techniques. After mapping the target on the planning CT, margins are given ranging from 0–5 mm to the target to get the PTV volume. The critical organs must be delineated, and a dose prescription of classically 25 to 30 Gy in a single fraction is advised. It is ideally planned using a Triple F beam. Delivery is possible with image guidance using stereotactic-capable equipment—a linear accelerator or CyberKnife. Once the plan is approved with respecting the critical organ tolerances, the delivery is scheduled. It's a team approach, and the radiation oncologist and electrophysiologist have to be present while delivering the plan. The ICD must be on during the treatment to diffuse any arrhythmias during the procedure. Also, it's advisable to stop amiodarone and start steroids 1–2 days prior to SBRT. The intracardiac probes can guide as fiducials for imaging and tracking during the delivery of treatment (Fig. 30.1).

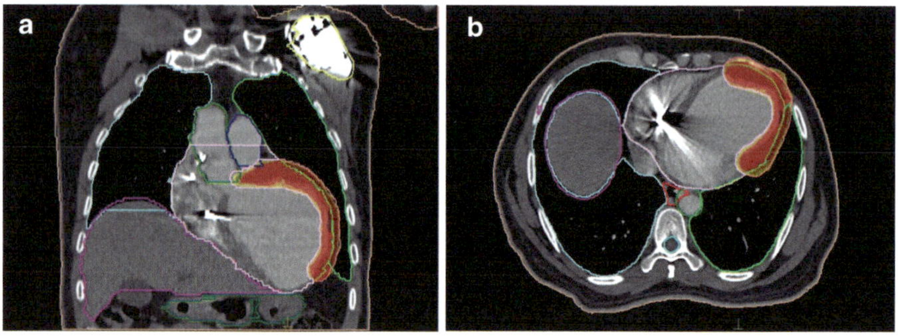

Fig. 30.1 Dose colour wash of SBRT plan for VT

30.1.5 Review of Literature and Case Studies

Dr. Cuculich and the team at Washington University published the data for five patients treated with 25 Gy single-fraction cardiac SBRT for VT. The arrhythmogenic scar was identified by anatomical imaging (SPECT/cardiac MRI) and noninvasive electrocardiographic imaging while the patient was on VT with an ICD. Planning CT was acquired with an immobilization technique using a vacuum-assisted device and 4-dimensional CT. Radiotherapy was delivered using image-guided radiotherapy-capable linear accelerator. ICD interrogations were carried out frequently, every 2 weeks for 2 months, monthly for the next 4 months, and then yearly thereafter treatment. The intent was to monitor the VT recurrence and to also taper and stop the medications as per the drop in events. The 5 patients had an aggregate of 6577 episodes of VT in the 3 months prior to SBRT. The blanking period is the window where patients could experience higher VT due to oedema post radiation. There were 680 episodes of VT during the blanking period of 6 weeks, following which there were only 4 episodes of VT recorded in the entire 46 patient months following SBRT (99.9% drop from baseline) [5].

A similar study from the Czech Republic by Neuwirth et al. in 2019 studied ten patients treated with 25 Gy SBRT using the CyberKnife system for delivery. The target was identified using electro anatomical mapping. No margin was added to the target for planning. Tracking was done using ICD leads as the surrogate for the markers. 212 episodes of VT were observed prior to SBRT, and an average of 26 episodes of VT in the blanking period set as 3 months in this study. Post-blanking period, there was a significant drop in the VT episodes, with the first episode requiring antiarrhythmic pacing at 6.5 months [7].

Lloyd et al. treated ten patients with heart failure who were deemed to have recurrent VT following intervention. The patients were eligible if they fulfilled 2 of the 3 criteria, that being: failed at least 2 antiarrhythmic drugs; failed at least 1 RF ablation defined as 1 inducible VTs after ablation; and failed 1 adjunctive therapy such as mechanical support or sympathetic blockade. The patient received 25 Gy single-fraction SBRT to the target defined by electro-anatomical mapping and imaging. In the eight patients that were eligible for analysis, there was a significant drop in the ant tachycardia pacing (ATP) from 17.3 to 8.9, a 48% reduction post SBRT. There was also a reduction in ICD shocks after SBRT by 68% [8].

30.1.6 Toxicity Profile and Strategies to Minimize Risks

SBRT in VT is commonly practiced in a subset of highly comorbid individuals who are already in cardiac failure, and there are many overlapping issues medically. The common toxicities across studies have been pneumonitis, pericarditis, and pericardial effusion attributed to SBRT directly. Heart failure worsening post-SBRT remains the most common cause of death, amounting to roughly one third of the deaths. Mortality is higher in the first 3 months post-SBRT, with many noncardiac deaths mostly due to the poor general condition of the patient [7].

Few studies recommend the use of steroids during and post-SBRT to reduce the effects of cardiac oedema. Also, across studies, amiodarone was stopped prior to SBRT to reduce the incidence of pneumonitis.

30.1.7 Future Directions and Conclusion

SBRT is still recommended in clinical trial settings alone, but with available data, it's a reasonable option when conventional methods have failed. Also, there is a need to study this approach closely in the future to understand better the long-term effects of radiotherapy on the irradiated normal heart tissues and how to mitigate the same. The exact demarcation of the target and the methodology for delivery vary across studies and need to be standardized. There are studies considering atrial arrhythmias, and results are awaited.

30.2 Prevention of Restenosis in CAD

30.2.1 Background

In-stent restenosis (ISR) following percutaneous coronary intervention (PCI) is conventionally defined as a reduction of 50% or more in the luminal diameter within the previously stented segment or in the adjacent vessel segments extending up to 5 mm proximal or distal to the stent edges. However, with the advent of intravascular imaging, the definition has been updated to consider ISR as a re-narrowing of ≥75% of the reference vessel area upon cross-sectional evaluation.

In the era of bare metal stents (BMS), intravascular brachytherapy (IVBT) emerged as a valuable tool in reducing restenosis rates. However, its use significantly declined following widespread adoption of drug-eluting stents (DES).

Despite the widespread adoption of DES, restenosis continues to pose a clinical concern, with incidence rates, though reduced, still ranging between 5% and 10% at one year. Moreover, the treatment of complex ISR, especially in cases involving multiple overlapping layers of DES, remains a significant therapeutic challenge. In this setting, IVBT has regained attention. IVBT may offer therapeutic value in patients with recurrent or refractory DES-related ISR. Recent studies suggest a potential niche for IVBT in modern interventional cardiology, particularly for cases where conventional therapies fall short [9, 10].

30.2.2 Pathogenesis

Stents used in PCI can cause vessel wall injury, which triggers neointimal hyperplasia. Preventing this process is the primary goal of radiation therapy.

Vessel injury leads to the migration of smooth muscle cells and fibroblasts from the media to the intima in response to various stimuli, a process akin to scar formation. Radiation has been shown to be effective in treating fibro-proliferative disorders such as keloids, which led to the extension of a similar theory for the prevention of re-stenosis.

Although the precise biological basis remains unclear, it is believed that radiation targets immature fibroblasts, disrupting cell cycle-regulating proteins and thereby preventing cell proliferation.

30.2.3 Role of Radiation Therapy (RT)

During the era of BMS, restenosis rates were frequently reported to be around 30%. Multiple randomized trials reported better outcomes with the combination of BMS and IVBT in both de novo and restenosis settings [11–14]. With the advent of DES, its role has been diminishing or rather redefined. DES replaced IVBT owing to its superior clinical outcomes and procedural simplicity.

However, target vessel revascularization (TVR) rates following DES implantation remain at approximately 5–8% at one year and 13–17% at five years [15]. There is no established consensus on treatment strategies for restenosis following DES implantation. Management options include balloon angioplasty, drug-coated balloons (DCB), repeat DES implantation, IVBT, and coronary artery bypass grafting (CABG).

In the current era, the role of IVBT has been redefined to focus on managing recurrent multilayered DES restenosis. Although there are no randomized trials investigating its role in the DES era, a few retrospective studies and meta-analyses have explored its effectiveness in recurrent DES restenosis and have shown favorable outcomes [9, 10, 16].

30.2.4 Radiation Technique

Two primary types of catheter-based radiation delivery systems have been extensively studied for the treatment of restenosis: gamma and beta radiation devices. Gamma-based devices utilize iridium-192 ribbons that emit photons, allowing for stable seed placement and a small catheter diameter. However, they penetrate over 10 mm of tissue and necessitate extensive shielding. On the other hand, beta-based devices use strontium/yttrium-90 radioisotopes that emit electrons, providing a wide energy range and penetrating only 2–3 mm of tissue. These devices feature shorter dwell times but require intermittent fluoroscopic confirmation during delivery to ensure proper seed positioning.

The US Food and Drug Administration has approved two such devices for clinical use: the Novoste™ Beta-Cath system (beta radiation) and the Cordis Checkmate™ system (gamma radiation).

The IVBT procedure involves a pretreatment phase designed to optimize lesion preparation before radiation is administered. This may include balloon angioplasty, laser atherectomy, or rotational atherectomy, depending on lesion morphology and the degree of stent restenosis.

For gamma radiation, the radiation catheter is navigated over a guidewire to the target lesion. An iridium-192 ribbon with a predetermined dose is inserted into the delivery catheter to cover the target area. The ribbon remains in place for an average dwell time of 12 to 20 minutes, based on the vessel diameter.

In beta-radiation therapy, a radioactive source wire is placed into a closed catheter with the assistance of a centering balloon and then advanced to the target site. The goal is to deliver a specific dose of radiation within a set distance (typically 2 mm) from the balloon-centered source wire. The average dwell time is between 3 and 5 minutes.

Across various studies, the prescribed radiation dose has ranged between 18 and 25 Gy, typically measured at a depth of 2 mm from the radiation source center at the site of ISR.

30.2.5 Toxicity Profile and Strategies to Minimize Risks

In the early trials, late thrombosis occurred in 3–10% of patients, typically developing within 1 to 9 months following treatment. However, more recent studies have shown that extending antiplatelet therapy for 6 to 12 months significantly reduces the incidence of late thrombosis, bringing it down to less than 1% [16]. This extension of therapy has proven to be an effective strategy for mitigating the risk of thrombotic events following the procedure. Edge restenosis, often referred to as the "candy wrapper effect," can occur at the treatment boundaries due to several factors, including geographical miss and insufficient radiation dose to the injured lesion margins. To minimize the occurrence of this phenomenon, it is essential to carefully assess the extent of vessel injury and ensure that the radiation source provides an adequate margin of coverage around the lesion edges. Employing precise techniques to map the lesion's boundaries and delivering targeted radiation to these areas can significantly reduce the risk of edge restenosis. The late catch-up phenomenon, characterized by lumen loss that develops after one year, has been observed in long-term follow-up studies. This delayed progression can complicate treatment outcomes, highlighting the need for potentially more aggressive interventions in patients after the initial treatment.

30.2.6 Review of Literature

Multiple randomized, placebo-controlled trials have demonstrated improved outcomes when IVBT was combined with BMS. Key pivotal trials utilizing gamma radiation include the SCRIPPS [11], Gamma-one [12], WRIST [13], and Long WRIST [14]. These trials reported favorable results, showing a reduction in target lesion revascularization (TLR) by 43–88% at 6–12 months. Similarly, beta-radiation-based studies such as Beta WRIST, START [17], and INHIBIT [18] also showed a reduction in TLR by 34–63% over the same time frame. This significant reduction in TLR contributed to the approval of the Beta-**Cath** system and the Checkmate system by the U.S. FDA during the BMS era.

The introduction of DES swiftly transformed the treatment landscape, casting doubt on the role of IVBT. Randomized trials, such as TAXUS [19], INDEED [20], and SISR [21], comparing DES with IVBT in the context of ISR, clearly demonstrated the superior efficacy of DES. As a result, the use of IVBT has been discontinued in many centers, as DES became the preferred option for managing ISR due to its enhanced performance and reduced restenosis rates.

Managing recurrent ISR remains a significant challenge, with limited treatment options available. Despite the lack of randomized studies specifically evaluating the role of IVBT in cases of multiple ISR, several retrospective studies suggest favorable outcomes with IVBT, particularly in cases involving two or more stent layers [9, 16]. A meta-analysis by Megaly et al. highlighted that the treatment of recurrent DES ISR with IVBT was associated with a 29.2% incidence of target vessel revascularization (TVR) over a 2-year follow-up period [10]. These findings suggest that IVBT may still offer benefit in select cases of recurrent ISR, though further prospective studies are needed to solidify its role in such scenarios.

30.2.7 Future Directions

One key advantage of radiation over more targeted pharmacological therapies is its nonspecific mechanism of action, effectively halting cell proliferation even in the presence of multiple proliferative stimuli. Understanding the underlying biology of ISR, particularly recurrent ISR, and defining the role of IVBT remain an area that warrants further research. Direct comparative studies of various treatment modalities, including IVBT, in cases of multi-layer ISR are required for establishing a comprehensive treatment algorithm. Additionally, determining the optimal radiation dose and identifying the patient subgroups that would benefit most from IVBT are essential areas for future research.

30.3 Conclusion

ISR remains a clinical challenge, although its incidence has decreased over the past few decades. The introduction of IVBT significantly reduced restenosis rates during the era of BMS. However, its role in the era of DES continues to evolve. Multi-layer or recurrent in-stent restenosis, a particularly complex clinical scenario, appears to benefit from IVBT, as indicated by several retrospective studies. Nevertheless, the specific patient population that would derive the most benefit from IVBT still requires further evaluation.

References

1. Al-Khatib SM, Stevenson WG, Ackerman MJ, Bryant WJ, Callans DJ, Curtis AB, et al. 2017 AHA/ACC/HRS guideline for management of patients with ventricular arrhythmias and the prevention of sudden cardiac death: a report of the American College of Cardiology/American Heart Association Task Force on Clinical Practice Guidelines and the Heart Rhythm Society. J Am Coll Cardiol. 2018;72(14):e91–220.
2. Kalra A, Jose AP, Prabhakaran P, Kumar A, Agrawal A, Roy A, et al. The burgeoning cardiovascular disease epidemic in Indians - perspectives on contextual factors and potential solutions. Lancet Reg Health Southeast Asia. 2023;12:100156.
3. Kiani S, Kutob L, Schneider F, Higgins KA, Lloyd MS. Histopathologic and ultrastructural findings in human myocardium after stereotactic body radiation therapy for recalcitrant ventricular tachycardia. Circ Arrhythm Electrophysiol. 2020;13(11):e008753.
4. Tokuda M, Kojodjojo P, Tung S, Tedrow UB, Nof E, Inada K, et al. Acute failure of catheter ablation for ventricular tachycardia due to structural heart disease: causes and significance. JAHA [Internet]. 2013 [cited 2025 Apr 22];2(3):e000072. Available from: https://www.ahajournals.org/doi/10.1161/JAHA.113.000072
5. Cuculich PS, Schill MR, Kashani R, Mutic S, Lang A, Cooper D, et al. Noninvasive cardiac radiation for ablation of ventricular tachycardia. N Engl J Med. 2017;377(24):2325–36.
6. Chowdhary A, Garg P, Das A, Nazir MS, Plein S. Cardiovascular magnetic resonance imaging: emerging techniques and applications. Heart. 2021;107(9):697–704.
7. Neuwirth R, Cvek J, Knybel L, Jiravsky O, Molenda L, Kodaj M, et al. Stereotactic radiosurgery for ablation of ventricular tachycardia. Europace. 2019;21(7):1088–95.
8. Lloyd MS, Wight J, Schneider F, Hoskins M, Attia T, Escott C, et al. Clinical experience of stereotactic body radiation for refractory ventricular tachycardia in advanced heart failure patients. Heart Rhythm [Internet]. 2020 [cited 2025 Apr 22];17(3):415–22. Available from: https://www.sciencedirect.com/science/article/pii/S1547527119309038
9. Varghese MJ, Bhatheja S, Baber U, Kezbor S, Chincholi A, Chamaria S, et al. Intravascular brachytherapy for the management of repeated multimetal-layered drug-eluting coronary stent restenosis. Cardiovasc Intervent [Internet]. 2018 [cited 2025 Mar 28];11(10):e006832. Available from: https://www.ahajournals.org/doi/10.1161/CIRCINTERVENTIONS.118.006832

10. Megaly M, Glogoza M, Xenogiannis I, Vemmou E, Nikolakopoulos I, Omer M, et al. Coronary intravascular brachytherapy for recurrent coronary drug-eluting stent in-stent restenosis: a systematic review and meta-analysis. Cardiovasc Revascular Med [Internet]. 2021 [cited 2025 Mar 28];23:28–35. Available from: https://www.sciencedirect.com/science/article/pii/S1553838920305042
11. Teirstein Paul S, Vincent M, Shirish J, Popma Jeffrey J, Mintz Gary S, Russo Robert J, et al. Catheter-based radiotherapy to inhibit restenosis after coronary stenting. N Engl J Med [Internet]. 1997 [cited 2025 Apr 13];336(24):1697–703. Available from: https://www.nejm.org/doi/full/10.1056/NEJM199706123362402
12. Leon Martin B, Teirstein Paul S, Moses Jeffrey W, Prabhakar T, Lansky Alexandra J, Shirish J, et al. Localized Intracoronary Gamma-Radiation Therapy to Inhibit the Recurrence of Restenosis after Stenting. New Engl J Med [Internet]. 2001 [cited 2025 Apr 13];344(4):250–6. Available from: https://www.nejm.org/doi/full/10.1056/NEJM200101253440402
13. Waksman R, Bhargava B, White L, Chan RC, Mehran R, Lansky AJ, et al. Intracoronary β-radiation therapy inhibits recurrence of in-stent restenosis. Circulation [Internet]. 2000 [cited 2025 Apr 13];101(16):1895–8. Available from: https://www.ahajournals.org/doi/10.1161/01.CIR.101.16.1895
14. Waksman R, Cheneau E, Ajani AE, White RL, Pinnow E, Torguson R, et al. Intracoronary radiation therapy improves the clinical and angiographic outcomes of diffuse in-stent restenotic lesions. Circulation [Internet]. 2003 [cited 2025 Apr 13];107(13):1744–9. Available from: https://www.ahajournals.org/doi/10.1161/01.CIR.0000060497.91775.6D
15. Kawamoto H, Ruparelia N, Latib A, Miyazaki T, Sato K, Mangieri A, et al. Drug-coated balloons versus second-generation drug-eluting stents for the management of recurrent multimetal-layered in-stent restenosis. JACC Cardiovasc Interv. 2015;8(12):1586–94.
16. Negi SI, Torguson R, Gai J, Kiramijyan S, Koifman E, Chan R, et al. Intracoronary brachytherapy for recurrent drug-eluting stent failure. JACC: Cardiovascular Interventions. 2016;9(12):1259.
17. Suntharalingam M, Laskey W, Lansky AJ, Waksman R, White L, Teirstien P, et al. Clinical and angiographic outcomes after use of 90Strontium/90Yttrium beta radiation for the treatment of in-stent restenosis: results from the Stents and Radiation Therapy 40 (START 40) registry. Int J Radiat Oncol Biol Phys [Internet]. 2002 [cited 2025 Apr 13];52(4):1075–82. Available from: https://www.sciencedirect.com/science/article/pii/S0360301601027122
18. Shirai K, Lansky AJ, Mintz GS, Costantini CO, Cristea E, Fahy M, et al. Feasibility and efficacy of tandem positioning on angiographic and clinical outcomes in the Intimal Hyperplasia Inhibition with Beta In-Stent Trial. Am J Cardiol [Internet]. 2003 [cited 2025 Apr 13];91(9):1113–5. Available from: https://www.ajconline.org/article/S0002-9149(03)00160-7/abstract
19. Stone GW, Ellis SG, O'Shaughnessy CD, Martin SL, Satler L, McGarry T, et al. Paclitaxel-eluting stents vs vascular brachytherapy for in-stent restenosis within bare-metal stents: the TAXUS V ISR randomized trial. JAMA. 2006;295(11):1253–63.
20. Park SW, Lee SW, Koo BK, Park DW, Lee SW, Kim YH, et al. Treatment of diffuse in-stent restenosis with drug-eluting stents vs. intracoronary beta-radiation therapy: INDEED Study. Int J Cardiol. 2008;131(1):70–7.
21. Holmes DR, Teirstein P, Satler L, Sketch M, O'Malley J, Popma JJ, et al. Sirolimus-eluting stents vs vascular brachytherapy for in-stent restenosis within bare-metal stents: the SISR randomized trial. JAMA. 2006;295(11):1264–73.

31 Castleman Disease

S. Abhijith, Rambha Pandey, Anjali V Ramdulari, and T. Balamurugan

31.1 Introduction

Castleman disease (CD) was named after Dr. Benjamin Castleman, who described 13 cases of localized mediastinal lymph node hyperplasia in 1956 [1]. In 1969, Flendrig and Schillings identified a plasma cell-rich variant, which Keller et al. further defined in 1972 by distinguishing the "hyaline-vascular type (HV)" from the less common "plasma cell type (PC)," associated with systemic signs and symptoms [2]. Multicentric lymphadenopathies with constitutional symptoms and histologic features like those seen in unicentric types of Castleman's disease (CD) were later described by other authors [3–6]. A decade later, a novel human herpes virus associated with Kaposi sarcoma, known as human herpes virus 8 (HHV-8) or Kaposi sarcoma herpes virus (KSHV), was discovered. HHV-8 was subsequently identified in primary effusion (or body-cavity-based) lymphomas and multicentric CD, particularly in HIV-positive individuals [7, 8].

By the mid-1980s, CD was divided into unicentric CD (UCD), which involved a single enlarged lymph node or region of lymph nodes, and multicentric CD (MCD), which involved multiple lymph node stations [4]. Co-occurrence between plasma cell (PC) neoplasm, polyneuropathy, organomegaly, endocrinopathy, monoclonal plasma cell disorder, and skin changes (POEMS syndrome) with MCD was noted in the 1980s and 1990s [9]. Monoclonal PCs causing POEMS were proposed to cause MCD. HHV8 was identified as the driver of all HIV+ and some HIV− MCD cases in the 1990s [7]. In the 2010s, Takai et al. recognized a severe form of HHV8− or idiopathic MCD (iMCD) characterized by a constellation of abnormal laboratory tests and clinical features known as TAFRO syndrome: thrombocytopenia, ascites,

S. Abhijith · R. Pandey (✉) · A. V. Ramdulari
Department of Radiation Oncology, AIIMS, New Delhi, India

T. Balamurugan
Department of Pathology, AIIMS, New Delhi, India

K. Sood Sharma (ed.), *Radiation Therapy for Benign Disorders*,
https://doi.org/10.1007/978-981-95-6635-8_31

anasarca, reticulin fibrosis, and organomegaly [10]. UCD is managed by complete surgical resection. In contrast, MCD is managed by a combination of anti-IL-6 monoclonal antibody, anti-CD20 antibody, high-dose steroids, and combination chemotherapy, depending on the severity of the disease [11].

31.2 Etiopathogenesis

31.2.1 Viral Infections

The clinicopathological similarity of CD patients with chronic viral infections steered initial research for a viral pathogen. Conclusive data emerged from a study by Miller et al., using computational analysis from next-generation sequencing (NGS) to identify any viral or viroid genome in patients of CD, suggesting active viral infection is unlikely to be a pathological driver of UCD or iMCD [12].

31.2.2 Interleukin-6 (IL-6)

Yoshizaki et al. (1989) demonstrated IL-6 production within germinal centers of lymph nodes in both unicentric plasma cell variant (U-PCV) and MCD [13]. Subsequent clinical studies further confirmed that serum IL-6 concentrations were markedly elevated during symptomatic episodes of MCD—at levels rarely observed in other diseases—and typically normalized with effective treatment [13–17].

IL-6, also called B-cell differentiation factor (BCDF or BSF-2), induces final maturation of B-cells into immunoglobulin-producing cells. Its production is augmented by antigenic stimuli and causes cell growth and differentiation, inducing cytokines, immunoglobulins, and acute-phase protein production. IL-6 signaling is mediated by an IL-6 receptor (IL-6R) and signal-transducing receptor glycoprotein, gp130, which binds the IL-6/IL-6R complex. IL-6 signaling can happen either via a classical signal using a membrane-bound IL-6 receptor (mIL-6R) coupled with gp130 or a soluble IL-6 receptor (sIL-6R) coupled with gp130, which mediates the trans signal pathway. Soluble IL 6 (sIL 6) was found to be an agonist of the signaling pathway that increases in inflammatory states, while soluble gp130 (sgp130) is an antagonist of the signaling pathway, preventing the IL-6/sIL-6R complex from binding the gp130. This postulated the creation of a humanized anti-IL-6R antibody, which would inhibit IL-6 binding on mIL-6R in the classical pathway and on sIL-6R in the trans signal pathway.

Although IL-6 is the driver of iMCD pathogenesis in some patients, IL-6 is not universally elevated in iMCD, and approximately one-half of iMCD patients do not respond to IL-6 inhibition, suggesting alternative drivers and signaling pathways. Sheila et al. identified CXCL13 as the most upregulated cytokine during flare, and it was strongly expressed in germinal centers of affected lymph nodes, suggesting a key role in disease activity and B-cell homing [18]. Clear proteomic differences were observed between iMCD subtypes: Patients of iMCD-TAFRO showed poor response to anti-IL-6 therapies and enrichment of complement activation and PI3K/Akt/mTOR signaling pathways, whereas iMCD-NOS patients more often responded to anti-IL-6 therapy and had different proteomic patterns, including increased VEGF signaling [19]. IL-1, IL-2, and TNF have also been shown to play a role in the pathogenesis of iMCD [20].

31.2.3 UCD

Li et al. reported platelet-derived growth factor receptor β (PDGFRB) Asn666Ser mutations in 17% of patients with UCD. These mutations have been localized to non-hematopoietic CD45-negative stromal cells, supporting the theory of a stromal cell-driven neoplastic process, likely the follicular dendritic cell (FDC) [21].

31.2.4 MCD

Castleman disease (CD), particularly iMCD, has traditionally been viewed as a polyclonal lymphoproliferative disorder driven by cytokine dysregulation—notably IL-6. Recent evidence suggests that clonality and cytogenetic abnormalities may play a role in at least a subset of patients [22]. Given that JAK1 is a key mediator in the IL-6/IL-6 receptor/gp130 signaling pathway, the V310I mutation is hypothesized to cause a conformational alteration that functionally activates the protein, potentially increasing the cell's sensitivity to IL-6, even at physiologic levels. Goodman et al. identified novel somatic alterations in UCD and iMCD. The study found no definitive oncogenic driver, or clonal lymphoid neoplasm in iMCD samples, but somatic alterations like TNS3-ALK fusion and chromosomal rearrangements in some UCD cases could suggest the potential for neoplastic transformation [23].

31.2.5 HHV-8 MCD

Human herpesvirus 8 (HHV-8) plays a central role in the pathogenesis of HHV-8-associated multicentric Castleman disease (MCD), primarily through infection of B cells and plasmablasts, which can be identified via immunohistochemical staining for latency-associated nuclear antigen-1 (LANA-1) [24]. They uniquely express high levels of cytoplasmic IgM lambda, reflecting the virus's preferential tropism for tonsillar IgM lambda–expressing B cells. These cells lack somatic hypermutation of immunoglobulin genes, suggesting an origin from naïve or IgM memory B cells. HHV-8-infected plasmablasts are atypical and detectable in peripheral blood, highlighting the key role of B cells, further evidenced by the effectiveness of B-cell–depleting therapy with rituximab [25]. Viral IL-6 (vIL-6), secreted during lytic and latent infection, activates gp130 without the need for IL-6Rα (gp80), potentially affecting a broader range of cells. HHV-8 is also implicated in primary effusion lymphoma and germinotropic lymphoproliferative disorder, though co-infection with EBV is common in these entities, unlike in HHV-8-associated MCD and plasmablastic lymphoma [26].

31.2.6 POEMS

Monoclonal plasma cells (PCs) are considered the primary etiologic drivers of POEMS-associated multicentric Castleman disease (POEMS-MCD). While the exact differences in cellular and cytokine profiles between POEMS-MCD and classic POEMS syndrome remain unclear, it is well established that excessive production of VEGF and IL-12—driven by somatic mutations in PCs—is central to the pathogenesis of classic POEMS [27]. A comprehensive genetic analysis of PCs from 20 patients with classic POEMS syndrome identified 20 mutations across seven recurrently mutated genes: KLHL6, LTB, EHD1, EML4, HEPHLI, HIPK1, and PCDH10. Interestingly, VEGFA expression was not elevated in the plasma cells of these POEMS patients. However, in contrast, Wang et al. reported that in patients with POEMS syndrome, bone marrow CD138+ plasma cells exhibited higher VEGF mRNA expression compared to CD138− cells [28–30].

31.3 Histopathology

Definitive diagnosis of CD requires excisional lymph node biopsy, as preserved LN architecture is essential for characterization. The histopathological findings in CD can be seen in other reactive and neoplastic conditions, underlining the need for a clinicopathological diagnosis complemented with laboratory findings. This is most necessary for MCD, which can resemble a plethora of conditions like autoimmune diseases (rheumatoid arthritis, SLE, adult-onset Still disease), IgG4-related diseases, infectious diseases (acute EBV infection, acute HIV infection), and malignancies (Hodgkin lymphoma, non-Hodgkin lymphoma, follicular dendritic cell sarcoma).

UCD HV-type constitutes the majority of UCD. Histologically involved lymph nodes can show varying degrees of follicular and interfollicular changes. Follicles are usually round or irregular with germinal centers depleted of lymphocytes but with increased FDCs (identified on CD21 immunostaining). There is increased vascularity with hyalinization of the vessel wall in the interfollicular area. Arrangement of mature lymphocytes around germinal centers in concentric circles produces a mantle zone with an onion skin appearance (Fig. 31.1). These concentric mantle zones and penetrating blood vessels in germinal centers produce a lollipop appearance. Twinning, due to a combination of two germinal centers and surrounded by mantle zone lymphocytes, is also occasionally seen. In approximately one-fourth of cases, atypical dendritic cells can be found, often multinucleated and resembling Warthin-Finkeldey cells. These cells are positive for follicular dendritic cell markers such as CD21 and CXCL13. PC-type accounts for less than 30% of UCD cases. Infiltrating plasma cells are generally polyclonal [30], but may exhibit light chain restriction, predominantly lambda expression [31–33] (Figs. 31.2 and 31.3).

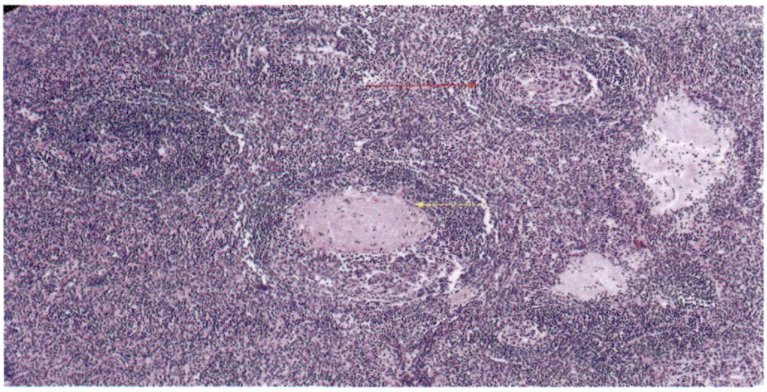

Fig. 31.1 Hyaline vascular type Castleman disease: Atretic germinal centers traversed by sclerotic penetrating vessels (yellow arrow). Mantle zones are thickened with lymphocytes arranged in layers—onion skin appearance (red arrow)

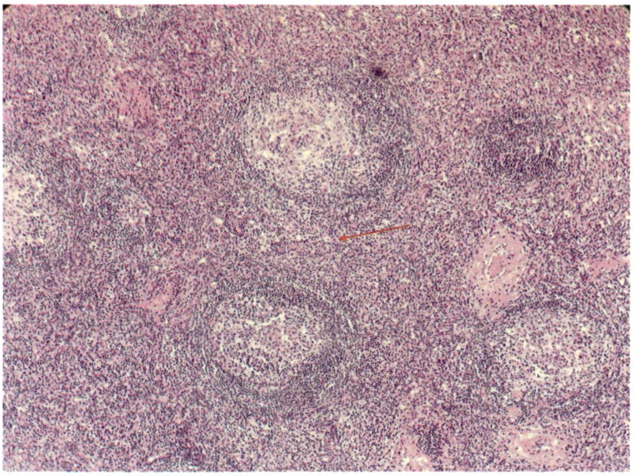

Fig. 31.2 Plasma cell-rich type Castleman disease—interfollicular region showing increased plasma cells (red arrow)

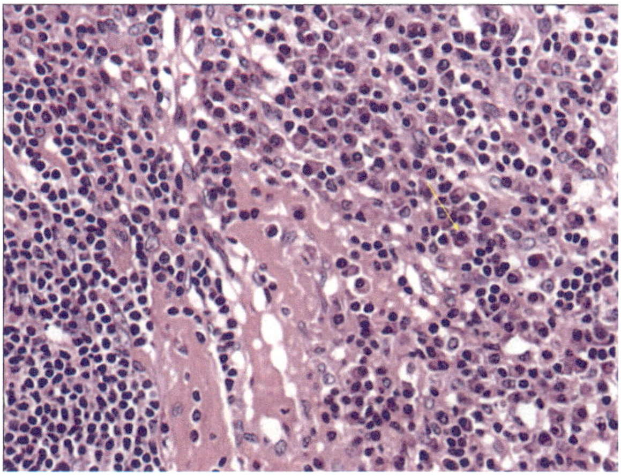

Fig. 31.3 High magnification highlighting the plasma cells (yellow arrow)

HHV-8-Associated MCD Lymph nodes (LN) are characterized by preserved LN architecture, increased follicle size, and abundant polyclonal plasmacytosis in the interfollicular area [34]. They are distinguished from the PC-type by the presence of KSHV-infected cells, which are positive on immunostaining for HHV8 (monoclonal antibodies to the LANA-1), and a subset of these express KSHV lytic genes, including the one encoding vIL-6 [35–37] These KSHV/HHV8-infected plasmablasts express lambda-restricted IgM [38]. A plasmablastic variant (plasma cells with promyelocytic features) is seen almost exclusively in HHV-8–MCD.

Idiopathic MCD iMCD is a heterogeneous group of disorders, with each subtype having clinicopathological differences. Histologically, iMCD can be divided into PC-type and Hyper-V-type, with the latter often presenting with TAFRO symptoms. iMCD-TAFRO is characterized by minimal LN enlargement and histological features such as marked vascular proliferation with plump endothelial cells in the interfollicular areas, with less plasmacytosis [39]. This histology is called Hyper-Vascular (Hyper-V) type which can show some similarities with HV-UCD but can be distinguished based on their clinical presentation. Bone marrow samples of iMCD-TAFRO show megakaryocytic hyperplasia and reticulin fibrosis. PC-type iMCD-TAFRO is often associated with positive autoantibodies such as anti-cardiolipin and anti-SS-A and can represent a potentially ill-defined autoimmune disease [39].

iMCD—Not Otherwise Specified (iMCD-NOS) Often presents as PC-type with sheet-like proliferation of mature plasma cells in the interfollicular region [39]. IL-6 is strongly positive in plasma cells in interfollicular areas and in B cells in germinal centers. Clinically, overproduction of IL-6 results in polyclonal hypergammaglobulinemia with high serum IgG4 levels and IgG4-positive plasma cells, differentiation between IgG4-related diseases difficult.

CD-Variant of POEMS Syndrome Characterized by clinical features of POEMS syndrome and CD-like histology but do not have an underlying clonal plasma cell proliferation disorder. Prominent plasma cell proliferation and hypervascularization in the interfollicular area are observed. Lambda (λ) light chain restriction is seen in all cases [39]. VEGF staining may be performed in suspected POEMS.

31.4 Clinical Features and Diagnostic Criteria

The Castleman Disease Collaborative Network (CDCN) proposes a classification system for CD based on etiological drivers and phenotypes of the disease (Fig. 31.4).

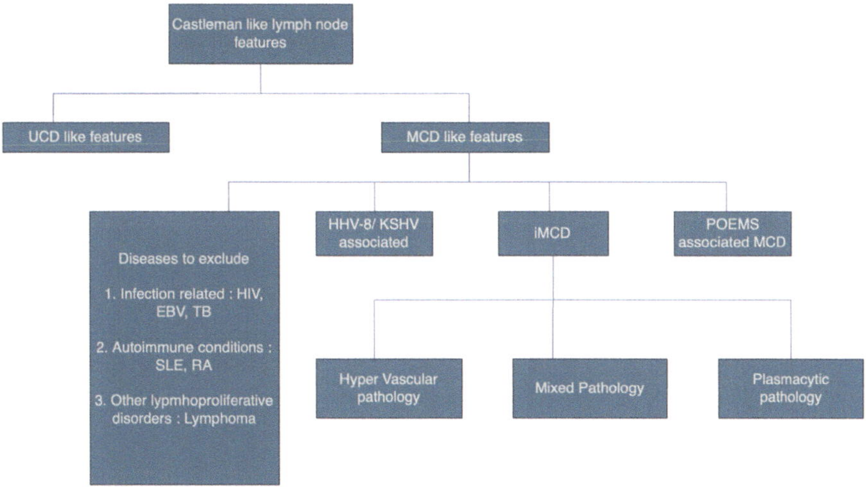

Fig. 31.4 Algorithmic approach for assessment of lymph node with features of CD. (Adapted from Dispenzieri and Fajgenbaum [27])

31.4.1 UCD

In patients with isolated lymphadenopathy and histopathological features of CD, the diagnosis of UCD is considered established if the patient is asymptomatic. However, the presence of constitutional symptoms (e.g., fevers, night sweats, weight loss), cutaneous findings, dyspnea, or neuropathy warrants further diagnostic evaluation to establish a clinical baseline and to exclude paraneoplastic pemphigus (PNP), bronchiolitis obliterans, or POEMS syndrome [40]. Patients with UCD typically present either with symptoms due to mass effect—such as dyspnea, dysphagia, or abdominal discomfort—or with incidental discovery of an enlarged lymph node during imaging for unrelated indications [27]. Laboratory studies are frequently normal, though anemia, hypergammaglobulinemia, or elevated inflammatory markers (e.g., ESR) may be present. Histologically, the hyaline-vascular (HV) subtype predominates, accounting for 70% to 90% of UCD cases [40]. UCD most commonly affects mediastinal, cervical, and intra-abdominal or pelvic nodal regions, though any lymph node basin may be involved [27]. While most patients have an indolent course, serious complications such as paraneoplastic pemphigus (PNP), polyneuropathy, pulmonary dysfunction, and autoimmune hemolytic anemia have been reported.

31.4.2 MCD

Multicentric Castleman disease (MCD) is characterized by generalized lymphadenopathy involving two or more lymph node regions, accompanied by a diverse and often relapsing-remitting spectrum of systemic symptoms and laboratory abnormalities (Table 31.1). Common presenting features include constitutional

Table 31.1 Clinical features of Castleman's disease (±, rarely present ; +, sometimes present; ++, often present; +++, very often present AIHA - autoimmune hemolytic anemia; DAT - direct antiglobulin test; MG - monoclonal gammopathy; PN - peripheral neuropathy; PNP - paraneoplastic pemphigus; cART - combined anti retroviral therapy. * : Fever, sweats, weight loss, malaise, effusions, autoimmune, and respiratory symptoms)

	UCD	iMCD-NOS	iMCD-TAFRO	MCD-POEMS	HHV-8 ass MCD
Age (decades)	4	5–6	5	5	5
Systemic symptoms	None or compressive	++ Occasional PN	+++ Anasarca	++	+++ Associated Kaposi sarcoma
Lymphadenopathy	Centrally, bulky	Peripheral and central, but small LN	Peripheral and central, but small LN	Peripheral and central,	Peripheral and central, but small LN
Organomegaly	±	++	+++	+++	+++
Inflammatory markers	±	+++	+++	++	+++
Hypergammaglobulinemia*	±	+++	±	+, small M spike	+++
Renal dysfunction	–	+	++	+	++
Autoimmune phenomenon	Rare, but PNP can be seen	++, AIHA, PNP, Interstitial lung disease	±	±	Positive DAT and MG
Pathologic features	Usually, HV variant	Usually, PC variant	Usually mixed or hypervascular type	Usually mixed or PC type	Usually, PC variant and often plasmablastic
Therapy	Surgery	IL-6 targeted therapy	IL-6 targeted therapy + calcineurin	Myeloma type therapy and localized radiation	IL-6 targeted therapy + cART
Clinical course	Benign	Variable	Very aggressive	Aggressive	Aggressive

Adapted from Fajgenbaum DC et al., *American Journal of Hematology*. 2020;95 (11):1353–1364
* Fever, sweats, weight loss, malaise, effusions, autoimmune, and respiratory symptoms
± rarely present, + sometimes present, ++ often present, +++ very often present
AIHA autoimmune hemolytic anemia, *DAT* direct antiglobulin test, *MG* monoclonal gammopathy, *PN* peripheral neuropathy, *PNP* paraneoplastic pemphigus, *cART* combined anti retroviral therapy

symptoms (e.g., fever, night sweats, weight loss), peripheral edema or effusions, cytopenia, and evidence of hepatic and renal dysfunction [27]. The lymphadenopathy can be present in any anatomic nodal basin, and affected nodes are often hypervascular and avid on fluorodeoxyglucose (FDG) PET imaging [41].

MCD may also be associated with a variety of systemic manifestations, including immune-mediated, inflammatory, or idiopathic cytopenia; hepatosplenomegaly; renal involvement (secondary amyloidosis); peripheral neuropathy (PN); and pulmonary abnormalities such as infiltrates, restrictive lung disease, lymphoid interstitial pneumonitis, or bronchiolitis obliterans. Dermatologic findings—such as rash, hyperpigmentation, cherry hemangiomatosis, paraneoplastic pemphigus (PNP), and Kaposi sarcoma—can also occur [27].

Evaluation at diagnosis should include testing for HIV and assessment for human herpesvirus-8 (HHV8) in lymph node tissue to differentiate HHV8-associated MCD from idiopathic MCD (iMCD), as HHV8 serologic testing lacks both sensitivity and specificity. A comprehensive diagnostic workup should also include serum and urine protein electrophoresis with immunofixation and neurologic assessment to evaluate for concurrent POEMS syndrome.

31.4.3 HHV8-Associated Multicentric Castleman Disease (HHV8-MCD)

A diagnosis of HHV8-MCD is established in the presence of multicentric lymphadenopathy, histopathological features consistent with CD, and detection of HHV8 in lymph node tissue, via latent nuclear antigen-1 (LANA-1) staining [24]. Baseline plasma HHV8 quantification may assist with disease monitoring. Hemophagocytic syndrome is a frequent complication with approximately three-quarters of patients requiring intensive care support due to hemodynamic instability or neurologic decline.

Clinical differences have been noted between HIV-positive and HIV-negative individuals with HHV8-MCD. HIV-positive patients tend to present at a younger age (median 42 vs. 65 years), are more often male and white, and are more likely to have fever, splenomegaly, and hemophagocytic syndrome. Conversely, HIV-negative patients more commonly exhibit monoclonal gammopathy and a positive direct antiglobulin test (DAT) [42].

31.4.4 Idiopathic Multicentric Castleman Disease (iMCD)

Idiopathic MCD (iMCD) shares many clinical and pathological features with HHV8-MCD but lacks evidence of HHV8 infection. Compared to HHV8-MCD, iMCD is more frequently associated with autoimmune phenomena, arthritis, renal dysfunction, cutaneous involvement, and lupus-like features [27]. The clinical presentation and laboratory abnormalities are heterogeneous (Table 31.1), reflecting the systemic nature of the disease.

The diagnostic criteria for iMCD include histopathologic confirmation of compatible lymph node findings and lymphadenopathy in at least two distinct nodal regions, and fulfillment of at least two minor criteria, one of which must be a laboratory abnormality. Importantly, alternative etiologies—such as infections, autoimmune conditions, and malignancies—must be excluded through appropriate clinical, histologic, and laboratory assessments.

iMCD can be further subclassified based on clinical phenotype. The iMCD-TAFRO variant (characterized by thrombocytopenia, anasarca, fever, reticulin fibrosis, renal dysfunction, and organomegaly) typically presents with a more aggressive and fulminant course. Patients without this constellation of features are categorized under iMCD-NOS (not otherwise specified).

31.4.5 iMCD-TAFRO

iMCD-TAFRO represents a distinct and clinically aggressive subtype of idiopathic multicentric Castleman disease (iMCD), characterized by thrombocytopenia, anasarca (typically presenting as ascites), reticulin fibrosis of the bone marrow, renal dysfunction, and organomegaly [43]. Lymph nodes in iMCD-TAFRO demonstrate marked vascular proliferation, resembling the hyaline-vascular (HV) histologic pattern commonly seen in unicentric CD (UCD), suggesting shared underlying angiogenic pathways.

Patients with iMCD-TAFRO often exhibit thrombocytopenia and either normal or only mildly elevated immunoglobulin levels. Given the severity of this subtype, evaluation should include assessment for disseminated intravascular coagulation and fibrinolysis. In addition, bone marrow biopsy is recommended to evaluate for reticulin fibrosis and megakaryocytic hyperplasia, which are characteristic findings in iMCD-TAFRO.

31.4.6 POEMS-MCD

A subset of patients with HHV-8–negative multicentric Castleman disease (MCD) also meet diagnostic criteria for POEMS syndrome and are thought to result from a common clonal population of pathogenic plasma cells driving both disease processes [44]. POEMS syndrome is a rare paraneoplastic disorder, most frequently associated with osteosclerotic myeloma. The acronym "POEMS" reflects several hallmark features: Peripheral neuropathy, Organomegaly (typically hepatosplenomegaly), endocrinopathy, monoclonal gammopathy (IgA or IgG with λ light chain restriction), and skin changes. Additional defining features not captured by the acronym include osteosclerotic bone lesions, papilledema, extravascular volume overload, thrombocytosis, lymphadenopathy, and pulmonary dysfunction [27].

A diagnosis of POEMS is a prerequisite for the diagnosis of POEMS-MCD and requires the presence of both polyradiculoneuropathy and a monoclonal plasma cell disorder, along with at least one of the following: a sclerotic bone lesion, elevated serum vascular endothelial growth factor (VEGF), or lymph node histopathology consistent with Castleman disease. Prognosis in POEMS-MCD is influenced by the presence of bone lesions; patients without osteosclerotic lesions generally have a worse clinical course.

Diagnostic evaluation should include imaging (particularly CT or PET/CT) for sclerotic bone lesions and comprehensive evaluation for monoclonal gammopathy via serum and urine protein electrophoresis with immunofixation. Additional workup should include detailed endocrine assessment (evaluating thyroid, adrenal, pituitary, and gonadal axes), bone marrow biopsy for clonal plasma cells and megakaryocytic atypia or hyperplasia, pulmonary function testing, and formal neurologic evaluation.

31.5 Management

31.5.1 UCD

The management of unicentric Castleman disease (UCD) is fundamentally influenced by the location, resectability, and symptomatology associated with the lymph node mass. Complete surgical excision is the preferred and potentially curative treatment for resectable UCD in both adults and children. This approach typically leads to resolution of both local and systemic manifestations. Dispenzieri et al. reported a 5-year overall survival (OS) rate of 91% in a cohort of 53 patients with unicentric Castleman disease (UCD) who underwent surgical resection at the Mayo Clinic and the University of Nebraska [45]. Similarly, Talat et al. conducted a retrospective analysis of 278 surgically treated UCD patients and observed a comparable OS exceeding 90%, with follow-up extending up to a decade. Mortality due to disease occurred in only 1.5% (1 of 68) of patients with peripheral lymphadenopathy versus 6.1% (9 of 148) in those with central lymphadenopathy, a difference that reached statistical significance [46]. The presence of unresectable disease was the sole factor predictive of disease-related mortality in that cohort. Given the size and vascularity of many UCD lesions, preoperative embolization may be considered to reduce intraoperative bleeding risk, particularly in large or centrally located lesions.

Infrequently, UCD lesions are deemed unresectable due to anatomical constraints, such as proximity to critical mediastinal structures. Observation with periodic surveillance is an acceptable strategy for asymptomatic patients with unresectable UCD. For patients experiencing local compressive symptoms, several strategies, such as rituximab with or without corticosteroids and partial debulking surgery, can be considered if complete excision is not feasible. In select cases, embolization may serve as an adjunct. There is limited prospective data, but case series suggest that some patients receiving medical therapy may subsequently become candidates for definitive surgical resection [47].

Patients exhibiting systemic inflammatory symptoms or laboratory markers of inflammation should be considered for anti–IL-6 therapy with siltuximab or tocilizumab before considering extensive surgery or radiotherapy. Any persisting lymphadenopathy should be surgically resected, if feasible. Patients who become asymptomatic can be safely observed, whereas those with ongoing troublesome symptomatology should be considered for radiotherapy.

31.5.2 Role of Radiation Therapy in Management of Castleman Disease

In patients with ongoing symptoms despite appropriate medical therapy and persistent unresectable disease, radiotherapy is a treatment option. Chronowski et al. described a series of four patients with unresectable unicentric Castleman disease treated with radiotherapy, three of whom achieved complete remission following doses around 4000 cGy [48]. In a separate review, Chan et al. compiled 17 reported cases of unresectable UCD managed with comparable radiotherapy regimens. Of these, 13 patients experienced disease control—seven with partial responses and six with complete responses. At a median follow-up of 20 months, only one patient had succumbed to disease progression [49]. Though well tolerated, late sequelae of side effects and increased risk of secondary malignancies in young individuals remain a concern. Although a definitive correlation between radiation dose and tumor control or symptom relief has not been established, it is hypothesized that radiation therapy administered at doses ranging from 2700 to 4500 cGy may result in complete or partial remission in most cases.

Recurrence following complete surgical resection is rare but has been reported [50]. When recurrence occurs, management should follow the same principles as initial therapy, with re-excision preferred if feasible. Longitudinal follow-up with annual CT imaging is recommended for at least 5 years postoperatively, after which surveillance may be symptom-driven.

Algorithm for management of UCD (Fig. 31.5)

31.5.3 HHV-8-Positive MCD

Rituximab monotherapy is a preferred first-line treatment for HIV-associated multicentric Castleman disease (MCD), supported by data from two phase II studies [51, 52]. In one prospective trial, four weekly doses of rituximab enabled 22 of 24 patients with relapsed/refractory, chemotherapy-dependent disease to become chemotherapy-independent, with sustained symptom control and disease stability in the majority at 2 years. Another phase II study involving patients with plasmablastic MCD reported symptomatic remission in 20 of 21 patients, with a 67% radiologic response rate and 2-year OS and DFS rates of 95% and 79%, respectively. Reactivation or flare of occult Kaposi sarcoma (KS), common in HHV8-positive

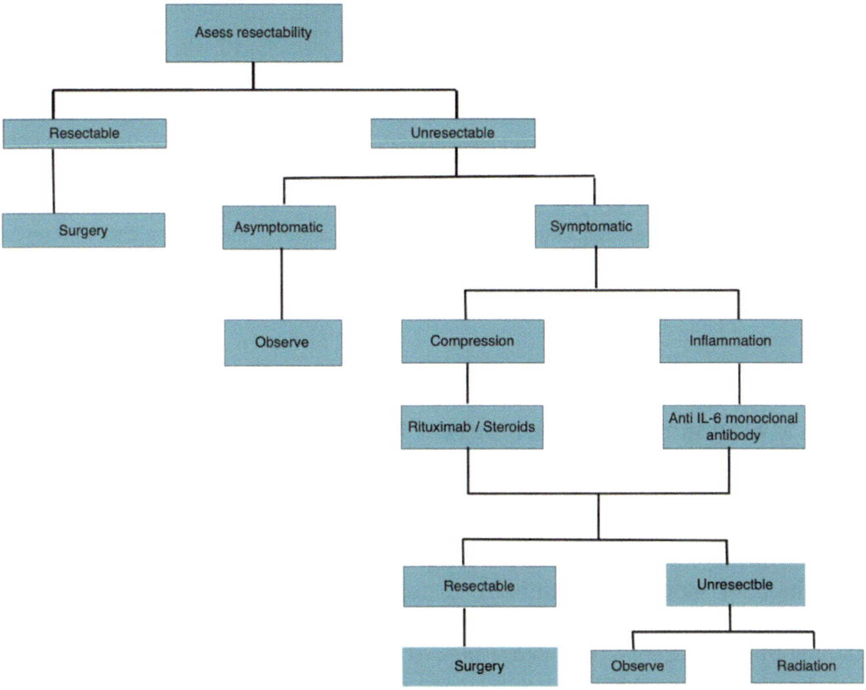

Fig. 31.5 Algorithm for management of UCD. (Adapted from van Rhee F et al., Blood Adv. 2020; 4(23):6039–50)

disease, may occur with rituximab or corticosteroids; however, combining rituximab with liposomal doxorubicin may reduce this risk and is especially beneficial in patients with concurrent KS [53]. Combination antiretroviral therapy (cART) is essential for all HIV-1–positive patients. Antiviral approaches, such as high-dose zidovudine with valganciclovir or ganciclovir, have also shown activity in HHV8-associated MCD, with modest progression-free survival but notable clinical responses in pilot studies. Rituximab-based regimens (with prednisone or liposomal doxorubicin) and zidovudine with antivirals remain key options in first-line therapy [54, 55].

31.5.4 iMCD

The clinical presentation of iMCD ranges from mild systemic symptoms to severe, life-threatening multiorgan dysfunction. To aid in treatment decision-making, a CDCN-endorsed severity classification system stratifies patients as *nonsevere* or *severe* based on performance status and organ dysfunction (Table 31.2).

Table 31.2 CDCN severity classification for rapid assessment and allocation of therapy

Severe iMCD
ECOG PS > 2
Stage IV Renal Dysfunction (eGFR < 30, serum creatinine > 3)
Anasarca and/or ascites and/or pleural/pericardial effusion
Hemoglobin ≤ 8 g/dl
Pulmonary involvement/interstitial pneumonitis with dyspnea

CDCN severity classification for rapid assessment and allocation of therapy. Patients with severe iMCD must have at least 2 of the 5 criteria listed above. Patients should be classified as having nonsevere iMCD if the above criteria are not met. *ECOG* Eastern Cooperative Oncology Group; *eGFR* estimated glomerular filtration rate

31.5.5 Management of Non-severe MCD

Nonsevere iMCD refers to patients without evidence of organ dysfunction or life-threatening disease but who often display constitutional symptoms and laboratory abnormalities reflective of an IL-6–mediated inflammatory process.

Anti–IL-6 monoclonal antibody therapy—siltuximab (11 mg/kg IV every 3 weeks)—is the standard of care for nonsevere iMCD. In a pivotal randomized, double-blind, placebo-controlled trial, 79 patients with idiopathic multicentric Castleman disease (iMCD) were assigned to receive either siltuximab ($n = 53$) or placebo ($n = 26$). Treatment with siltuximab resulted in a significantly higher rate of durable tumor and symptomatic response compared to placebo (34% vs. 0%; $P = 0.0012$) [56]. Subsequent long-term follow-up, with a median duration of 6 years, confirmed the sustained efficacy and favorable safety profile of siltuximab in this population. Progression-free survival (PFS) was also significantly improved in the siltuximab group, with median PFS not reached versus 15 months in the placebo group ($P = 0.0001$). Grade ≥ 3 adverse events were observed in 60% of patients receiving siltuximab, the most frequent being hypertension (13%), fatigue (8%), nausea (7%), neutropenia (7%), and vomiting (5%). Benefit of siltuximab was seen with all histologies.

Discontinuation of therapy is associated with relapse, and indefinite maintenance therapy is generally advised for responders, although dosing intervals may be extended (e.g., to every 6 weeks) in stable patients. In settings where siltuximab is unavailable or not approved, tocilizumab serves as an appropriate alternative. Like siltuximab, tocilizumab is well tolerated, with the most common adverse effects being mild cytopenia, hyperlipidemia, and pruritus [57].

While corticosteroid monotherapy is not recommended due to high relapse rates and lack of durable responses, they may serve as adjuncts to anti–IL-6 therapy, especially in patients with high inflammatory burden or symptomatic flares. Corticosteroids should be discontinued as early as clinically feasible to minimize long-term toxicity [58].

For patients with milder inflammatory phenotypes or when anti–IL-6 therapy is contraindicated or unavailable, rituximab may be considered as an alternative first-line. Response rates for rituximab monotherapy or rituximab-cyclophosphamide-based regimens have been variable. However, progression-free survival is generally inferior to that achieved with siltuximab [59–64].

31.5.6 Management of Severe MCD

Prompt initiation of high-dose corticosteroids, combined with siltuximab, is recommended. An intensified weekly dosing schedule of siltuximab for the first month may be employed to achieve rapid therapeutic levels. Patients demonstrating an immediate response should continue siltuximab at standard 3-week intervals with gradual steroid tapering [45]. It is important to recognize that severe iMCD may not respond immediately to corticosteroids or anti–IL-6 monoclonal antibodies (mAbs), as steady-state drug levels can take weeks to establish. Furthermore, a subset of patients may fail to respond altogether. In such cases, early initiation of multiagent cytotoxic chemotherapy is warranted, particularly if clinical deterioration occurs or there is no response to siltuximab within 1 week. The goal of chemotherapy is to suppress the hyperactivated immune system and control the cytokine storm driving disease severity.

Various chemotherapy regimens have been utilized, including lymphoma-based protocols such as R-CHOP (rituximab, cyclophosphamide, doxorubicin, vincristine, prednisone), CVAD (cyclophosphamide, vincristine, doxorubicin, dexamethasone), and CVP (cyclophosphamide, vincristine, prednisone). Combination chemotherapy is appropriate for patients with poor performance status, including those in intensive care units, as rapid control of the cytokine storm can be lifesaving. Although cytotoxic chemotherapy achieves the highest overall response rate, its significant toxicity profile and frequent relapses limit its use to the most severe cases [48, 65, 66].

Severe iMCD frequently manifests as the TAFRO subtype. In an analysis of 49 published cases with treatment data, corticosteroids, anti–IL-6 mAbs, cytotoxic chemotherapy, and cyclosporine A were the most used agents. While initial efficacy parallels that seen in other iMCD subtypes, higher rates of treatment failure and relapse are observed. Treatment of iMCD-TAFRO should follow the general severity-based algorithm, initiating therapy with anti–IL-6 mAbs ± corticosteroids. For anti–IL-6-refractory cases, cyclosporine A has demonstrated utility, particularly in managing refractory ascites and thrombocytopenia [67, 68]. The Japanese TAFRO research group endorses high-dose steroids, tocilizumab, and cyclosporine A for this population [69]. Emerging evidence from a treatment-refractory iMCD-TAFRO patient highlighted upregulation of the mTOR pathway, with sustained remission achieved using sirolimus. Proteomic analyses suggest distinct chemokine and cytokine profiles between classical and TAFRO-iMCD, supporting heterogeneity in disease pathogenesis and therapeutic targets [70].

In patients with multicentric Castleman disease (MCD) associated with POEMS syndrome, therapeutic efforts should be directed toward the underlying plasma cell dyscrasia, employing regimens typically used in the management of multiple myeloma. High-dose chemotherapy followed by autologous stem cell rescue (HDT/ASCR) has been associated with durable responses and may be particularly effective.

31.5.7 Refractory/Progressive Disease

Nonresponse or progressive disease should prompt a thorough re-evaluation of the diagnosis to exclude mimicking conditions, such as lymphoma, autoimmune disease, or infection. In patients with relapsed or refractory disease, biopsy is recommended to exclude histologic transformation to diffuse large B-cell lymphoma (DLBCL), as well as to assess for the emergence of secondary malignancies or opportunistic infections [45].

For patients with HHV8-positive multicentric Castleman disease (MCD) without evidence of organ failure, single-agent antiviral therapy with ganciclovir or valganciclovir is preferred. In contrast, individuals presenting with organ dysfunction are best managed with combination chemotherapy, with or without rituximab. Acceptable agents for single-agent therapy include etoposide (oral or intravenous), vinblastine, liposomal doxorubicin (particularly in HHV8-positive disease), siltuximab (in HHV8-negative disease), and the mTOR inhibitor sirolimus. Recommended second-line chemotherapy regimens include CHOP, CVAD, and CVP, with liposomal doxorubicin ± rituximab specifically noted for use in HHV8-positive disease complicated by organ failure. For HHV8-positive patients who respond to initial treatment, maintenance therapy with valganciclovir or active observation may be considered [45].

For patients who experience further progression after second-line therapy, alternative single-agent or combination regimens should be considered. Tocilizumab may be effective in individual's refractory to rituximab and conventional chemoimmunotherapy. Other treatment options, supported primarily by case reports and small series, include bortezomib ± rituximab, thalidomide ± rituximab, lenalidomide ± rituximab, high-dose zidovudine with valganciclovir, and the IL-1 receptor antagonist anakinra. Autologous and allogeneic stem cell transplantation have been reported in a limited number of cases, with mixed outcomes, and be considered as last resort [71–74].

Algorithm for management of iMCD (Fig. 31.6)

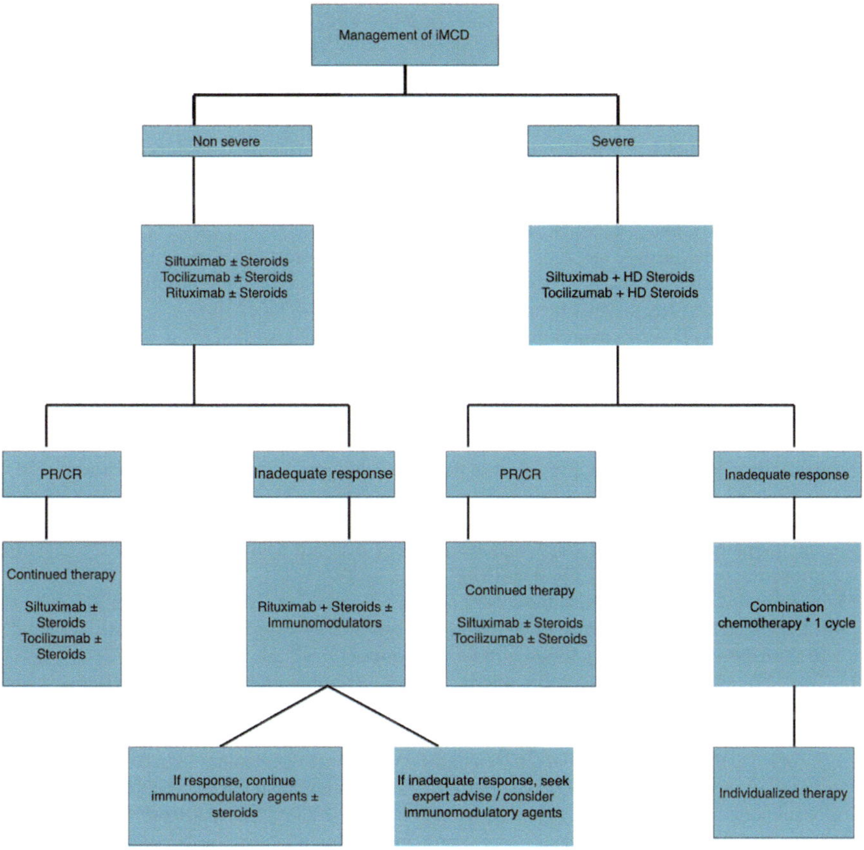

Fig. 31.6 Algorithm for management of iMCD. PR Partial response, CR Complete response. (Adapted from van Rhee F et al., Blood. 2018;132(20):2115–24)

References

1. Castleman B, Iverson L, Menendez VP. Localized mediastinal lymphnode hyperplasia resembling thymoma. Cancer. 1956;9(4):822–30. https://doi.org/10.1002/1097-0142(195607/08)9:4<822::aid-cncr2820090430>3.0.co;2-4.
2. Keller AR, Hochholzer L, Castleman B. Hyaline-vascular and plasma-cell types of giant lymph node hyperplasia of the mediastinum and other locations. Cancer. 1972;29(3):670–83. https://doi.org/10.1002/1097-0142(197203)29:3<670::aid-cncr2820290321>3.0.co;2-#
3. Flendrig JA, Schillings PHM. Benign giant lymphoma: the clinical signs and symptoms. Folia Med Neerl. 1969;12:119–20.
4. Frizzera G, Banks PM, Massarelli G, Rosai J. A systemic lymphoproliferative disorder with morphologic features of Castleman's disease. Pathological findings in 15 patients. Am J Surg Pathol. 1983;7(3):211–31. https://doi.org/10.1097/00000478-198304000-00001.

5. Gaba AR, Stein RS, Sweet DL, Variakojis D. Multicentric giant lymph node hyperplasia. Am J Clin Pathol. 1978;69(1):86–90. https://doi.org/10.1093/ajcp/69.1.86.
6. Martin JM, Bell B, Ruether BA. Giant lymph node hyperplasia (Castleman's disease) of hyaline vascular type. Clinical heterogeneity with immunohistologic uniformity. Am J Clin Pathol. 1985;84(4):439–46. https://doi.org/10.1093/ajcp/84.4.439.
7. Soulier J, Grollet L, Oksenhendler E, Cacoub P, Cazals-Hatem D, Babinet P, d'Agay MF, Clauvel JP, Raphael M, Degos L. Kaposi's sarcoma-associated herpesvirus-like DNA sequences in multicentric Castleman's disease. Blood. 1995;86(4):1276–80.
8. Du MQ, Liu H, Diss TC, Ye H, Hamoudi RA, Dupin N, Meignin V, Oksenhendler E, Boshoff C, Isaacson PG. Kaposi sarcoma-associated herpesvirus infects monotypic (IgM lambda) but polyclonal naive B cells in Castleman disease and associated lymphoproliferative disorders. Blood. 2001;97(7):2130–6. https://doi.org/10.1182/blood.v97.7.2130.
9. Dispenzieri A. POEMS syndrome: update on diagnosis, risk-stratification, and management. Am J Hematol. 2023;98(12):1934–50. https://doi.org/10.1002/ajh.27081.
10. Takai K, Nikkuni K, Shibuya H, Hashidate H. Rinsho ketsueki. Jpn J Clin Hematol. 2010;51(5):320–5.
11. Fajgenbaum DC, Uldrick TS. Castleman disease (Chapter 103). In: DeVita, Hellman, and Rosenberg's cancer: principles & practice of oncology. 11th ed. Wolters Kluwer; 2021. p. 1771–82.
12. Miller I, Mumau MD, Shyamsundar S, et al. No evidence for active viral infection in unicentric and idiopathic multicentric Castleman disease by viral-track analysis. Sci Rep. 2025;15:1676. https://doi.org/10.1038/s41598-025-85193-x.
13. Yoshizaki K, Matsuda T, Nishimoto N, Kuritani T, Taeho L, Aozasa K, Nakahata T, Kawai H, Tagoh H, Komori T, et al. Pathogenic significance of interleukin-6 (IL-6/BSF-2) in Castleman's disease. Blood. 1989;74(4):1360–7. PMID: 2788466.
14. Beck JT, Hsu SM, Wijdenes J, Bataille R, Klein B. Brief report: alleviation of systemic manifestations of Castleman's disease by monoclonal anti-interleukin-6 antibody. N Engl J Med. 1994;330(9):602–5.
15. Brandt SJ, Bodine DM, Dunbar CE, Nienhuis AW. Dysregulated interleukin 6 expression produces a syndrome resembling Castleman's disease in mice. J Clin Invest. 1990;86(2):592–9.
16. Nishimoto N, Yoshizaki K, Tagoh H, Monden M, Kishimoto S, Kishimoto T. Elevation of serum interleukin 6 prior to acute phase proteins on the inflammation by surgical operation. Clin Immunol Immunopathol. 2000;96(1):115–8.
17. Oksenhendler E, Boutboul D, Fieschi C, Meignin V, Meignin V, Galicier L. Interleukin-6 in HIV-infected patients with multicentric Castleman's disease. AIDS. 2000;14(2):221–2.
18. Pierson SK, Katz L, Williams R, Mumau M, Gonzalez M, Guzman S, Rubenstein A, Oromendia AB, Beineke P, Fosså A, van Rhee F, Fajgenbaum DC. CXCL13 is a predictive biomarker in idiopathic multicentric Castleman disease. Nat Commun. 2022;13(1):7236. https://doi.org/10.1038/s41467-022-34873-7. PMID: 36433996; PMCID: PMC9700691.
19. Pierson SK, Stonestrom AJ, Shilling D, Ruth J, Nabel CS, Singh A, Ren Y, Stone K, Li H, van Rhee F, Fajgenbaum DC. Plasma proteomics identifies a 'chemokine storm' in idiopathic multicentric Castleman disease. Am J Hematol 2018;93(7):902–912. https://doi.org/10.1002/ajh.25123. Epub 2018 May 16. PMID: 29675946.
20. Gherardi RK, Bélec L, Fromont G, Divine M, Malapert D, Gaulard P, Degos JD. Elevated levels of interleukin-1 beta (IL-1 beta) and IL-6 in serum and increased production of IL-1 beta mRNA in lymph nodes of patients with polyneuropathy, organomegaly, endocrinopathy, M protein, and skin changes (POEMS) syndrome. Blood. 1994;83(9):2587–93. PMID: 8167341.
21. Li Z, Lan X, Li C, Zhang Y, Wang Y, Xue W, Lu L, Jin M, Zhou Z, Wang X, Li L, Zhang L, Li X, Fu X, Sun Z, Wu J, Zhang X, Yu H, Nan F, Chang Y, Yan J, Wu X, Wang G, Zhang D, Zhang Y, Young KH, Zhang M. Recurrent PDGFRB mutations in unicentric Castleman disease. Leukemia. 2019;33(4):1035–8. https://doi.org/10.1038/s41375-018-0323-6. Epub 2019 Jan 3. PMID: 30607019; PMCID: PMC6484698.

22. Chang KC, Wang YC, Hung LY, et al. Monoclonality and cytogenetic abnormalities in hyaline vascular Castleman disease. Mod Pathol. 2014;27:823–31. https://doi.org/10.1038/modpathol.2013.202.
23. Kanai K, Sawai S, Sogawa K, Mori M, Misawa S, Shibuya K, Isose S, Fujimaki Y, Noto Y, Sekiguchi Y, Nasu S, Nakaseko C, Takano S, Yoshitomi H, Miyazaki M, Nomura F, Kuwabara S. Markedly upregulated serum interleukin-12 as a novel biomarker in POEMS syndrome. Neurology 2012;79(6):575–82. https://doi.org/10.1212/WNL.0b013e318263c42b. Epub 2012 Jul 25. PMID: 22843279.
24. Dupin N, Diss TL, Kellam P, Tulliez M, Du MQ, Sicard D, Weiss RA, Isaacson PG, Boshoff C. HHV-8 is associated with a plasmablastic variant of Castleman disease that is linked to HHV-8-positive plasmablastic lymphoma. Blood. 2000;95(4):1406–12. PMID: 10666218.
25. Gonzalez-Farre B, Martinez D, Lopez-Guerra M, Xipell M, Monclus E, Rovira J, Garcia F, Lopez-Guillermo A, Colomo L, Campo E, Martinez A. HHV8-related lymphoid proliferations: a broad spectrum of lesions from reactive lymphoid hyperplasia to overt lymphoma. Mod Pathol 2017;30(5):745–760. https://doi.org/10.1038/modpathol.2016.233. Epub 2017 Jan 13. PMID: 28084335.
26. Bülbül G, Gül G, Özcan MA, Özkal S. HHV-8 and EBV positive lymphoproliferative disease: a challenging case. Turk Patoloji Derg. 2022;38(2):142–7. https://doi.org/10.5146/tjpath.2021.01540. PMID: 34514570; PMCID: PMC9999693.
27. Dispenzieri A, Fajgenbaum DC. Overview of Castleman disease. Blood 2020;135(16):1353–64. https://doi.org/10.1182/blood.2019000931. PMID: 32106302.
28. Nagao Y, Mimura N, Takeda J, Yoshida K, Shiozawa Y, Oshima M, Aoyama K, Saraya A, Koide S, Rizq O, Hasegawa Y, Shiraishi Y, Chiba K, Tanaka H, Nishijima D, Isshiki Y, Kayamori K, Kawajiri-Manako C, Oshima-Hasegawa N, Tsukamoto S, Mitsukawa S, Takeda Y, Ohwada C, Takeuchi M, Iseki T, Misawa S, Miyano S, Ohara O, Yokote K, Sakaida E, Kuwabara S, Sanada M, Iwama A, Ogawa S, Nakaseko C. Genetic and transcriptional landscape of plasma cells in POEMS syndrome. Leukemia. 2019;33(7):1723–35. https://doi.org/10.1038/s41375-018-0348-x. Epub 2019 Jan 11. PMID: 30635632.
29. Wang C, Huang XF, Cai QQ, Cao XX, Cai H, Zhou D, Li J. Remarkable expression of vascular endothelial growth factor in bone marrow plasma cells of patients with POEMS syndrome. Leuk Res. 2016;50:78–84. https://doi.org/10.1016/j.leukres.2016.09.017. Epub 2016 Sep 26. PMID: 27697660.
30. Frizzera G. Castleman's disease and related disorders. Semin Diagn Pathol. 1988;5(4):346–64. PMID: 2464187.
31. Hall PA, Donaghy M, Cotter FE, Stansfeld AG, Levison DA. An immunohistological and genotypic study of the plasma cell form of Castleman's disease. Histopathology. 1989;14:333–46.
32. Hsi ED, Lorsbach RB, Fend F, Dogan A. Plasmablastic lymphoma and related disorders. Am J Clin Pathol. 2011;136:183–94.
33. Radaszkiewicz T, Hansmann ML, Lennert K. Monoclonality and polyclonality of plasma cells in Castleman's disease of the plasma cell variant. Histopathology. 1989;14:11–24.
34. Chadburn A, Said J, Gratzinger D, et al. HHV8/KSHV-positive lymphoproliferative disorders and the spectrum of plasmablastic and plasma cell neoplasms: 2015 SH/EAHP workshop report-part 3. Am J Clin Pathol. 2017;147:171–87.
35. Du MQ, et al. Kaposi sarcoma-associated herpesvirus infects monotypic (IgM lambda) but polyclonal naive B cells in Castleman disease and associated lymphoproliferative disorders. Blood. 2001;97:2130–6.
36. Chadburn A, et al. Immunophenotypic analysis of the Kaposi sarcoma herpesvirus (KSHV; HHV-8)-infected B cells in HIV+ multicentric Castleman disease (MCD). Histopathology. 2008;53:513–24.
37. Dupin N, Fisher C, Kellam P, et al. Distribution of human herpesvirus-8 latently infected cells in Kaposi's sarcoma, multicentric Castleman's disease, and primary effusion lymphoma. Proc Natl Acad Sci USA. 1999;96:4546–51.

38. Wu D, Lim MS, Jaffe ES. Pathology of Castleman disease. Hematol Oncol Clin North Am. 2018;32:37–52.
39. Nishimura MF, Nishimura Y, Nishikori A, Yoshino T, Sato Y. Historical and pathological overview of Castleman disease. J Clin Exp Hematop. 2022;62(2):60–72. https://doi.org/10.3960/jslrt.21036. Epub 2022 Apr 27. PMID: 35474035; PMCID: PMC9353854.
40. Hoffmann C, Oksenhendler E, Littler S, Grant L, Kanhai K, Fajgenbaum DC. The clinical picture of Castleman disease: a systematic review and meta-analysis. Blood Adv. 2024;8(18):4924–35. https://doi.org/10.1182/bloodadvances.2024013548. PMID: 38985311; PMCID: PMC11421328.
41. Jiang Y, Hou G, Zhu Z, Huo L, Li F, Cheng W. 18F-FDG PET/CT imaging features of patients with multicentric Castleman disease. Nucl Med Commun. 2021;42(7):833–838. https://doi.org/10.1097/MNM.0000000000001404. PMID: 33741858; PMCID: PMC8191470.
42. Fajgenbaum DC, van Rhee F, Nabel CS. HHV-8-negative, idiopathic multicentric Castleman disease: novel insights into biology, pathogenesis, and therapy. Blood. 2014;123(19):2924–33. https://doi.org/10.1182/blood-2013-12-545087. Epub 2014 Mar 12. PMID: 24622327.
43. Williams C, Phillips A, Aggarwal V, Slonim LB, Fajgenbaum DC, Karmali R. TAFRO syndrome and elusive diagnosis of idiopathic multicentric Castleman disease treated with empiric anti-interleukin-6 therapy. Case Rep Oncol. 2021;14(3):1359–65. https://doi.org/10.1159/000518079. PMID: 34720942; PMCID: PMC8525304.
44. Fajgenbaum DC, Uldrick TS, Bagg A, Frank D, Wu D, Srkalovic G, Simpson D, Liu AY, Menke D, Chandrakasan S, Lechowicz MJ, Wong RS, Pierson S, Paessler M, Rossi JF, Ide M, Ruth J, Croglio M, Suarez A, Krymskaya V, Chadburn A, Colleoni G, Nasta S, Jayanthan R, Nabel CS, Casper C, Dispenzieri A, Fosså A, Kelleher D, Kurzrock R, Voorhees P, Dogan A, Yoshizaki K, van Rhee F, Oksenhendler E, Jaffe ES, Elenitoba-Johnson KS, Lim MS. International, evidence-based consensus diagnostic criteria for HHV-8-negative/idiopathic multicentric Castleman disease. Blood. 2017;129(12):1646–57. https://doi.org/10.1182/blood-2016-10-746933. Epub 2017 Jan 13. PMID: 28087540; PMCID: PMC5364342.
45. van Rhee F, Oksenhendler E, Srkalovic G, Voorhees P, Lim M, Dispenzieri A, Ide M, Parente S, Schey S, Streetly M, Wong R, Wu D, Maillard I, Brandstadter J, Munshi N, Bowne W, Elenitoba-Johnson KS, Fössa A, Lechowicz MJ, Chandrakasan S, Pierson SK, Greenway A, Nasta S, Yoshizaki K, Kurzrock R, Uldrick TS, Casper C, Chadburn A, Fajgenbaum DC. International evidence-based consensus diagnostic and treatment guidelines for unicentric Castleman disease. Blood Adv. 2020;4(23):6039–50. https://doi.org/10.1182/bloodadvances.2020003334. PMID: 33284946; PMCID: PMC7724917.
46. Talat N, Belgaumkar AP, Schulte KM. Surgery in Castleman's disease: a systematic review of 404 published cases. Ann Surg. 2012;255(4):677–84. https://doi.org/10.1097/SLA.0b013e318249dcdc. PMID: 22367441.
47. Mohan M, Meek JC, Meek ME, Broadwater RL, Stone K, Greenway A, Alapat D, van Rhee F. Treatment of unresectable unicentric Castleman disease with therapeutic embolization. Blood. 2018;132(Supplement 1):2415. https://doi.org/10.1182/blood-2018-99-119820.
48. Chronowski GM, Ha CS, Wilder RB, Cabanillas F, Manning J, Cox JD. Treatment of unicentric and multicentric Castleman disease and the role of radiotherapy. Cancer. 2001;92:670–6. https://doi.org/10.1002/1097-0142(20010801)92:3<670::AID-CNCR1369>3.0.CO;2-Q.
49. Chan KL, Lade S, Prince HM, Harrison SJ. Update and new approaches in the treatment of Castleman disease. J Blood Med. 2016;7:145–58.
50. Ren N, Ding L, Jia E, Xue J. Recurrence in unicentric castleman's disease postoperatively: a case report and literature review. BMC Surg. 2018;18(1):1. https://doi.org/10.1186/s12893-017-0334-7. PMID: 29301533; PMCID: PMC5755032.
51. Gerard L, Berezne A, Galicier L, et al. Prospective study of rituximab in chemotherapy-dependent human immunodeficiency virus associated multicentric Castleman's disease: ANRS 117 CastlemaB Trial. J Clin Oncol. 2007;25:3350–6. Available at: https://www.ncbi.nlm.nih.gov/pubmed/17664482

52. Bower M, Powles T, Williams S, et al. Brief communication: rituximab in HIV-associated multicentric Castleman disease. Ann Intern Med. 2007;147:836–9. Available at: https://www.ncbi.nlm.nih.gov/pubmed/18087054
53. Gerard L, Michot JM, Burcheri S, et al. Rituximab decreases the risk of lymphoma in patients with HIV-associated multicentric Castleman disease. Blood. 2012;119:2228–33. Available at: https://www.ncbi.nlm.nih.gov/pubmed/22223822
54. Ramaswami R, Lurain K, Polizzotto MN, et al. Characteristics and outcomes of KSHV-associated multicentric Castleman disease with or without other KSHV diseases. Blood Adv. 2021;5:1660–70. Available at: https://www.ncbi.nlm.nih.gov/pubmed/33720337
55. Uldrick TS, Polizzotto MN, Aleman K, et al. High-dose zidovudine plus valganciclovir for Kaposi sarcoma herpesvirus-associated multicentric Castleman disease: a pilot study of virus-activated cytotoxic therapy. Blood. 2011;117:6977–86. Available at: https://www.ncbi.nlm.nih.gov/pubmed/21487108
56. van Rhee F, Wong RS, Munshi N, et al. Siltuximab for multicentric Castleman's disease: a randomised, double-blind, placebo-controlled trial. Lancet Oncol. 2014;15(9):966–74.
57. Nishimoto N, Kanakura Y, Aozasa K, et al. Humanized anti-interleukin-6 receptor antibody treatment of multicentric Castleman disease. Blood. 2005;106(8):2627–32.
58. Bowne WB, Lewis JJ, Filippa DA, et al. The management of unicentric and multicentric Castleman's disease: a report of 16 cases and a review of the literature. Cancer. 1999;85(3):706–17.
59. Ocio EM, Sanchez-Guijo FM, Diez-Campelo M, et al. Efficacy of rituximab in an aggressive form of multicentric Castleman disease associated with immune phenomena. Am J Hematol. 2005;78(4):302–5.
60. Ide M, Ogawa E, Kasagi K, Kawachi Y, Ogino T. Successful treatment of multicentric Castleman's disease with bilateral orbital tumour using rituximab. Br J Haematol. 2003;121(5):818–9.
61. Gholam D, Vantelon JM, Al-Jijakli A, Bourhis JH. A case of multicentric Castleman's disease associated with advanced systemic amyloidosis treated with chemotherapy and anti-CD20 monoclonal antibody. Ann Hematol. 2003;82(12):766–8.
62. Ide M, Kawachi Y, Izumi Y, Kasagi K, Ogino T. Long-term remission in HIV-negative patients with multicentric Castleman's disease using rituximab. Eur J Haematol. 2006;76(2):119–23.
63. Mian H, Leber B. Mixed variant multicentric Castleman disease treated with rituximab: case report. J Pediatr Hematol Oncol. 2010;32(8):622.
64. Adam Z, Szturz P, Koukalová R, et al. PET-CT documented remission of multicentric Castleman disease after treatment with rituximab: case report and review. Vnitr Lek. 2015;61(3):251–9.
65. Seo S, Yoo C, Yoon DH, et al. Clinical features and outcomes in patients with human immunodeficiency virus-negative, multicentric Castleman's disease: a single medical center experience. Blood Res. 2014;49(4):253–8.
66. Zhu SH, Yu YH, Zhang Y, Sun JJ, Han DL, Li J. Clinical features and outcome of patients with HIV-negative multicentric Castleman's disease treated with combination chemotherapy: a report on 10 patients. Med Oncol. 2013;30(1):492.
67. akasawa N, Sekiguchi Y, Takahashi T, Muryoi A, Satoh J, Sasaki T. A case of TAFRO syndrome, a variant of multicentric Castleman's disease, successfully treated with corticosteroid and cyclosporine A [published online ahead of print 14 July 2014]. Mod Rheumatol. https://doi.org/10.1080/14397595.2016.1206243.
68. Yamaga Y, Tokuyama K, Kato T, et al. Successful treatment with Cyclosporin a in tocilizumab-resistant TAFRO syndrome. Intern Med. 2016;55(2):185–90.
69. Masaki Y, Kawabata H, Takai K, et al. Proposed diagnostic criteria, disease severity classification and treatment strategy for TAFRO syndrome, 2015 version. Int J Hematol. 2016;103(6):686–92.

70. Fajgenbaum D, Shilling D, Partridge HL, et al. Prolonged remission achieved in a relapsing idiopathic multicentric castleman disease patient with a novel, targeted treatment approach [abstract]. Blood. 2017;130(suppl 1):Abstract 3593.
71. Jerkeman M, Lindén O. Long-term remission in idiopathic Castleman's disease with tocilizumab followed by consolidation with high-dose melphalan--two case studies. Eur J Haematol. 2016;96(5):541–3.
72. Tal Y, Haber G, Cohen MJ, et al. Autologous stem cell transplantation in a rare multicentric Castleman disease of the plasma cell variant. Int J Hematol. 2011;93(5):677–80.
73. Ogita M, Hoshino J, Sogawa Y, et al. Multicentric Castleman disease with secondary AA renal amyloidosis, nephrotic syndrome and chronic renal failure, remission after high-dose melphalan and autologous stem cell transplantation. Clin Nephrol. 2007;68(3):171–6.
74. Angenendt L, Kerkhoff A, Wiebe S, et al. Remissions of different quality following rituximab, tocilizumab and rituximab, and allogeneic stem cell transplantation in a patient with severe idiopathic multicentric Castleman's disease. Ann Hematol. 2015;94(7):1241–3.

GPSR Compliance

The European Union's (EU) General Product Safety Regulation (GPSR) is a set of rules that requires consumer products to be safe and our obligations to ensure this.

If you have any concerns about our products, you can contact us on ProductSafety@springernature.com

In case Publisher is established outside the EU, the EU authorized representative is:

Springer Nature Customer Service Center GmbH
Europaplatz 3
69115 Heidelberg, Germany

Batch number: 10732076

Printed by Printforce, the Netherlands